ASSESSMENT
AND CARE
OF THE WELL
NEWBORN

ASSESSMENT AND CARE OF THE WELL NEWBORN

SECOND EDITION

Patti J. Thureen, MD
Associate Professor, Department of Pediatrics
University of Colorado School of Medicine
The Children's Hospital and University Hospital
Denver, Colorado

Jane Deacon, RNC, MS, NNP
Neonatal Nurse Practitioner
The Children's Hospital and University Hospital
Denver, Colorado

Jacinto A. Hernandez, MD, MHA
Professor, Department of Pediatrics
University of Colorado School of Medicine
The Children's Hospital and University Hospital
Denver, Colorado

Daniel M. Hall, MD
Medical Director, Newborn Center
Associate Professor, Department of Pediatrics
University of Colorado School of Medicine
The Children's Hospital
Denver, Colorado

ELSEVIER
SAUNDERS

ELSEVIER
SAUNDERS

An Imprint of Elsevier

11830 Westline Industrial Drive
St. Louis, Missouri 63146

ASSESSMENT AND CARE OF THE WELL NEWBORN
Copyright © 2005, Elsevier (USA). All rights reserved.

NOTICE

Medicine is an ever-changing field. Standard safety precautions must be followed, but as new research and clinical experience broaden our knowledge, changes in treatment and drug therapy may become necessary or appropriate. Readers are advised to check the most current product information provided by the manufacturer of each drug to be administered to verify the recommended dose, the method and duration of administration, and contraindications. It is the responsibility of the licensed prescriber, relying on experience and knowledge of the patient, to determine dosages and the best treatment for each individual patient. Neither the publisher nor the author assumes any liability for any injury and/or damage to persons or property arising from this publication.

Previous edition copyrighted 1999

ISBN-13: 978-0-7216-0393-3
ISBN-10: 0-7216-0393-9

Executive Editor: Michael S. Ledbetter
Developmental Editor: Amanda Sunderman Politte
Publishing Services Manager: John Rogers
Senior Project Manager: Helen Hudlin
Designer: Amy Buxton

Printed in the United States of America

Last digit is the print number: 9   8   7   6   5

We dedicate this book to the Network for International Collaboration on Health Education (NICHE), a foundation committed to improving the care of newborns throughout the world.

Contributors

Mark J. Abzug, MD
Professor
Department of Pediatrics
University of Colorado School of Medicine
The Children's Hospital and University
    Hospital
Denver, Colorado
Bacterial Infections; Viral Infections

Robyn E. Berryman, RNC, MS, NNP
Neonatal Nurse Practitioner
Aurora Regional Medical Center
Denver, Colorado
Routine Care

Jill K. Davies, MD
Assistant Professor
Department of Obstetrics and Gynecology
University of Colorado School of Medicine
Denver, Colorado
Maternal Factors Affecting the Newborn

Jane Deacon, RNC, MS, NNP
Neonatal Nurse Practitioner
The Children's Hospital and University
    Hospital
Denver, Colorado
*Parental Preparation; Discharge Assessment;
    Postdischarge Care*

Meica M. Efird, MD
Instructor of Pediatrics
University of Colorado School of Medicine
The Children's Hospital and University
    Hospital
Denver, Colorado
Birth Injuries

Ruth Evans, RNC, MS, NNP
Neonatal Nurse Practitioner
The Children's Hospital and
    University Hospital
Denver, Colorado
*Adaptation to Extrauterine Life and
    Management During Normal and
    Abnormal Transition*

Lucy Fashaw, RNC, BSN
Professional Research Assistant
University of Colorado School of
    Medicine
Denver, Colorado
*Adaptation to Extrauterine Life and
    Management During Normal and
    Abnormal Transition*

Sharon M. Glass, RNC, MS, NNP
Neonatal Nurse Practitioner
The Children's Hospital and University
    Hospital
Denver, Colorado
*Physical Assessment of the Newborn; Feeding
    the Newborn; Routine Care; Genetic
    Screening; Circumcision; Immunizations;
    Legal Issues*

Anne Gross, RNC, MS, NNP
Neonatal Nurse Practitioner
The Children's Hospital and University
    Hospital
Denver, Colorado
*Recognition and Management of Neonatal
    Emergencies*

Daniel M. Hall, MD
Medical Director, Newborn Center
Associate Professor
Department of Pediatrics
University of Colorado School of
    Medicine
The Children's Hospital
Denver, Colorado
Fetal Assessment, Labor, and Delivery;
    Bacterial Infections

Jacinto A. Hernandez, MD, MHA
Professor
Department of Pediatrics
University of Colorado School of
    Medicine
The Children's Hospital and University
    Hospital
Denver, Colorado
Adaptation to Extrauterine Life and
    Management During Normal and
    Abnormal Transition; Birth Injuries;
    Physical Assessment of the Newborn

John C. Hobbins, MD
Professor and Chief of Obstetrics
Department of Obstetrics and
    Gynecology
University of Colorado School
    of Medicine
Denver, Colorado
Maternal Factors Affecting the Newborn; Fetal
    Assessment, Labor, and Delivery

Janis J. Johnson, MD
Clinical Assistant Professor
Department of Pediatrics
University of Colorado School of
    Medicine
Unit Medical Director
Swedish Medical Center
Pediatrix Medical Group
Denver, Colorado
Plethora and Pallor; Perinatal Drug
    Exposure

Sharon Langendoerfer, MD
Associate Professor
Department of Pediatrics
University of Colorado School of Medicine
Denver Health Medical Center
Denver, Colorado
Perinatal Drug Exposure

Annette LeBel, RN, BSN
Clinical Nurse
Women's and Infants' Services
University of Colorado Hospital
Denver, Colorado
Maternal Factors Affecting the Newborn

Susan Niermeyer, MD
Professor
Department of Pediatrics
University of Colorado School
    of Medicine
The Children's Hospital and University
    Hospital
Denver, Colorado
Resuscitation of the Newborn Infant;
    Recognition and Management of Neonatal
    Emergencies

Jan Paisley, MD
Senior Instructor
Department of Pediatrics
University of Colorado School of Medicine
Denver, Colorado
Director, Special Care Nursery
Poudre Valley Hospital
Fort Collins, Colorado
Viral Infections

Elizabeth H. Thilo, MD
Associate Professor
Department of Pediatrics
University of Colorado School of Medicine
The Children's Hospital and University
    Hospital
Denver, Colorado
Neonatal Jaundice

Patti J. Thureen, MD
Associate Professor
Department of Pediatrics
University of Colorado School of Medicine
The Children's Hospital and University
    Hospital
Denver, Colorado
Maternal Factors Affecting the Newborn;
    Bacterial Infections; Viral Infections;
    Isolation Procedures

Susan F. Townsend, MD
Associate Clinical Professor
Department of Pediatrics
University of Colorado School of Medicine
Memorial Hospital
Colorado Springs, Colorado
Approach to the Infant at Risk for
    Hypoglycemia; The Large-for-Gestational-
    Age and Small-for-Gestational-
    Age Infant

Preface

The field of Neonatology has experienced a tremendous growth over the past thirty years. Most textbooks on Neonatology focus primarily on the care of the sick newborn and new modalities of treatment. Frequently the approach to care of the normal newborn is given very little space and attention.

As authors on this project, our intent was to create a handbook for all levels of hospital neonatal caregivers, which can be used as a guide in caring for the well newborn. To accomplish this goal, this book must include an explanation of the events surrounding delivery, the processes necessary to identify newborns who deviate from normal, and the immediate interventions and care required in these situations as well as routine care considerations frequently encountered in caring for these infants. In developing the text along these lines, we divided it into the following sections:

Obstetric Considerations in the Management of the Well Newborn
Delivery Room Management
Evaluation and Care of the Newborn Infant During the Transitional Period and Beyond
Post-Transition Care
Warning Signs of Common Problems of the Well Newborn
Management of the Infant at Risk for Perinatal Infections
Discharge Planning and Follow-Up Care

In the appendices, we include information sheets, which can be copied for distribution to parents, geared toward facilitating parent education in the care of their newborn.

We are proud that any royalties from the sale of this book will be used to fund projects under the non-profit organization we created as NICHE (Network for International Collaboration on Health Education). NICHE was formed to serve as a conduit of funding and educational resources for maternal-neonatal health education projects in developing countries.

Patti J. Thureen
Jane Deacon
Jacinto A. Hernandez
Daniel M. Hall

Contents

Color Plates

Color Plates

PLATE 1 ● Vernix caseosa.

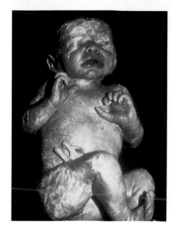

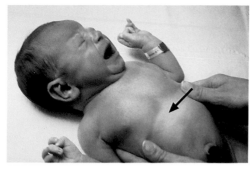

PLATE 2 ● Plethora contrasted to normal-appearing color of compressed skin *(arrow)*.

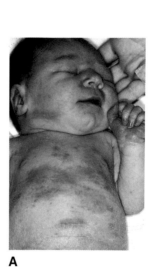

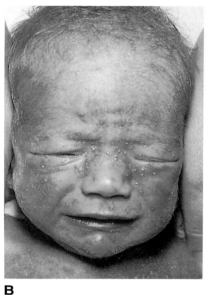

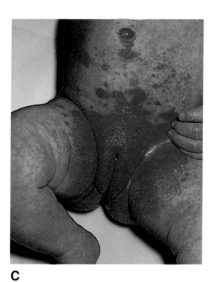

A

B

C

PLATE 3 ● **A** and **B,** Erythema toxicum. **C,** *Candida* dermatitis. (*B* and *C* from Beischer NA, Mackey EV, Colditz PB: *Obstetrics and the newborn,* ed 3, Philadelphia, WB Saunders, 1997.)

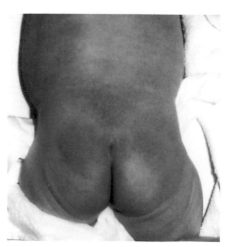

PLATE 4 ● Mongolian spot.

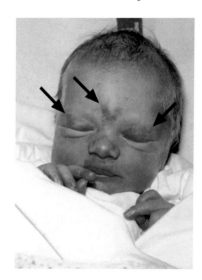

PLATE 5 ● Nevus flammeus *(arrows)*. (From Beischer NA, Mackey EV, Colditz PB: *Obstetrics and the newborn,* ed 3, Philadelphia, WB Saunders, 1997.)

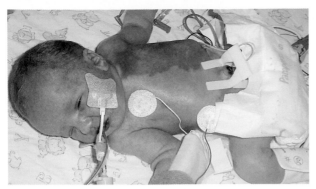

PLATE 6 ● Harlequin sign.

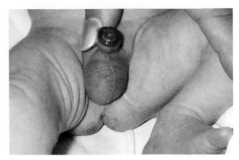

PLATE 7 ● Plastibell circumcision.

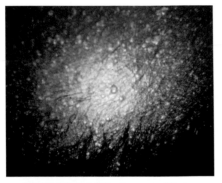

PLATE 8 ● Miliaria crystallinia.

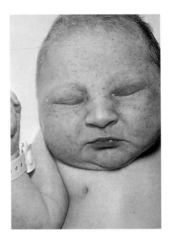

PLATE 9 ● Facial petechiae. (From Beischer NA, Mackey EV, Colditz PB: *Obstetrics and the newborn,* ed 3, Philadelphia, WB Saunders, 1997.)

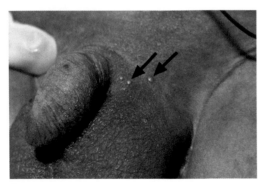

A

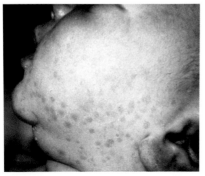

B

PLATE 10 ● **A,** Benign pustules. This type of lesion may also be the first stage of pustular melanosis. **B,** Pustular melanosis.

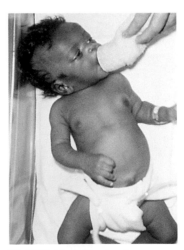

PLATE 11 ● Benign breast enlargement due to maternal hormone stimulation.

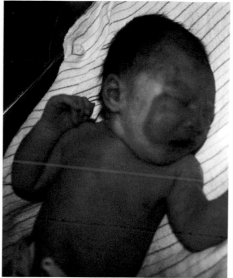 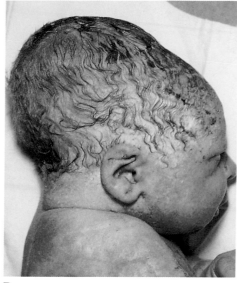

A B

PLATE 12 ● **A,** Molding of the head; also facial bruising secondary to facial application of vacuum. **B,** Molding of the head. (*B* from Beischer NA, Mackey EV, Colditz PB: *Obstetrics and the newborn,* ed 3, Philadelphia, WB Saunders, 1997.)

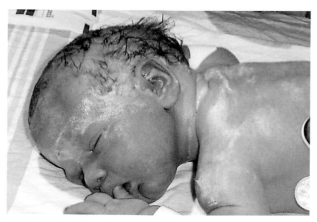

PLATE 13 ● Breech head and vernix.

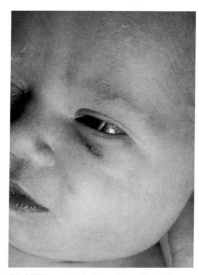

PLATE 14 ● Subconjunctival hemorrhage. (From Beischer NA, Mackey EV, Colditz PB: *Obstetrics and the newborn,* ed 3, Philadelphia, WB Saunders, 1997.)

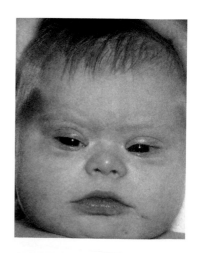

PLATE 15 ● Infant with Down syndrome.

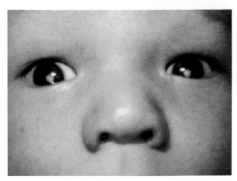

PLATE 16 ● Cataracts.

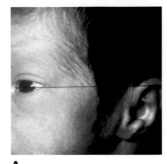

A

B

PLATE 17 ● Ear position. **A,** Normal ear position. **B,** Low-set ear.

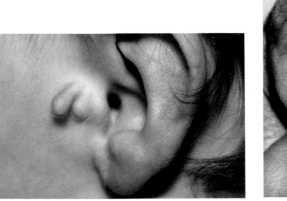

PLATE 18 ● Preauricular skin tags.

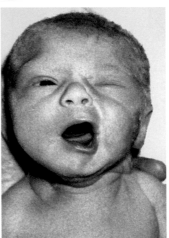

PLATE 19 ● Facial palsy.

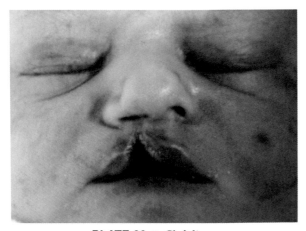

PLATE 20 ● Cleft lip.

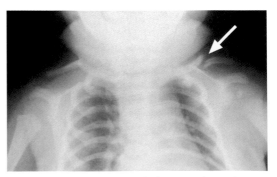

PLATE 21 ● Clavicle fracture *(arrow)*.

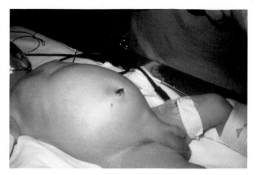

PLATE 22 ● Abdominal distention.

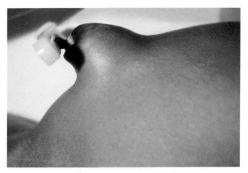

PLATE 23 ● Umbilical hernia.

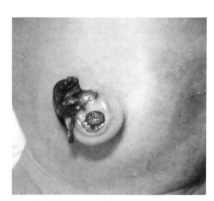

PLATE 24 ● Patent urachus.

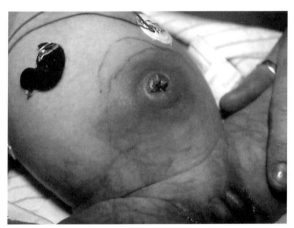

PLATE 25 ● Omphalitis.

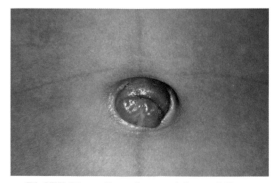

PLATE 26 ● Granuloma of the umbilicus.

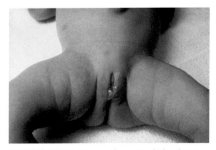

PLATE 27 ● Normal vaginal discharge.

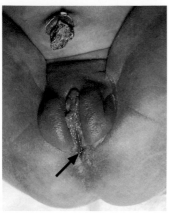

PLATE 28 ● Anteriorly placed (perineal) anus *(arrow)*. (From Beischer NA, Mackey EV, Colditz PB: *Obstetrics and the newborn,* ed 3, Philadelphia, WB Saunders, 1997.)

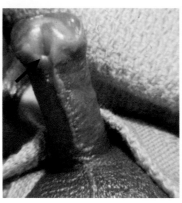

PLATE 29 ● Hypospadias *(arrow).*

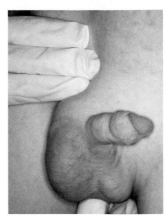

PLATE 30 ● Right-sided inguinal hernia.

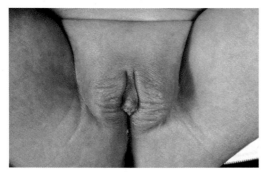

PLATE 31 ● Ambiguous genitalia in congenital adrenal hyperplasia.

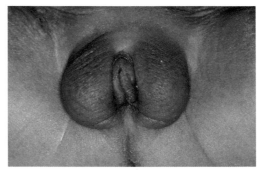

PLATE 32 ● Ambiguous female genitalia.

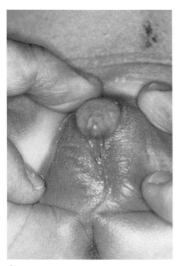

A

PLATE 33 ● **A** and **B,** Ambiguous genitalia.

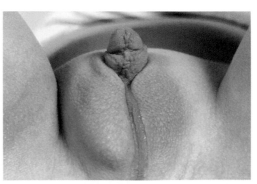

B

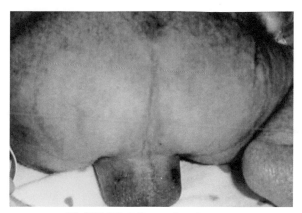

PLATE 34 ● Imperforate anus.

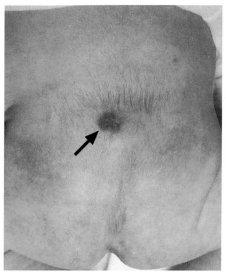

PLATE 35 ● Small meningomyelocele *(arrow)*. (From Beischer NA, Mackey EV, Colditz PB: *Obstetrics and the newborn*, ed 3, Philadelphia, WB Saunders, 1997.)

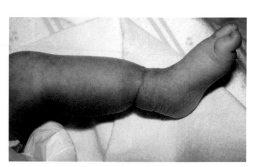

PLATE 36 ● Amniotic band.

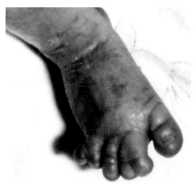

PLATE 37 ● Syndactyly of second and third toes and polydactyly with a sixth toe.

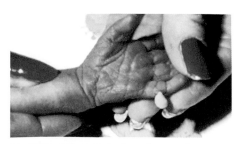

PLATE 38 ● Polydactyly with extra digit tied off with a ligature.

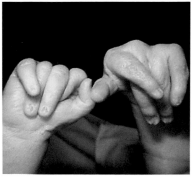

PLATE 39 ● Bilateral clinodactyly in Trisomy 18.

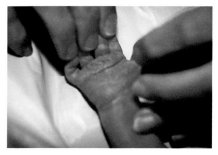

PLATE 40 ● Simian crease.

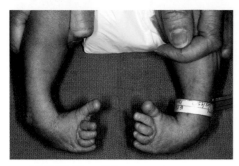

PLATE 41 ● Talipes equinovarus.

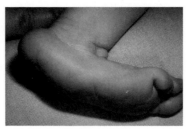

PLATE 42 ● Rocker-bottom foot.

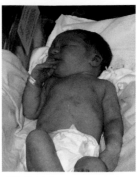

PLATE 43 ● Erb palsy.

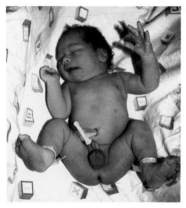

PLATE 44 ● Infant posture after a breech delivery.

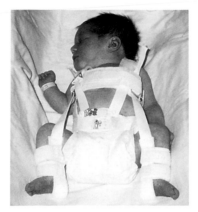

PLATE 45 ● Pavlik harness for congenital hip dislocation.

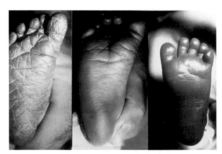

PLATE 46 ● Plantar surface of the foot.

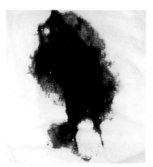

A

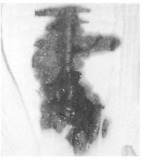

B

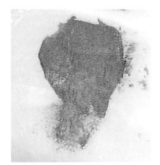

C

PLATE 47 ● Newborn stools. **A,** Meconium. **B,** Breast-fed. **C,** Formula fed. (From Nichols FH, Zwelling E: *Maternal-newborn nursing: theory and practice,* Philadelphia, WB Saunders, 1997.)

Obstetric Considerations in the Management of the Well Newborn

A basic understanding of maternal conditions and the process of labor and delivery is essential for those who care for newborns. This section focuses on the most common maternal health issues encountered during pregnancy and their implications for the fetus and newborn, as well as providing a background in labor and delivery management.

1 Maternal Factors Affecting the Newborn

Patti J. Thureen, MD ▪ *Jill K. Davies*, MD ▪ *Annette LeBel*, RN, BSN ▪ *John C. Hobbins*, MD

MATERNAL HISTORY

Approximately 75% of perinatal risk factors for an adverse pregnancy outcome can be identified before labor. Because of this, consistent, well-documented prenatal care is essential to ensure fetal well-being. A fetus's status can change from very low risk to high risk at any time during the pregnancy. However, a thorough maternal history helps to identify conditions that threaten the health of the mother and/or fetus. Once problematic conditions and risk factors are identified, they can be evaluated and treatment options can be discussed early in the pregnancy, optimally at the first prenatal visit.

   A. **Past Obstetric History:** Whenever possible, a complete history (including records) of the mother's prior pregnancies and deliveries should be reviewed, particularly when a previous pregnancy involved a maternal, fetal, or newborn complication. Pertinent questions include asking about prior history of:
   1. Infertility: Document hormonal therapy for infertility (at risk for multiple gestation pregnancy), uterine surgery, or abnormal uterine structure (may be at increased risk for prematurity or cesarean section delivery).
   2. Recurrent spontaneous abortions
      a. In general, an abortus is defined as a fetus delivered at <20 weeks and with a weight <500 g; however, states may differ in their definition and required reporting processes.
      b. Reasons for recurrent abortions should be ascertained and documented and may include hormonal inadequacy, chromosomal abnormality, infectious diseases, immunologic disorders, coagulation disorders (both inherited and acquired), collagen vascular disease, uterine abnormality, incompetent cervix.
   3. Stillbirth and/or perinatal death
      a. Stillbirth = fetal death and is defined as fetal demise at >20 weeks gestation.
      b. Neonatal death is death occurring after delivery but before 29 days of age.
      c. Perinatal death is fetal/infant death after 20 weeks gestation but before 29 days after birth.
      d. In all situations, cause of death needs to be determined for future pregnancy counseling and possible therapy; autopsy should be offered.

4. High parity: Five or more prior births can contribute to rapid labor, hypertension, and placenta previa.
5. Abnormal pregnancy duration
   a. Preterm labor or delivery: Preterm delivery is defined as delivery <37 weeks gestation. One or more previous episodes of preterm labor increases the risk for another preterm delivery. The risk for recurrent preterm delivery for women whose first delivery was preterm is increased threefold over women whose first delivery was at term (Cunningham et al., 1997).
   b. Prolonged pregnancy
      (1) Defined by the World Health Organization (1977) and the International Federation of Gynecology and Obstetrics (1986) as pregnancy >294 days from the last menstrual period (42 weeks) or >280 days from the time of ovulation.
      (2) Occurs in 12% of pregnancies based on menstrual dating criteria. However, when dates are calculated on the basis of second trimester ultrasound information, only 2.6% of pregnancies go beyond 42 weeks (Boyd et al., 1988); thus a significant number of pregnancies that were thought to be prolonged were not dated accurately.
      (3) Previous history of a prolonged pregnancy carries a 50% chance for a recurrence.
      (4) Fetal problems may include cord accidents due to decreased amniotic fluid, growth restriction, fetal distress, meconium aspiration, and perinatal death.
6. Infant or fetus with congenital anomalies: Antenatal consultation with a perinatologist or postnatal consultation with a genetics specialist as early as possible is recommended. Three generations of family history should be evaluated, including photographs, medical records, and reproductive history (including frequent spontaneous abortions). With some fetal anomalies, such as neural tube defects, delivery by cesarean section is best.
7. Rh or other isoimmune disease: History should include any spontaneous or therapeutic abortions and fetal or neonatal deaths. A history of transfusions, as well as the paternity history, should be elicited. Subsequent fetuses have a 2% to 16% increased risk for developing Rh disease depending on the ABO-compatibility status of the mother and infant (Tabsh and Theroux, 1992).
8. Abruptio placenta and placenta previa (Benedetti, 2002)
   a. Abruptio placenta is the premature separation of the normally implanted placenta from the uterus (ranging from slight to major separation), resulting in decreased blood supply to the fetus. The primary cause is unknown, but predisposing factors include maternal hypertension, blunt trauma to the abdomen (which may be caused by domestic violence), inherited thrombophilias (e.g., Factor V Leiden deficiency), smoking, illicit drug use, and medication use. Incidence is 1 in 86 to 206 births, with a recurrence risk for abruption ranging from 5% to 17%. Early delivery in a tertiary center should be considered if abruptio placenta has occurred previously. Increased perinatal morbidity and

mortality occur with abruption, with fetal/neonatal death rate as high as 25% to 30% in some studies.

    b. Placenta previa is the implantation of the placenta over the cervical os. Usually presenting as painless vaginal bleeding, it is the primary cause of hemorrhage in the third trimester. It is thought to be due to bleeding secondary to disruption of the attachment to the lower part of the uterus as this area thins in preparation for labor. Incidence is 1 in 200 births. Risk factors include prior cesarean delivery (primary risk factor, with an incidence of 1% to 4%, and increasing risk proportional to the number of prior cesarean deliveries), maternal age >35 years, and race (African-American or other minority races). Placental ultrasound should be performed in subsequent pregnancies to rule out recurrent previa. Mode of delivery depends on degree of previa, gestational age, and amount of bleeding, as well as other factors.

  9. Macrosomic infant (over 4000 g in the presence of maternal diabetes, 4500 g in the absence of diabetes): Evaluation for diabetes should be done early in prenatal care. Careful measurements of the fundal height of the uterus and ultrasound should be used to follow the growth of the fetus.

  10. Pregnancy-induced hypertension (PIH): Hypertension in pregnancy follows along a continuum from gestational hypertension to preeclampsia to eclampsia. The incidence of PIH is commonly reported to be 5%, although numerous variations are reported. Predisposing factors include nulliparity, familial history of preeclampsia or eclampsia, multiple fetuses, diabetes, chronic vascular disease, renal disease, hydatidiform mole, and fetal hydrops (Cunningham et al., 1977). Approximately one third of women who have had PIH previously will develop it again in subsequent pregnancies (Ferris, 1988).

  11. Cesarean section (C/S) and/or vaginal birth after cesarean section (VBAC)

    a. After C/S, risk for uterine rupture with labor in subsequent pregnancies is low (1% after low transverse and 6% after classical incisions).

    b. With classical scar, C/S is indicated before onset of labor.

    c. After low transverse scar, trial of labor with intended vaginal delivery is offered; appropriate monitoring of the uterus and fetus during labor is vital. Induction of labor with a prior C/S is discouraged because of the increased risk over spontaneous labor (Lydon-Rochelle, 2001).

B. History of Current Pregnancy: A history of previous uncomplicated pregnancies does not mean a women has no risk for developing risk factors in her current pregnancy. The history of the current pregnancy should include the following:

  1. Pregnancy dating: The estimated date of confinement (EDC) or due date can be established from the menstrual history or by ultrasound.

    a. Nagele's rule for dating by menstrual history: subtract 3 months and add 7 days to the first day of the last normal menstrual period. This may not be accurate with spotting or bleeding or with long or short menstrual cycles.

    b. Ultrasound is most accurate if done in the first trimester.

  2. Pregnancy number and status

a. Gravity is the total number of pregnancies in a patient, no matter what the outcome (e.g., G_3 = three pregnancies; a first pregnancy, even with twins, is G_1, not G_2).

b. Parity is the number of pregnancies carried to ≥20 weeks period (e.g., P_2 = two pregnancies carried to >20 weeks and includes the current pregnancy if ≥20 weeks).

c. For more information, spontaneous abortions (SAB), therapeutic abortions (TAB), and living children may be included (e.g., $G_7P_3SAB_2TAB_2LC_4$ implies seven pregnancies, three pregnancies carried to ≥20 weeks, two spontaneous abortions, two therapeutic abortions, and four living children; thus one pregnancy must have resulted in twins). Others may record parity simply as four numbers (e.g., P_{3044}, signifying full-term pregnancies [≥37 weeks gestation], preterm pregnancies [20 to <37 weeks gestation], abortions [<20 weeks gestation], and living children, respectively).

3. Prenatal lab results (Table 1-1)
4. Maternal age
    a. Age 15 years or younger: Greater risk for PIH, poor nutrition and weight gain, and socioeconomic problems, including substance abuse and domestic violence. Increased risk for preterm labor possibly due to immaturity of the uterus and cervix.
    b. Age 35 years or older: Increased risk for PIH, medical diseases including diabetes and chronic hypertension, and infant with Down syndrome.
5. Multiple gestation: Increased risk for perinatal morbidity and mortality, preeclampsia, placenta previa, intrauterine growth retardation, gestational diabetes, twin-twin transfusion, monochorionic twins, prolapsed cord, and congenital malformations. More common in infertile patients who become pregnant. Increased fetal surveillance is recommended with serial ultrasound studies to monitor growth and antepartum surveillance after 32 to 34 weeks.
6. Presentation: The size of the maternal pelvis, location of the placenta, and position of the fetus are important to ascertain prior to labor since disorders of dilation and descent occur with increased frequency in cases of abnormal presentation.
7. Amniotic fluid
    a. Polyhydramnios
        (1) Excessive amniotic fluid
        (2) May be associated with multiple gestation, Rh disease, maternal diabetes, anencephaly, fetal gastrointestinal tract abnormalities, or idiopathic etiology
        (3) Can be associated with cord prolapse and placental abruption, as well as malpresentation
    b. Oligohydramnios
        (1) Marked decrease in amniotic fluid
        (2) Has been associated with rupture of membranes, Potter syndrome, fetal growth retardation, chromosomal abnormalities (trisomies

● TABLE 1-1
● **Prenatal Screening Tests**

Test	Reason for Screening Test
Blood type, Rh, antibody screen	Identifies fetuses at risk for isoimmune disease
Hemoglobin or hematocrit	Baseline lab, rule out anemia, thalassemia, or high-risk groups; usually repeated in early third trimester
Rubella antibody screen	Identifies women susceptible to acquiring rubella during pregnancy; susceptible women should be immunized *after* delivery
Tuberculin skin testing	Identifies infected women for treatment
Hepatitis B surface antigen (HBsAg)	Identifies women whose offspring can be treated at birth to prevent hepatitis B infection
Serologic test for syphilis (VDRL or RPR)	Treatment reduces fetal/neonatal morbidity; mandated by law in most states
Human immunodeficiency virus status	Identifies women for treatment and perinatal therapy to decrease transmission to the fetus
Urinalysis	
Glucose, ketones, protein	Screen for diabetes, pregnancy-induced hypertension, renal disease
Red cells, white cells, bacteria	Possible urinary tract infection
Diabetes screen (24-28 weeks)	Fasting and glucose tolerance tests to evaluate for gestational diabetes
Pap smear	Identifies cervicitis and precancerous/cancerous lesions
Gonorrhea and chlamydia* probe	Identifies treatable sexually transmitted diseases, most of which can cause fetal or neonatal morbidity
Triple or quad screen (maternal serum for α-fetoprotein [AFP], human chorionic gonadotropin, estriol, inhibin A)	Done at 16-20 weeks at mother's discretion after counseling; AFP screens for neural tube defects, Down's syndrome; combination of multiple tests very sensitive in identifying Down syndrome with low false-positive rate
Other†	

*Some centers also screen for *Mycoplasma hominis* and group B streptococcus colonization.
†Lab tests may vary from one center to another. Certain tests may be ordered if patient is at specific risk (e.g., hemoglobin electrophoresis to evaluate for thalassemia and sickle cell disease in an African-American patient whose status is unknown or with a family history). Ultrasound is considered by some to be a screening tool for congenital anomalies. Cystic fibrosis testing is recommended for all couples planning a pregnancy, particularly for those ethnic groups at highest risk (e.g., Caucasians and Ashkenazi Jews).
Adapted from *Clinic Protocol for Department of Obstetrics and Gynecology*, University of Colorado Health Sciences Center.

13 and 18 most commonly), umbilical cord compression during labor, fetal genitourinary abnormalities, pulmonary hypoplasia, and positional deformities of the fetus.

8. Fetal growth abnormalities
   a. Intrauterine growth restricted (IUGR) fetus: Growth parameters less than 10% for gestational age (also see Chapters 16 and 17)
     (1) *Symmetric* growth retardation

(a) Body length, weight, and head circumference of the fetus are all similarly affected.

(b) Common causes are genetic abnormalities or intrauterine infection.

(2) *Asymmetric* growth retardation

(a) Head circumference, body length, and body weight are not equally diminished in size (usually weight is disproportionately affected). The abdominal circumference lags compared with head and/or long bone parameters.

(b) Generally secondary to utero-placental insufficiency associated with maternal hypertension, smoking, drug use, medical illnesses, severe malnutrition, or placental abnormalities.

b. Large for gestational age fetus (also see Chapters 16 and 17)

(1) Refers to fetus >90% for gestational age

(2) If later in pregnancy, may be due to maternal diabetes (known or unidentified)

(3) At risk for neonatal hypoglycemia, birth trauma, and asphyxia

9. Preterm premature rupture of membranes (PPROM)

a. Rupture of membranes prior to 37 weeks gestation

b. Delivery should be considered if the pregnancy is advanced and/or the fetal lungs are mature by antenatal amniotic fluid testing.

c. If immature lungs, frequent evaluation for intrauterine infection is essential (maternal fever, elevated white blood cell count, fetal tachycardia, foul-smelling vaginal discharge, uterine tenderness), with timely delivery once intrauterine infection is suspected.

10. Maternal substance abuse (see Chapter 18 for more details and specific effects of individual drugs)

a. In one study of women entering prenatal care, the prevalence of positive urine toxicology screens for cocaine, marijuana, alcohol, or heroin was 16% in the public health care system and 13% in private obstetric care (Chasnoff et al., 1990).

b. Ongoing abuse during pregnancy puts both maternal and fetal/neonatal health at risk.

11. Maternal exposure to teratogenic medications (Table 1-2). Questions regarding specific teratogens can be answered through the Organization of Teratology Information Services (OTIS; *www.otispregnancy.org*), an organization with member Teratogen Information Service (TIS) centers throughout the United States and Canada. Each TIS center is designed to serve a particular population in a geographic area.

12. Any other maternal health problems, including those discussed below.

MATERNAL CONDITIONS AFFECTING THE NEWBORN

A. **Maternal Infections** (see Chapters 19 and 20 for more detail): Many infections that are chronic, asymptomatic, or trivial to the healthy adult, such as rubella

● TABLE 1-2
Drugs Associated With Congenital Malformations in Human Beings

Drugs	Fetal Factor, Organ System Involved								
	Fetal growth	Growth retardation	Mental retardation	Central nervous system	Cardio-vascular	Musculo-skeletal	Urogenital	Eye and ear	Thyroid
Antimicrobials									
Tetracycline									
Streptomycin						X	X		
Quinine							X		
Antineoplastics									
Methotrexate	X	X		X		X			
Bisulfan, chlorambucil, cyclophosphamide				X		X	X	X	
Central nervous system drugs									
Morphine, methadone, heroin	X	X							
Thalidomide						X			
Anticonvulsants									
Phenytoin		X	X			X		X	
Barbiturates			X		X	X			
Trimethadione			X		X	X		X	
Valproic acid				X					
Steroid hormones									
Androgens							X		
Diethylstilbestrol							X		
Estrogen, progestins							X		
Iodine, propylthiouracil									X
Warfarin		X				X		X	
Propranolol		X							
Alcohol		X	X		X	X	X	X	
Tobacco smoking	X	X							
Isotretinoin			X	X		X		X	

From Aranda JV, Hales BF, Rieder MF: Developmental pharmacology. In Fanaroff AA, Martin RJ, editors, *Neonatal-perinatal medicine: diseases of the fetus and infant*, ed 7, 2002, St Louis, Mosby.

and cytomegalovirus, can be devastating to the fetus. Infection during the first 4 months of gestation can cause major malformations and/or widespread damage to the already formed but rapidly developing organs. Additionally, infections contribute to premature labor, can be introduced to the fetus and newborn in a variety of ways, and come in a variety of forms. High fever, for example, has been implicated in causing neural tube defects.

1. TORCH infections (Table 1-3)
   a. TORCH is an acronym for five infectious diseases: *t*oxoplasmosis, *o*thers (e.g., parvovirus), *r*ubella, *c*ytomegalovirus (CMV) and *h*erpes simplex virus (HSV).
   b. Still commonly referred to, but infrequently used as a diagnostic grouping. Most often mentioned when these infections are considered as part of the differential diagnosis in neonates who are born with severe growth restriction, microcephaly, hepatosplenomegaly, or petechiae.
   c. Each may cross the placenta and adversely affect the fetus.
   d. Immunity to rubella is part of the standard prenatal panel.
2. Sexually transmitted diseases (STDs) (Table 1-4)
   a. Sexually transmitted diseases are transmitted from one person to another during sexual intercourse through contact with the genitalia, mouth, or rectal area.
   b. 12 million cases of STDs occur each year, most in persons under 25 years.
   c. Sexually transmitted diseases that may affect the newborn include human immunodeficiency virus (HIV), chlamydia, gonorrhea, human papillomavirus (HPV), syphilis, trichomonas, and candidiasis.
3. Other communicable diseases (Table 1-5)
   a. Effect of infection varies depending on the disease, but in each case both the mother and the fetus must be considered.
   b. Common communicable diseases of concern include measles, mumps, chickenpox, influenza, mononucleosis, tuberculosis, and parvovirus.
4. Chorioamnionitis
   a. Chorioamnionitis is an infection of the chorion, amnion, and the amniotic fluid and is a major cause of perinatal morbidity and mortality.
   b. Usually associated with premature rupture of membranes, prolonged labor, or being GBS-positive; has also been demonstrated in patients with intact membranes.
   c. Typically, this is an ascending infection of endogenous lower genital tract flora into the uterus. Bacteria such as *E. coli*, group B streptococcus, anaerobic streptococci, and *Bacterioides* are frequently involved in chorioamnionitis. However, organisms such as *N. gonorrhea*, *L. monocytogenes*, herpes simplex virus, and cytomegalovirus have also been identified as the causative agents in chorioamnionitis.
5. Group B streptococcus (see Chapter 19)
   a. Of all pregnant women, 15% to 40% will be culture positive for group B streptococci when cultures of the lower genital tract are done between

TABLE 1-3
TORCH Infections

Infection/ Incubation	Transmission	Detection	Maternal Effects	Neonatal Effects	Incidence and Prevention
Cytomegalovirus (CMV) Incubation: unknown	Maternal infection via intimate contact with infected secretions Transplacentally infects fetus in utero; worst neonatal effects occur with maternal primary infection Neonatal infection at or immediately after birth from cervical secretions or breast milk; usually does not cause infant illness	Viral isolation from culture; presumptive diagnosis from 4-fold increase in antibody titer PCR certain labs	Clinically "silent"; only 1%–5% develop symptoms: low-grade fever, malaise, arthralgia, hepatomegaly	Infection most likely to occur with maternal primary infection 90% of infected infants are asymptomatic at birth, but 5%–15% of these may have long-term sequelae; 10% have severe involvement at birth: IUGR, microcephaly, periventricular calcification, deafness, blindness, chorioretinitis, mental retardation, hepatosplenomegaly	Primary infection occurs in 1%–2% of pregnant women 90% of adult population in the U.S. is seropositive Rigorous personal hygiene throughout pregnancy to prevent infection if CMV-negative
Herpes simplex virus (HSV) Incubation: 2–10 days	Intimate mucocutaneous exposure Passage through an infected birth canal Ascending infection, especially with rupture of membranes	Suspect with vesicles on cervix, vagina, or external genital area; painful lesions Presumptive diagnosis by	Painful genital lesions Primary infection is commonly associated with fever, malaise, myalgias	Rare transplacental transmissions have resulted in miscarriages 33%–50% risk for neonatal infection if mother has primary genital infection and	Estimated 300,000 new cases per year 1 in 3000–20,000 live births with perinatal trans- mission

(Continued)

● TABLE 1-3
TORCH Infections—cont'd

Infection/Incubation	Transmission	Detection	Maternal Effects	Neonatal Effects	Incidence and Prevention
	Transplacentally (rare) if initial infection occurs during pregnancy	fluorescent antibody or Papanicolaou smear on vesicular fluid Confirm diagnosis by vesicle culture	Numbness, tingling, burning, itching, and pain with lesions Lymphadenopathy Urinary retention	vaginal birth; 5% risk for neonatal infection with reactivation infection Severe neurologic sequelae may occur with CNS infection Disseminated disease involves multiple organs, especially liver and lungs Approximately 1/3 each CNS, disseminated, surface infections	Up to 80% of women delivering infected infants have no history of genital herpes; C/S if known active infection Avoid genital contact when male has penile lesions; use condoms
Rubella Incubation 14–23 days, usually 16–18 days	Nasopharyngeal secretions postnatally Transplacentally	Rubella-specific IgM usually indicates congenital or recent infection; rubella-specific	Pink maculopapular rash on face, neck, arms, and legs lasting 3 days Lymph node enlargement,	Fetal infection rate greatest before 11 weeks and after 35 weeks, but severe sequelae occurs with first trimester	Since introduction of vaccine in late 1960s, rubella is rare Occurs more commonly in

Organism/Incubation	Mode of Transmission	Maternal Signs/Symptoms	Diagnosis	Fetal/Newborn Effects	Comments
		fever, malaise, headache / History of exposure 3 weeks earlier	IgG with stable or increasing titer indicates congenital infection / Virus isolation from nasal or other specimens	infection; this includes deafness (60%–70%), eye defects (10%–30%), CNS anomalies (10%–25%), congenital heart disease (10%–20%)	springtime / Vaccine contraindicated during pregnancy; vaccinate susceptible women postpartum
Toxoplasmosis (protozoa, Toxoplasma gondii) Incubation: 7 days, with range 4–21 days	Eating raw meat containing T. gondii / Ingesting T. gondii cysts secreted in feces of infected cats; contaminated water / Transplacentally / Not transmitted human-to-human since the infecting organisms are tissue-bound and are not excreted	90% of women are asymptomatic / Posterior cervical lymphadenopathy / Malaise / Premature labor and delivery	Best tested by specialized labs assessing serologic antibody testing / Rarely, congenital infection can be detected prenatally by detecting parasite in fetal blood or amniotic fluid	Severity varies with gestational age (usually, earlier infection results in more severe effects) / Neurologic, ophthalmologic, and cognitive sequelae are variable / IUGR / Hydrocephalus / Microcephaly	Incidence varies throughout world (1–4 infants per 1000 live births) / 20%–30% of U.S. women have been exposed / Incidence of congenital toxoplasmosis infection in U.S is 1 in 1000–8000 / Reduce contact with cats during pregnancy

● TABLE 1-4
Sexually Transmitted Diseases

Infection/Agent/Incubation	Detection	Maternal Effects	Neonatal Effects	Incidence
Human immune deficiency virus (HIV)–acquired immunodeficiency syndrome (AIDS) is the most severe form of HIV. Incubation: usually 12–18 months in untreated perinatal infection	For screening of pregnant women, a rapid HIV antibody test is available; positive screens need follow-up confirmatory tests		13%–39% chance of transmission to newborn from untreated HIV seropositive mother; most-critical factor is maternal viral load. Worldwide, 1/3–1/2 of mother-to-infant infections may occur via breastfeeding	1% of all U.S. AIDS cases occur in children (this incidence has been reduced almost by half over last decade by maternal treatment with antiretroviral therapy during pregnancy and by new treatment options for infected children)
Chlamydia bacteria: *Chlamydia trachomatis*. Incubation: variable, but is usually >1 week	Endocervical and urethral culture, nucleic acid amplification tests (e.g., PCR), or antigen tests (EIA, DFA) on swab specimens	Most asymptomatic. Mucopurulent cervicitis. Frequently associated with other sexually transmitted diseases. Occasionally, premature rupture of membranes, preterm labor, IUGR, infertility, chorioamnionitis	30%–40% of exposed infants develop conjunctivitis; 3%–8% develop pneumonia	Most common reportable sexually transmitted disease in the U.S. Prevalence in pregnant women 6%–12%; may be higher in pregnant teens. 70% of infections may be asymptomatic
Gonorrhea bacteria: *Neisseria gonorrhoea*, gram-negative diplococcus. Incubation: 2–7 days	Endocervical, oral, or rectal cultures. Genital or blood cultures. Gram stain of lesions. Nucleic acid amplification tests becoming more commonly used on endocervical/urethral swabs	60%–80% of those infected are asymptomatic. Occasionally, pelvic peritonitis, premature rupture of membranes, postpartum endometritis, chorioamnionitis, increased infertility, ectopic pregnancy	Purulent conjunctivitis is most common. Disseminated disease with sepsis and meningitis or focal abscess can occur	Estimated 650,000 cases are reported in U.S. each year. Highest rates are in adolescents 16–19 years of age
Human papillomavirus (HPV)	Most diagnosed on clinical exam	Significant number of lesions enlarge during	Potential transmission of laryngeal papillomata	Estimated 40–60 million persons infected

Incubation: unknown but probably 3 months to several years	Definitive diagnosis based on detection of viral DNA or RNA	pregnancy Usually multicentric in pregnancy	Very rare (less than 1 in 1000–1500 pregnancies in which mothers have genital condyloma)	worldwide Anogenital HPV the most common sexually transmitted disease in the U.S. (40% are sexually active adolescent females) HPV lesions probably more frequent in pregnant women because of increased hormone levels Associated with other STDs
Syphilis spirochete: *Treponema pallidum* Incubation: 3 weeks on average (range of 10–90 days)	Definitive diagnosis with spirochetes seen on darkfield exam or by DFA on exudate or tissue Nontreponemal tests include VDRL, RPR (rapid plasma reagin), or ART (automated reagin test) Treponemal tests include FTA-ABS and TP-PA tests	Primary chancre: painless ulcerative lesion Secondary syphilis: fever and malaise, red macules on palms or soles of feet Generalized lymphadenopathy Early latent syphilis (positive serology <1 year duration) Latent (cardiovascular) syphilis Neurosyphilis	Vary depending on gestation Stillbirth IUGR Nonimmune hydrops Premature labor	70%–100% fetal transmission rate in primary maternal disease In untreated pregnancies, 40% end in spontaneous abortion Transmission to the fetus can occur with any stage, but 60%–100% of transmission is during secondary syphilis
Trichomonas protozoa: *Trichomonas vaginalis* Incubation: 4–28 days	"Wet prep" saline examination Papanicolaou smear Urinalysis	Malodorous, discoloured vaginal discharge Dysuria	Infant contact through infected vagina Usually asymptomatic	Not reported to CDC but estimated in as many as 20% of pregnancies Estimates of 10%–15% of all cases of vaginitis

● TABLE 1-5
Other Communicable Diseases

Infection/Agent/ Incubation	Mode of Transmission	Maternal Effects	Neonatal Effects	Incidence and Prevention
Influenza virus Incubation: 24–72 hours	Respiratory secretions	Usually brief but incapacitating disease Death occurs from secondary bacterial pneumonia	Any risk of malformation has been confined to first trimester Most studies fail to support teratogenicity	Killed virus vaccine Vaccine during pregnancy is indicated if mother is at medical risk because of other diseases
Mumps paramyxovirus Incubation: 16–18 days	Respiratory secretions	Spontaneous abortion rate increased 2-fold	Teratogenicity unknown	Avoid pregnancy for 3 months after vaccination
Parvovirus B19 (fifth disease) DNA virus Incubation: 4–14 days	Respiratory secretions Percutaneous exposure to blood Mother-to-fetus transmission	Erythema Elevated temperature Arthralgia	Spontaneous abortions Can cause fetal hydrops and death but is not proven cause of congenital anomalies Risk for fetal death 2%–6%, greater in first half of pregnancy	Risk for fetal infection in women with primary infection during first 20 weeks of pregnancy is 15%–17%
Hepatitis B virus Incubation: 45–160 days	Sexually Perinatally Transplacentally Blood, stool, and saliva transmission	Fever, jaundice, malaise, hepatosplenomegaly Premature labor	Increased stillbirth rate Infected infants usually asymptomatic at birth	200,000–300,000 cases in the U.S. each year Risk for HBV infection 70%–90% for infant born to mother who is HBsAg- and HBeAg-positive; 5%–20% if mother is HBeAg-negative
Varicella (chickenpox) Varicella-zoster virus Incubation: 10–21 days (usually 14–16 days)	Probably by aerosolized respiratory droplets Portal of entry is respiratory tract Transplacentally	Severe in adults Risk for premature labor due to high temperature Risk for varicella pneumonia appears to be increased during pregnancy	2% of infants with maternal infection in first trimester have cutaneous scarring, eye abnormalities, and retardation At risk if maternal rash onset 5 days before to 2 days after delivery; severe disseminated neonatal disease may develop, and one third die	95% of women are immune In U.S. occurs in <0.1% of pregnancies

23 and 26 weeks (Cunningham et al., 1997; AAP Red book, 2003). Maternal colonization group B streptococcus (GBS) can be intermittent or constant during pregnancy. The rectal reservoir for GBS cannot be eradiated with antepartum antibiotics, so intrapartum treatment is recommended.

   b. Maternal-infant transmission of GBS can occur before delivery (ascending colonization or infection after rupture of membranes), during delivery, or after delivery by direct contact.

   c. Prior to the recommendation for use of intrapartum antibiotic to mothers to prevent neonatal GBS disease in infants, the incidence of neonatal disease was 1 to 4 cases per 1000 live births. With intrapartum chemoprophylaxis, the incidence of early-onset disease has decreased by 70% (Centers for Disease Control and Prevention, 2002).

B. Hypertension in Pregnancy (Roberts, 1989): The incidence of hypertension in pregnancy ranges from 10% to 40% depending on the population studied. This includes a variety of hypertensive disorders that contribute to significant maternal and fetal/neonatal morbidity and mortality. Maternal hypertension is associated with maternal cerebral vascular accident, placental infarct, placental abruption, and fetal growth restriction.

  1. Classification

    a. Preeclampsia; also referred to as pregnancy-induced hypertension (PIH) or gestational hypertension

      (1) Generally occurs in third trimester

      (2) Diagnostic criteria: hypertension, proteinuria, with or without pathologic edema (face, hands, and feet)

      (3) Abnormalities range from mild to severe; severe preeclampsia includes some or all of the following:

        (a) Systolic blood pressure (BP) ≥160 mm Hg or diastolic BP ≥110 mm Hg on two measurements at bed rest and at least 6 hours apart

        (b) Proteinuria ≥5 g in 24 hours or ≥3+ by dipstick method on two urine specimens at least 4 hours apart

        (c) Oliguria of ≤400 mL urine in 24 hours

        (d) Cerebral or visual disturbances

        (e) Epigastric pain

        (f) Pulmonary edema or cyanosis

        (g) Fetal growth restriction or severe oligohydramnios

      (4) Accounts for 70% of the hypertension in pregnant women.

      (5) Although cause is not clear, hypertension resolves with delivery of the infant and placenta.

      (6) HELLP syndrome is a malignant form of preeclampsia associated with *h*emolysis, *e*levated *l*iver enzymes, and *l*ow *p*latelets; mortality is as high as 10%.

    b. Eclampsia: Preeclampsia plus seizures

    c. Chronic hypertension of any etiology

    d. Chronic hypertension with superimposed preeclampsia

    e. Late or transient hypertension, or "gestational hypertension": Refers to hypertension that develops during pregnancy and that is not associated with proteinuria.

  2. Management of pregnancy-induced hypertension depends on the gestational age at which the diagnosis is made.

    a. Mild PIH: Home bed rest, salt restriction, and frequent maternal-fetal evaluation is recommended at term.

    b. Unresponsive hypertension and/or proteinuria: Hospitalization for bed rest, fluid management, and monitoring of both mother and fetus. If estimated gestational age is <34 weeks, antenatal steroids are usually given because of the increased probability of premature delivery. Antenatal steroids are recommended if estimated gestational age is <34 weeks and mother and infant are sufficiently stable for possible delay of delivery.

    c. Severe hypertension: Antihypertensive medications and possibly delivery of the infant.

    d. Monitoring neurologic status is important because of the high maternal morbidity associated with eclamptic seizures. Assessment should include evaluation of deep tendon reflexes and clonus. Magnesium sulfate may be used for seizure prophylaxis in at-risk women with close supervision for signs and symptoms of toxicity.

  3. Fetal/neonatal effects: Associated with premature delivery, reduced birth weight, and perinatal death

C. Diabetes: Diabetes is a systemic disorder caused by a relative or absolute deficiency of insulin secretion that results in hyperglycemia. Diabetes is estimated to occur in 3% to 5% of pregnancies. Diabetes in pregnancy may be a preexisting condition, a chronic condition that is first detected in pregnancy, or a condition manifested only during pregnancy (gestational diabetes). Although both maternal and fetal mortality from this disorder have declined dramatically over the last century, maternal diabetes still has significant morbidity implications for both the mother and fetus. Outcome is closely related to diabetic control prior to conception and during pregnancy.

  1. Classification: A variety of classification systems have been developed, but that proposed by White in 1949 is still widely used for both clinical and prognostic purposes (Table 1-6).

  2. Maternal effects of preexisting diabetes

    a. Normal fertility but marked increase in incidence of spontaneous abortions with poor control (Coustan, 1988; Mills et al., 1988).

    b. Maternal mortality of diabetic patients is approximately 8 to 10 times higher than that of nondiabetic patients.

    c. At risk for hypoglycemia and ketoacidosis.

    d. Increased risk for preterm delivery.

    e. Increased risk for preeclampsia.

    f. More commonly have polyhydramnios, which increases the risk for premature rupture of the membranes.

    g. Patients with proliferative retinopathy may have progression of disease during pregnancy.

● TABLE 1-6
White Classification of Diabetes in Pregnancy

Class	Age of Onset (yr)		Duration (yr)	Vascular Disease	Insulin
A	Any		Any	0	Diet only
B	>20		<10	0	—
C	10–19	or	10–19	0	—
D	<10	or	>20	Benign retinopathy	—
F	Any		Any	Nephropathy	—
R	Any		Any	Proliferative retinopathy	—
H	Any		Any	Heart disease	—

From White P: Pregnancy complicating diabetes, *Am J Med* 7:609, 1949. Copyright 1949 by Excerpta Medica, Inc.

3. Fetal effects
   a. Increased incidence of fetal macrosomia secondary to chronic neonatal hyperglycemia and insulin growth effects.
   b. With significant maternal vascular disease (Class D and higher) up to 20% of infants are small for gestational age secondary to decreased placental function.
   c. Increased risk for fetal death, usually in the third trimester, and especially with maternal ketoacidosis.
   d. Incidence of major anomalies is 3% to 25% overall but is highest when maternal diabetic control is poor.
4. Neonatal disease (see Chapters 16 and 17)
   a. Neonatal problems may include labor-related trauma, increased C/S rate, perinatal asphyxia, hypoglycemia, hypocalcemia, hypomagnesemia, polycythemia, hyperbilirubinemia, respiratory distress syndrome, hypertrophic cardiomyopathy, and congenital anomalies.
   b. Prognosis appears to correlate with severity of maternal vascular disease and with maternal diabetic control; with very tight diabetic control during pregnancy, neonatal outcome may be similar to nondiabetics, regardless of the maternal diabetic class (Coustan et al., 1980).
5. Management of pregnancy, labor, and delivery
   a. Cornerstone of therapy is good diabetic control with glucose levels maintained in a tight range and avoidance of hypoglycemia and ketoacidosis.
   b. Close follow-up of renal function and eye disease.
   c. Fetal ultrasound:
      (1) In first trimester for dating purposes
      (2) At 16-18 weeks to rule out anomalies
      (3) Late pregnancy to estimate fetal size for delivery
   d. Maternal serum alpha-fetoprotein (AFP) at 16 to 20 weeks because of increased incidence of congenital anomalies
   e. Fetal surveillance (e.g., biophysical profile or non-stress test, see Chapter 2) every 1 to 2 weeks beginning in the third trimester. Onset of antepartum testing depends on degree of control; this ranges from testing

beginning around 32 weeks with good control to testing initiated at around 26 to 28 weeks with poor control.

    f. Optimal delivery time is based on fetal health and maternal disease control.

D. Thyroid Disorders

    1. Maternal hyperthyroidism

        a. Occurs in 0.2% of pregnancies, with severe disease (thyroid storm) rare but associated with up to 25% maternal mortality.

        b. Usually secondary to Graves disease (diffuse toxic goiter).

        c. Maternal treatment:

            (1) Medical management with thioamides (propylthiouracil [PTU] preferred over methimazole [Tapazole]) to block thyroid hormone synthesis

            (2) Partial surgical ablation of the thyroid if medical management fails.

            (3) Radioactive iodine ablation is reserved for the postpartum period and after breastfeeding is terminated (or delayed).

        d. Fetal effects can include:

            (1) Growth retardation, prematurity; approximately 1% of infants born to mothers with Graves disease develop thyrotoxicosis, with a mortality of 10% to 20%.

            (2) Because PTU crosses the placenta, may see transient neonatal hypothyroidism; or may see hyperthyroidism when the thyroid suppressive medications are gone from the newborn but the passively transferred thyroid-stimulating medications from the mother have stimulated the newborn's thyroid gland.

    2. Maternal hypothyroidism

        a. Rare

        b. Treated with thyroid replacement therapy

        c. Good fetal and maternal outcomes

        d. Untreated maternal hypothyroidism may lead to decreased IQ in their offspring.

E. Asthma

    1. Prevalence of asthma is increasing over time in the general population.

    2. Complications occur in approximately 1% of all pregnancies. Maternal effects of asthma and its treatment during pregnancy can include preeclampsia, asthma exacerbations, cesarean section delivery, and premature rupture of membranes.

    3. Associated fetal and neonatal complications can include increased perinatal mortality and spontaneous fetal abortion rates, prematurity, growth retardation, hypoxia, birth asphyxia, hypoadrenalism, and theophylline toxicity (Whitty and Dombrowski, 2002).

F. Blood Group Incompatibilities (also see Chapter 14).

    1. Maternal blood type, Rh status, and antibody screen should be part of prenatal lab tests.

    2. If antibody screen is positive, the specific antibody ("irregular antibody") should be identified.

3. Isoimmunization occurs when mother produces an antibody against fetal blood group antigens, which her body recognizes as foreign; these antibodies can cross the placenta and destroy fetal red blood cells, particularly in subsequent pregnancies.
4. Rh isoimmunization
   a. Most common type of isoimmunization
   b. Rh-negative mother, Rh-positive fetus
   c. Prevented by Rh immune globulin (RhoGAM) administered at 28 weeks gestation; decreases exposure to the Rh antigen in the maternal circulation, thereby preventing antibody formation. Repeat immunization is given after delivery with confirmation of Rh-positive child.
5. Isoimmunization from irregular antibodies
   a. Examples of red blood cell antigens to which irregular antibodies can form: Kell, Duffy, Kidd.
   b. Occurs in only 2% of isoimmunization situations but is on the rise because of the decline of Rh-D disease due to successful RhoGAM programs.
   c. If mother is irregular antibody–positive, father should be checked for the antigen. If father is negative, no further evaluation needed. If father is antigen-positive, further fetal assessment and surveillance need to be done in the form of serial antibody titers, ultrasound examinations, amniocentesis, and fetal blood sampling and transfusion.
6. Fetal effects: Untreated fetal isoimmunization may result in severe anemia, kernicterus, hydrops, and fetal death.

G. **Multiple-Gestation Pregnancy:** Multiple gestation is considered a "complication" of pregnancy because there is increased risk for maternal morbidity as well as increased risk for fetal/neonatal morbidity and mortality.
   1. Incidence: Varies with ethnicity and is increased with familial history of multiple pregnancy, increased maternal age, and increased parity.
   2. The use of fertility-stimulating therapies and assisted reproductive technologies has caused a marked increase in multiple births in the last 20 years. The number of multiple births in the United States exceeded 100,000 for the first time in 1993. The vast majority of these pregnancies are not monochorionic.
   3. The increase in multiple births is mainly seen among older Caucasian women with high educational status.
   4. Maternal morbidity
      a. Anemia
      b. Polyhydramnios
      c. Premature rupture of membranes
      d. Premature labor
      e. Hypertension, preeclampsia
   5. Fetal/neonatal morbidity
      a. Prematurity
      b. Vascular anastomoses
         (1) May be arterial, venous, or arteriovenous.

(2) Complications can include oligohydramnios/polyhydramnios, hydrops, fetal demise, and fetal malformations.

(3) Twin-twin transfusion syndrome results from ateriovenous anastomoses in monozygotic twins who are monochorionic-diamniotic. Usually, arterial blood goes from a donor twin to the recipient twin via the anastomosis to the vein of the recipient twin. Donor complications include hypovolemia, anemia, and undergrowth, whereas the recipient may develop hypervolemia, cardiomegaly, congestive heart failure, hyperviscosity, and polycythemia.

c. Growth retardation

d. Abnormal presentation

e. Placental abruption, placenta previa, cord prolapse

f. Congenital anomalies are increased in monochorionic pregnancies and chromosomal anomalies are increased in offspring of women of advanced maternal age.

6. Twins

a. Occur spontaneously in approximately 1:94 pregnancies in the United States (Cunningham et al., 1997).

b. Monozygotic (identical) twins (Figure 1-1, *A*): Occur when an egg divides after fertilization. Always the same sex. Depending on the timing of the egg division, the placenta may be:

(1) Diamniotic/dichorionic (division <3 days); most common type.

(2) Diamniotic/monochorionic (division occurs days 4 to 8).

(3) Monoamniotic/monochorionic (division after day 8); most morbidity occurs in this group.

c. Dizygotic (fraternal) twins (Figure 1-1, *B*): Twice as common as monogygotic twinning. Results from more than one egg being fertilized by

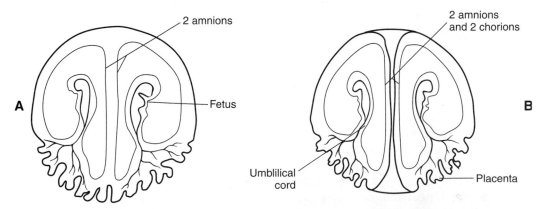

FIGURE 1-1 ● **A,** Monozygotic twins usually share one placenta and chorion and usually have individual amniotic sacs with two layers separating them. **B,** Dizygotic twins: each fetus has its own placenta, chorion, and amnion with four layers separating them. (From Beischer NA, Mackey EV, Colditz PB: *Obstetrics and the newborn,* ed 3, Philadelphia, 1997, WB Saunders.)

more than one sperm. There are two amnions, two chorions, and separate or fused placentas.

   d. Mean gestational age at delivery is 37 weeks.

  7. Triplets or more

   a. The majority of triplet and quadruplet pregnancies are complicated by the same problems characteristic of twin pregnancies. Triplet outcomes are reported at 95% infant survival.

   b. Virtually all triplet, quadruplet, and higher multiple pregnancies are delivered by C/S and prematurely.

MATERNAL PSYCHOSOCIAL CONSIDERATIONS

A. Mothers with Multiple-Gestation Pregnancies

  1. Approximately 50,000 women in the United States have multiple-gestation pregnancies.

  2. Psychosocial risks: Maternal stresses are significant and can include extended antepartum and neonatal hospital stays, exhaustion from caring for multiple infants, short- and long-term financial burden. These women are at increased risk for postpartum depression, problems with bonding, social isolation, substance use, and child abuse. Maternal problems are often overlooked secondary to the excitement surrounding multiple births.

  3. For women who undergo fetal reduction procedures or spontaneous partial loss of the pregnancy, there may be guilt, as well as grief and loss issues. Often these go unrecognized by family and health care professionals.

  4. Care provider implications: These include, but are not limited to, thorough pre- and postconception counseling, anticipatory discussion of maternal stresses, information about outpatient services and home care assistance as needed, perinatal loss support if applicable.

B. Teen Mothers

  1. At risk for pregnancy complications and preterm deliveries.

  2. Often come from high-risk backgrounds, the risk factors of which are likely to persist postnatally (e.g., unstable homes, divorce, domestic abuse, substance abuse).

  3. Often uninformed about pregnancy, hospitalization, infant care, and parenting.

  4. Care provider implications: Special services should be available, ideally from preconception to postdelivery. Do not discharge until thorough infant care teaching has been completed, clear follow-up has been established, and it is clear the infant is feeding well.

C. Developmentally Disabled Mothers

  1. Unfortunately, many women with developmental disabilities live in high-risk situations. They are often targets for abuse and victimization, typically lack education and safe housing, and are frequently involved with alcohol and drugs. They often put themselves in difficult situations, further promoting physical and emotional abuse.

  2. Without family or social service support, many of these women do not have basic knowledge about caring for their babies and small children.

Time permitting, it is important to spend as much time as possible with these mothers in basic care instructions and to have them return demonstrate their understanding of routine neonatal care.

3. It is known that many developmentally disabled mothers are less likely to be affectionate, responsive, and accommodating towards their children, characteristics that have been shown to be critical for optimal language, cognitive, and social development of children. Studies have shown that educational programs for these mothers can significantly improve maternal parenting skills, with demonstrable positive benefits in their children (Feldman et al., 1989; Feldman, 1992). Unfortunately, few hospital pre- or postnatal parental education services are geared to the developmentally disabled mother. It is recommended that local resources be identified, if available, and that the mother be connected with these programs prior to hospital discharge.

D. Postpartum Depression (PPD)

1. PPD is defined as the most common complication of pregnancy, with a substantial risk for morbidity and death. It affects 10% to 30% of all patients after delivery, and up to 50% of PPD cases have gone undiagnosed.

2. PPD is commonly used as a catch-all phrase for many postpartum emotional symptoms. The fourth edition of the *Diagnostic and Statistical Manual of Mental Disorders (DSM-IV)* defines PPD as an episode of depression beginning within 4 weeks after delivery, though onset can occur anytime in the first year after delivery. Without treatment, the average duration of PPD is 7 months.

3. Four postpartum mood disorders have been identified:
   a. Postpartum psychosis: Rare, occurring in 1 to 2 per 1000 births. Usually occurs within 2 weeks of delivery and can be associated with unusual hallucinations, delusions, agitation, bizarre irrational behavior, and extreme disorganization of thought.
   b. Postpartum obsessive compulsive disorder: Clinical signs and symptoms can include repetitive intrusive thoughts of harming baby, fear of being alone with the baby, or hypervigilance in protecting the baby.
   c. Postpartum-onset panic disorder: Acute onset of anxiety, fear, rapid breathing, palpation, and a sense of doom.
   d. Postpartum depression (PPD): Most common of the postpartum mood disorders. Clinical signs and symptoms include:
      (1) Period of at least 2 weeks of depressed mood or loss of interest in activities; withdrawn, flat affect, less responsive, and less affectionate to their infants than nondepressed mothers
      (2) Changes in appetite or weight
      (3) Feelings of worthlessness or guilt
      (4) Difficulty with concentrating or making decisions
      (5) Recurrent thought of death or suicidal ideation, plans, or attempts.

4. Significant predictors of PPD (Beck, 2002): History of prior depression, newborns with eating or sleeping difficulties, stressful life situations (e.g., divorce, marital dissatisfaction, financial problems, family illness),

fatigue, lack of emotional support from spouse or family, feelings of anxiety about being a parent during pregnancy, low self-esteem, periods of tearfulness and mood swings during the first week after delivery, unwanted pregnancy, history of prior pregnancy loss, and, occasionally, unplanned cesarean section.

5. Diagnosis and treatment: Early diagnosis and intervention are critical.
   a. The greatest obstacle to early diagnosis is failure of health care professionals to evaluate symptoms or question mothers during the postpartum period. Additionally, women fail to report symptoms or discount their feelings, blaming them on hormones.
   b. Treatment should depend on the severity of depression. Therapeutic options include antidepressants, support groups, and individual or group psychotherapy.
   c. Two organizations that can provide information and support regarding PPD:
      (1) Depression After Delivery, Inc: (800) 944-4PPD, *www.behavenet. com/dadinc*
      (2) Postpartum Support International: (805) 967-7636, *www.iup. edulan/postpartum*

REFERENCES

American Academy of Pediatrics: Group B streptococcal infections. In Pickering LK, editor: *Red book: report of the committee on infectious diseases,* ed 26, Elk Grove Village, IL, 2003, American Academy of Pediatrics, pp 584-591.

Beck CT: Revision of the postpartum depression predictors inventory, *JOGNN* 31: 394-402, 2002.

Benedetti TJ: Obstetric hemorrhage. In Gabbe SG, Niebyl JR, Simpson JL, editors: *Obstetrics: normal and problem pregnancies,* ed 4, Philadelphia, 2002, Churchill-Livingstone, pp 503-538.

Boyd ME, Usher RH, McLean FH, Kramer MS: Obstetric consequences of postmaturity, *Am J Obstet Gynecol* 158:334-338, 1988.

Campbell WA, Nochimson DJ, Vintzileos AM: Prolonged pregnancy. In Knuppel RA, Drukker JE, editors: *High-risk pregnancy: a team approach,* Philadelphia, 1993, WB Saunders.

Centers for Disease Control and Prevention: Prevention of perinatal group B streptococcal disease: revised guidelines from CDC, *MMWR* 51(RR-11):1-22, August 12, 2002.

Chasnoff IJ, Landress HJ, Barrett ME: The prevalence of illicit-drug or alcohol use during pregnancy and discrepancies in mandatory reporting in Pinellas County, Florida, *N Engl J Med* 322:1202-1206, 1990.

Comeau J, Shaw L, Marcel C, Lavery JP: Early placenta previa and delivery outcome, *Obstet Gynecol* 61:577-580, 1983.

Coustan DR, Berkowitz RL, Hobbins JC: Tight metabolic control over diabetes in pregnancy, *Am J Med* 68:845-852, 1980.

Coustan DR: Pregnancy in diabetic women, *N Engl J Med* 319:1663-1665, 1988 (editorial).

Cunningham G, McDonald P, Gant N, et al: *Williams obstetrics,* ed 20, Norwalk, CT, 1997, Appleton & Lange.

Feldman MA: Teaching child-care skills to mothers with developmental disabilities, *J App Behav Anal* 25:205-215, 1992.

Feldman MA, Case L, Rincover A, et al: Parent Education Project. III. Increasing affection and responsivity in developmentally handicapped mothers: component analysis, generalization, and effects on child language, *J App Behav Anal* 22:211-222, 1989.

Ferris TF: Toxemia and hypertension. In Burrow GN, Ferris TF, editors: *Medical complications during pregnancy*, ed 3, Philadelphia, 1988, WB Saunders, pp 1-33.

Hill DJ, Beischer NA: Placenta previa without antepartum hemorrhage, *Aust N Z J Obstet Gynecol* 20:21-23, 1980.

International Federation of Gynecology and Obstetrics (FIGO): *Report of the FIGO Subcommittee on Perinatal Epidemiology and Health Statistics* (following a workshop in Cairo, November 1984), London, 1986, International Federation of Gynecology and Obstetrics, p 54.

Lydon-Rochelle M, Hold VL, Easterling TR, et al: Risk of uterine rupture during labor among women with a prior cesarean delivery, *N Engl J Med* 345:3-8, 2001.

Mills JL, Simpson JL, Driscoll SG, et al: Incidence of spontaneous abortions among normal women and insulin-dependent diabetic women whose pregnancies were identified within 21 days of conception, *N Engl J Med* 319:1617-1623, 1988.

Ricci JM: Antepartum hemorrhage. In Hacker NF, Moore JG, editors: *Essentials of obstetrics and gynecology*, ed 2, Philadelphia, 1992, WB Saunders, pp 154-162.

Roberts JM: Pregnancy-related hypertension. In Creasy RK, Resnik R, editors: *Maternal-fetal medicine*, ed 2, Philadelphia, 1989, WB Saunders, pp 777-823.

Schrag SJ, Zell ER, Lynfield R: A population-based comparison of strategies to prevent early-onset group B streptococcal disease in neonates, *N Engl J Med* 347:233-239, 2002.

Tabsh K, Theroux N: Rhesus isoimmunization. In Hacker NF, Moore JG, editors: *Essentials of obstetrics and gynecology*, ed 2, Philadelphia, 1992, WB Saunders, pp 299-307.

Whitty DE, Dombrowski MP: Respiratory diseases in pregnancy. In Gabbe SG, Niebyl JR, Simpson JL, editors: *Obstetrics: normal and problem pregnancies*, ed 4, Philadelphia, 2002, Churchill-Livingstone, pp 1033-1064.

World Health Organization: Recommended definition, terminology and format for statistical tables related to perinatal period and rise of a new certification for cause of perinatal deaths (modification recommended by FIGO as amended, October 1976), *Obstet Gynecol Scand* 56:347, 1977.

2 Fetal Assessment, Labor, and Delivery

Daniel M. Hall, MD ■ *John C. Hobbins, MD*

FETAL ASSESSMENT

A. Fetal Heart Rate Monitoring (Figure 2-1)

1. Normal baseline is 120–160 beats per minute (BPM).
2. Bradycardia: <110–120 BPM.
    a. Heart rate (HR) of 100–120 with good variability (see below) may be normal, possibly mild hypoxia.
    b. HR <100 is most commonly associated with fetal asphyxia.
    c. Other causes can include fetal heart block and maternal drugs such as β-blocking agents or cocaine.
3. Tachycardia: >160 BPM.
    a. Causes include prematurity, maternal fever or infection (especially chorioamnionitis), mild hypoxia, fetal tachyarrhythmias, fetal anemia, fetal hyperthyroidism, and maternal drugs such as terbutaline and β-adrenergic agents.
    b. Tachycardia is of much more concern if poor variability is present.
4. Sinusoidal heart rate pattern
    a. Baseline between 120–160 with smooth undulations resembling a sine wave
    b. Associated with severe fetal anemia such as in isoimmunization or fetal-maternal hemorrhage and with maternal narcotic administration
5. Heart rate variability ("beat-to-beat variability")
    a. Normal variability
        (1) Short-term variability: Variation in rate between several sequential beats.
        (2) Long-term variability: Gradual increase or decrease in heart rate baseline over several minutes.
        (3) Presence of both short- and long-term variability makes hypoxia unlikely.
    b. Abnormal variability
        (1) Decreased variability: Heart rate variation of <6 beats over 1 minute.
        (2) Absent variability: "Flat" tracing.
        (3) Presence of either or both suggests hypoxia, heart block, maternal drugs (e.g., magnesium sulfate, narcotics, Valium), anencephaly.

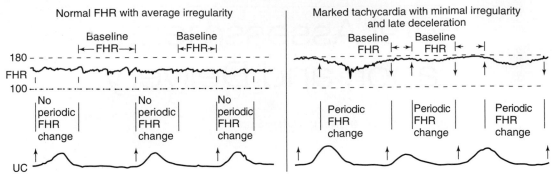

FIGURE 2-1 ● Evaluation of fetal heart rate (FHR) is subdivided into control (nonstressed or baseline) and stress (periodic) portions. The baseline rate may correspond to the time between contractions (UC), as shown at left, or may be only a short interval, as shown at right. (From Hon EH: *An atlas of fetal heart rate patterns*, New Haven, CT, 1968, Harty Press.)

    6. Periodic changes in fetal heart rate seen with labor and delivery
        a. Accelerations: Occur as a normal response to fetal movement or uterine contractions (Figure 2-2)
        b. Decelerations (Figure 2-3)
            (1) Early decelerations
                (a) Occur at the same time as uterine contractions and mirror the contraction intensity.
                (b) Heart rate rarely goes below 100 BPM.
                (c) Occurs secondary to vagal stimulation from head compression and mild transient hypoxia.
                (d) Benign and need no intervention.
            (2) Variable decelerations
                (a) Duration, depth, shape are variable.
                (b) Secondary to insufficient umbilical blood flow, which may be due to cord compression or vagal stimulation.
                (c) Often seen with oligohydramnios.
                (d) Severe variable decelerations are of concern if recurrent, prolonged, or associated with HR <60 BPM.
            (3) Late decelerations
                (a) Start well after contraction is underway, reach lowest point after peak of contraction has passed, and return to baseline after contraction is complete (late "mirror image").
                (b) Caused by uteroplacental insufficiency.
                (c) May result in fetal myocardial hypoxia and fetal distress.
                (d) Most ominous of the heart rate patterns; if recurrent and associated with absent heart rate variability or marked fetal bradycardia, immediate intervention (usually delivery) is indicated.
  B. Ultrasound Assessment In Labor and Delivery
    1. Assessing fetal gestational age (GA)

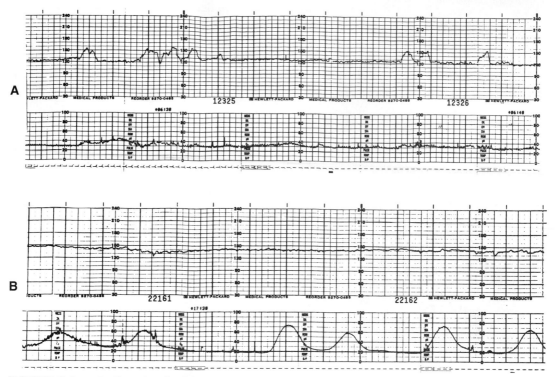

FIGURE 2-2 ● **A,** Reactive fetal heart rate pattern with accelerations in response to fetal stimulation. **B,** Nonreactive fetal heart rate pattern, with no accelerations. (From Simpson KR, Creehan PA, editors: *AWHONN perinatal nursing,* Philadelphia, 1996, Lippincott Raven, p 198.)

    a. GA determination by ultrasound is best done by serial measurements, with at least one during the second trimester. Dating by last menstrual period may be more reliable if first ultrasound is performed after 30 weeks gestation.

    b. Measurement techniques

       (1) Biparietal diameter (BPD)

          (a) Diameter at the widest point of the skull correlates with GA.

          (b) Most accurate for dates if performed between 12-18 weeks gestation; at term can be inaccurate if head is deep in pelvis.

       (2) Femur length (FL)

          (a) Most accurate when measured in 2nd trimester

          (b) May be inaccurate with chromosomal anomalies, abnormal fetal growth, or skeletal dysplasias.

2. Assessing fetal weight

    a. Estimated by combining BPD, FL, and measurement of abdominal circumference.

    b. At term, accuracy of measurements may vary depending on fetal position and amniotic fluid volume.

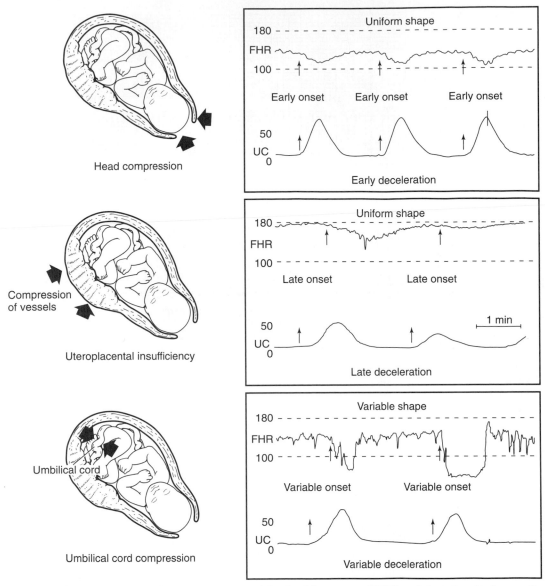

FIGURE 2-3 ● Deceleration patterns of the fetal heart rate (FHR) and their implied causative mechanisms. Intrauterine pressure (UC) is measured in millimeters of mercury. (From Hon EH: *An atlas of fetal heart rate patterns,* New Haven, CT, 1968, Harty Press.)

3. Confirming fetal presentation
4. Determining placental location
   a. Placenta previa (placental tissue on both sides of the internal os of the cervix); risk for severe maternal/fetal hemorrhage with labor and vaginal delivery.

      b. Placental abruption (premature separation of placenta from the uterus) can be confirmed by ultrasound in only a minority of cases; a normal study does *not* rule out a placental abruption.

  5. Assessing amniotic fluid volume

      a. Amniotic fluid index (AFI): Measures the maximal depth of pockets of fluid in four quadrants of the uterus.

      b. Oligohydramnios: AFI <5 cm

         (1) Can be seen with ruptured membranes, placental insufficiency (poor placental function), fetal renal anomalies, and postmature (>41 weeks) fetuses.

         (2) Oligohydramnios for several weeks or more may place the fetus at risk for developing pulmonary hypoplasia, limb contractures, or umbilical cord compression with compromise to fetal blood flow.

      c. Polyhydramnios: AFI >20 cm

         (1) Can be seen with maternal diabetes, fetal neurologic disorders (secondary to disordered swallowing), or intestinal obstructions (secondary to lack of fluid absorption by the fetal intestine).

         (2) Presence of polyhydramnios may place pregnancy at risk for preterm or dysfunctional labor and postpartum hemorrhage (secondary to uterine atony).

  6. Evaluating blood flow to the fetus by Doppler ultrasound

      a. Primarily used to evaluate blood flow velocity in the umbilical artery; decreased or reversed (toward the fetus) blood flow during diastole suggests diminished placental-fetal reserves and is a risk factor for poor fetal growth and fetal distress.

      b. Examining blood flow velocity in other fetal vessels (e.g., middle cerebral artery) is less common but can help in assessing fetal well-being.

C. Integrated Tests of Fetal Well-Being

  1. The nonstress test (NST)

      a. Used in late gestation (after 34 weeks) and combines monitoring of fetal heart rate with fetal activity.

      b. "Reactive" NST

         (1) Two or more spontaneous increases in fetal heart rate within a 20-minute period accompanying fetal movement.

         (2) Suggests a normal fetus.

      c. "Non-reactive" NST

         (1) No increase in fetal heart rate within a 20- minute period accompanying fetal movement.

         (2) May indicate hypoxia, but usually is due to fetal sleep state; maternal sedatives can also cause a nonreactive NST.

         (3) A complete biophysical profile or contraction stress test is done if the NST is nonreactive.

  2. The contraction stress test (CST; Figure 2-4)

      a. Monitors fetal heart rate during spontaneous or induced uterine contractions.

      b. "Positive" if late decelerations accompany uterine contractions, suggesting limited placental reserve.

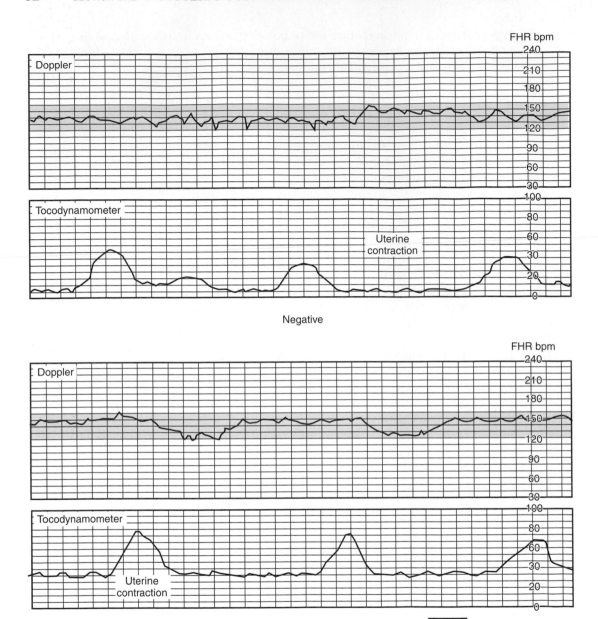

FIGURE 2-4 ● Negative results from a contraction stress test occur when no late or variable decelerations are recorded in response to stimulated contractions, which is a reassuring indication that the fetus can tolerate labor. Positive results occur when late decelerations are recorded with 50% or more of the contractions. (Negative tracing adapted from Freeman R, Garite T, Nageotte M: *Fetal heart rate monitoring*, ed 2, Baltimore, 1991, Lippincott, p 161; positive tracing from Parer JT: *Handbook of fetal heart rate monitoring*, Philadelphia, 1983, WB Saunders, p 188.)

c. "Suspicious" or equivocal tests show inconsistent late decelerations and require further fetal assessment and monitoring.

3. The biophysical profile (BPP; Table 2-1)

a. A 10-point scoring system assessing five measures of fetal well-being: Fetal breathing movements, heart rate reactivity, body movement, tone, and amniotic fluid volume.

b. BPP scores of 4 or less are associated with significant chronic fetal asphyxia, low Apgar scores, and fetal acidosis.

D. **Fetal Assessment of Oxygen and Acid-Base Status**

1. Fetal pulse oximetry is measured when FHR is confusing or nonreassuring.

a. Nonreassuring FHR includes persistent late decelerations, severe variables, loss of variability or accelerations, baseline bradycardia.

b. Abnormal saturation: <30% for 10 episodes or for longer than 10 minutes.

2. Scalp pH is measured when concern is high for fetal distress and acidosis.

a. pH of 7.20 to 7.25 is normal; follow patient closely.

b. pH <7.20 is an indication of fetal distress and need to expedite delivery.

c. Complications of scalp sampling are uncommon but include occasional infection at the sampling site and excessive bleeding.

d. Maternal HIV infection is considered by many to be a contraindication to fetal scalp monitoring.

● TABLE 2-1
Technique and Interpretation of Biophysical Profile Scoring

Biophysical Variable	Normal (Score = 2)	Abnormal (Score = 0)
Fetal breathing movements (FBM)	At least one episode of FBM of at least 30-sec duration in 30-minute observation	Absent FBM or no episode of >30 sec in 30 min
Gross body movement	At least three discrete body or limb movements in 30 min (episodes of active continuous movement considered as single movement)	Two or fewer episodes of body or limb movements in 30 min
Fetal tone	At least one episode of active extension with return to flexion of fetal limb(s) or trunk; opening and closing of hand considered normal tone	Either slow extension with return to partial flexion or movement of limb in full extension, absent fetal movement
Reactive fetal heart rate (FHR)	At least two episodes of FHR acceleration of >15 bpm and at least 15-sec duration associated with fetal movement in 30 min	Fewer than two episodes of acceleration of FHR or acceleration of >15 bpm in 30 min
Qualitative amniotic fluid (AF) volume	At least one pocket of AF that measures at least 1 cm in two perpendicular planes	Either no AF pockets or a pocket <1 cm in two perpendicular planes

From Manning FA, Harman CR: The fetal biophysical profile. In Eden RD, Boehm FH, Haire M, Jonas HS, editors: *Assessment and care of the fetus*, Norwalk, CT, 1990, Appleton & Lange, p 389, with permission.

3. Percutaneous umbilical blood sampling (PUBS) under ultrasound guidance.
   a. Used for measurements of fetal hemoglobin, platelet count, and acid base balance.
   b. Technique for administering packed red cell transfusions or medications directly and rapidly to fetus (e.g., in cases of severe fetal anemia or cardiac arrhythmia).
4. Umbilical cord gases (Table 2-2) should be obtained on all depressed newborns to help in determining the presence, duration, and extent of fetal compromise.

LABOR AND DELIVERY

A. **Management and Assessment of Labor**
   1. Labor is divided into three phases according to rate of dilation of the cervix.
      a. Latent phase: From the onset of labor to the increase in dilation rate
      b. Active phase: From approximately 3 cm to complete dilation (10 cm)
      c. Descent: From complete dilation to delivery of infant; also referred to as the "second stage of labor"
   2. Vaginal examination
      a. Determines progress toward delivery during each phase of labor; three parameters are followed:
         (1) Dilation of the cervix: Assessed by digital exam, from fully closed to completely dilated (10 cm)
         (2) Effacement of the cervix: Describes the gradual thinning of the cervix, from long and thick (0%) to fully effaced (100%)
         (3) Station or position of the fetus in the pelvis: Begins with "0" station, when the head first enters the pelvis, progressing to +1, +2, +3 (centimeters), as so on, as the baby descends into the pelvic outlet
      b. Assessment of possible complicating factors for delivery
         (1) Presentation: Presenting body part (e.g., cephalic, breech, transverse, brow, and shoulder)
         (2) Position: Describes the position of the head in relation to the pelvis in cephalic presentations (Figure 2-5)

● TABLE 2-2
Normal Cord Blood Gas Values

	Vein	Artery
pH	≥7.25	≥7.20
Po_2 (mm Hg)	≥30	≥15
Pco_2 (mm Hg)	<40	<50
HCO_3 (mMol/L)	≥19	≥18
BE (mMol/L)	<−6	<−8

Abstracted from Huch R, Huch A. In Beard RW, Nathanielsz PC, editors: *Fetal physiology and medicine*, New York, 1984, Marcel Dekker, with permission.

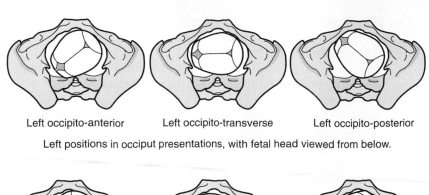

Left occipito-anterior   Left occipito-transverse   Left occipito-posterior

Left positions in occiput presentations, with fetal head viewed from below.

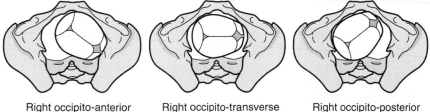

Right occipito-anterior   Right occipito-transverse   Right occipito-posterior

Right positions in occiput presentations.

Left mento-anterior   Right mento-anterior   Right mento-posterior

Left and right positions in face presentations.

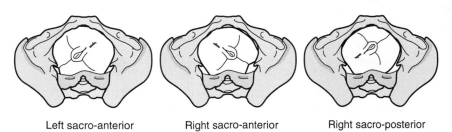

Left sacro-anterior   Right sacro-anterior   Right sacro-posterior

Left and right positions in breech presentations.

FIGURE 2-5 ● Positions in relation to various presentations, with fetus viewed from below. (From Pritchard JA, MacDonald PC, editors: *Williams' obstetrics*, ed 19, New York, 1993, Appleton-Century-Crofts.)

B. Complications of Labor and Delivery
1. Prolonged rupture of membranes (PROM)
    a. If membranes are ruptured for >12 to 18 hours without delivery of the infant, there is an increased risk for infection in the newborn; this risk increases substantially with PROM >24 hours.
    b. Antibiotic treatment may be given to asymptomatic mothers to prevent neonatal infection in high-risk situations (e.g., mother known to have a positive culture for group B streptococcus).
2. Umbilical cord prolapse
    a. Occurs when the cord falls below the presenting part and can be compressed between the presenting part and the pelvis or cervix.
    b. Predisposing factors include malposition of the fetus (such as transverse lie or breech), intrauterine growth retardation, polyhydramnios, multiple pregnancy, long cord, placenta previa, lack of engagement prior to labor (most common in multiparous women), cephalopelvic disproportion (large fetus for size of pelvis), and high station at the time of membrane rupture.
3. Prolonged second stage of labor
    a. Defined as second stage lasting >2 hours without adequate fetal descent; occurs in approximately 5% deliveries (Sokol et al., 1977).
    b. Commonly requires assistance at the time of delivery with forceps or vacuum extraction.
    c. Predisposing factors include large infant, abnormal fetal position, inadequate uterine contraction strength, ineffective pushing.
    d. Neonatal assessment after assisted delivery should include evaluation for bruising, cephalohematoma, eye involvement, and facial nerve damage.
4. Shoulder dystocia
    a. Occurs when there is inability to easily deliver the infant after delivery of the head.
    b. Occurs in approximately 1 in 300 births but increases in infants weighing >4000 g (Resnik, 1980).
    c. Predisposing factors include maternal obesity, excessive weight gain, oversized infant, history of large infants, maternal diabetes, and contracted pelvic outlet.
    d. Assessment of the newborn after delivery should include careful evaluation for brachial plexus injury, hypoxia, and fractured clavicle.
5. Shortened second stage (rapid labor) increases the risk in the newborn for abnormal transition, persistent pulmonary hypertension, and retained lung fluid.
6. Conditions that may require more rapid delivery and thus produce a shortened second stage include maternal cardiac disease, extreme maternal fatigue, and fetal distress.
7. Breech presentation
    a. Occurs when the infant presents with the head at the top of the uterus and the buttocks or feet at the cervix.
        (1) Frank breech: Buttocks presenting with both fetal thighs flexed and knees extended
        (2) Complete breech: Buttocks presenting with both fetal thighs flexed and one or both knees flexed

       (3) Incomplete or footling breech: One or both fetal thighs extended and one or both knees or feet lying below the buttocks

   b. Occurs in 3% to 4% of all pregnancies, decreasing with increased gestational age; 65% frank breech, 25% complete breech, and 10% incomplete breech (Shields and Medearis, 1992).

   c. Predisposing factors include high multiparity, polyhydramnios, uterine anomalies or masses, fetal anomalies, contracted pelvis, and premature delivery.

   d. Neonatal assessment should include observation for signs of asphyxia, which may occur secondary to delayed delivery of the fetal head, compression of the umbilical cord, aspiration of amniotic fluid or meconium, edema of external genitalia, and congenital hip dislocation.

8. Prolonged pregnancy (post-term pregnancy)

   a. Defined as gestation >294 days or 42 weeks.

   b. The ability of the placenta to adequately provide oxygen and nutrition to the fetus is thought to be compromised after this time.

   c. Occurs in 2.6% to 12% of pregnancies.

   d. Associated with cord accidents secondary to the relative oligohydramnios that may occur, growth retardation resulting from inadequate fetal oxygenation and nutrition secondary to a poorly functioning placenta, and fetal distress including meconium aspiration.

   e. Neonatal assessment should include evaluation for intrauterine growth retardation, birth asphyxia, meconium aspiration, and signs of postmaturity (long fingernails, parchment-like skin, decreased body fat, abundant hair growth, and meconium staining).

9. Meconium-stained fluid

   a. Signifies fetal passage of meconium in utero.

   b. May be a physiologic event, particularly if >40 weeks gestation; however, may be a sign of fetal distress, especially if accompanied by diminished amniotic fluid volume or abnormal fetal heart rate monitoring.

   c. Occurs in 8% to 25% of deliveries.

   d. Should be an alerting sign for possible neonatal depression.

   e. Clearing the airway and supporting ventilation are indicated in depressed infants; routine intubation and suctioning of the airway of a vigorous infant are not indicated.

10. Improper cord clamping: Timing of clamping can influence newborn hematocrit.

   a. Anemia can result from early clamping, cord accidents, and elevating the infant above the placenta (i.e., above the mother's body).

   b. Polycythemia can result from delayed clamping or lowering the infant below the level of the placenta,

11. Operative delivery (cesarean birth)

   a. Indications for cesarean birth include abnormalities of fetal presentation, fetal macrosomia, multiple gestation, active genital herpes infection, failure to progress in labor, severe preeclampsia or eclampsia, and severe fetal distress.

   b. Occurs in 5% to 30% of all births in the United States.

    c. Neonatal assessment should include evaluation for respiratory distress due to retained lung fluid, evidence of asphyxia, and/or complications related to the primary reason for the cesarean section.

C. Medications Used During Labor

  1. Oxytocin

    a. Used to induce labor by stimulation of the uterus; most women will achieve the active phase of labor within a few hours.

    b. The Bishop score evaluates cervical readiness for induction of labor as assessed by vaginal exam; total score of 9 is associated with successful induction of labor (Table 2-3).

    c. Maternal side effects: Can include uterine hypercontractility, water intoxication secondary to ADH-like effects, hypertension, uterine rupture, and amniotic fluid embolism

  2. Tranquilizers

    a. Used to reduce anxiety, provide muscle relaxation, and potentiate narcotics.

    b. Commonly used tranquilizers include benzodiazepines (Valium, Ativan, Versed).

    c. Neonatal assessment should include evaluation for hypotonia, hypoactivity, respiratory depression, and poor temperature control.

  3. Narcotics

    a. Used to increase woman's pain threshold during active labor.

    b. Commonly used narcotics include Demerol and Stadol.

    c. Maximal neonatal depression occurs if delivery is within 2 to 4 hours after maternal administration of narcotic.

    d. Neonatal assessment should include evaluation for respiratory depression, lethargy, poor temperature control, and impaired breast-feeding; respiratory depression at birth can be reversed with Narcan.

  4. Epidural anesthesia

    a. Used to block the nerves leaving the spinal cord by injection of local anesthesia into the epidural space.

● TABLE 2-3
Bishop Score for Assessing Readiness for Induction

Factor	Assigned Value			
	0	**1**	**2**	**3**
Cervical dilation	0	1–2 cm	3–4 cm	5 cm or more
Cervical effacement	0–30%	40–50%	60–70%	80% or more
Fetal station	−3	−2	−1, 0	+1, +2
Cervical consistency	Firm	Moderate	Soft	
Cervical position	Posterior	Midposition	Anterior	

From Bishop EH: Pelvic scoring for elective induction, *Obstet Gynecol* 24:266, 1964, with permission.

    b. May cause hypotension and subsequent decrease in uterine blood flow; maternal blood pressure and intravascular volume must be carefully monitored.

    c. Neonatal assessment should include evaluation for asphyxia related to maternal hypotension and birth injury if assisted delivery is required or poor pushing efforts are documented.

    d. Associated with maternal intrapartum fever and increased neonatal sepsis work-ups.

5. Local anesthesia

    a. Used to block the nerves at the pelvic outlet and perineum by pudendal and paracervical injection of local anesthetic

    b. Can be associated with fetal bradycardia

REFERENCES

Bennett BB: Shoulder dystocia: an obstetric emergency, *Obstet Gynecol Clin North Am* 3:445-458, 1999.

Devoe LD, editor: Antenatal fetal assessment, *Clin Perinatol* 21:(4), 1984.

Elzschig HK, Lieberman ES, Camann WR: Regional anesthesia and analgesia for labor and delivery, *NEJM* 4:319-332, 2003.

Garite TJ, Dildy GA, McNamara H, et al: A multicenter controlled trial of fetal pulse oximetry in the intrapartum management of non-reassuring fetal heart rate patterns, *Am J Obstet Gynecol* 183(5): 1049-1058, 2000.

Naef RW, Martin JN: Emergent management of shoulder dystocia, *Obstet Gynecol Clin North Am* 22(2):247-259, 1995.

Nahum GG: Detecting and managing fetal macrosomia, *Contemp OB/GYN* June 89-119, 2000.

Resnik R: Management of shoulder girdle dystocia, *Clin Obstet Gynecol* 23:559-564, 1980.

Satoh S, Nakano H: Clinical applications of the Doppler technique in monitoring the fetus, *Clin Perinatol* 26(4):853-868, 1999.

Shields JR, Medearis AL: Fetal malpresentations. In Hacker NF, Moore JG, editors: *Essentials of obstetrics and gynecology,* ed 2, Philadelphia, 1992, WB Saunders, pp 230-240.

Sokol RJ, Stojkov J, Chik L, Rosen MG: Normal and abnormal labor progress: I. A quantitative assessment and survey of the literature, *J Reprod Med* 18:47-53, 1977.

Delivery Room Management

Timely, skilled resuscitation of the newborn infant can prevent or reduce morbidity and mortality. The fundamental postnatal transitions from fluid-filled to air-filled lungs and from low to higher pulmonary blood flow require establishment of effective respirations immediately after birth. Thus much of neonatal resuscitation focuses on ventilation, oxygenation, and reversal of perinatal asphyxial insults. Anticipation and application of basic procedures are often the only measures required to successfully resuscitate a depressed infant. However, certain clinical conditions present special challenges in the delivery room and may require emergency procedures, such as umbilical vessel cannulation and chest tube placement, in their management.

The role of the health care provider responsible for the newborn infant extends to follow-up care and guidance for parents. Difficult decisions regarding an infant who is extremely premature, afflicted with lethal anomalies, or unresponsive to resuscitative measures require individualized counseling and choices but must be based on current, accurate information regarding treatment options and outcome.

3 Resuscitation of the Newborn Infant

Susan Niermeyer, MD

PREPARATION FOR RESUSCITATION

A. **Anticipation**: Use factors in the antepartum and intrapartum history to anticipate the need for resuscitation (Box 3-1).

B. **Equipment**
   1. Assemble, check, and prepare for use all equipment necessary for a complete resuscitation (Box 3-2).
   2. Multiple-gestation deliveries require a full set of equipment (and personnel) for each infant.

C. **Personnel**
   1. At every delivery, there should be at least one person responsible for the baby who is capable of initiating resuscitation.
   2. That person, or a second person who is immediately available, should be capable of performing a complete resuscitation.
   3. When asphyxia is anticipated, two persons should be present with responsibilities only for resuscitation of the infant; roles should be designated in advance.

D. **Knowledge**
   1. ABCs of resuscitation
      a. Airway
      b. Breathing
      c. Circulation
   2. Evaluation-decision-action cycle: The cycle of evaluating infant status, deciding on the next step, and taking action is repeated throughout resuscitation, whether uncomplicated or extended.

INITIAL STEPS AFTER DELIVERY

A. **Perform a Rapid Assessment**
   1. Within a few seconds after delivery, answer the following questions:
      a. Is the amniotic fluid clear of meconium?
      b. Is the baby breathing or crying?
      c. Is the muscle tone good?
      d. Is the color pink?
      e. Is the baby term?

● BOX 3-1
ANTEPARTUM/INTRAPARTUM FACTORS ASSOCIATED WITH POTENTIAL ASPHYXIA

Antepartum Factors
Age >35 years
Maternal diabetes
Pregnancy-induced hypertension
Chronic hypertension
Anemia or isoimmunization
Previous fetal or neonatal death
Bleeding in second or third trimester
Maternal infection
Hydramnios
Oligohydramnios
Premature rupture of membranes
Post-term gestation
Multiple gestation
Size-dates discrepancy
Drug therapy (e.g., lithium carbonate, magnesium, adrenergic blocking drugs)
Maternal substance abuse
Fetal malformation
Diminished fetal activity
No prenatal care

Intrapartum Factors
Emergency cesarean section
Breech or other abnormal presentation
Premature labor
Prolonged rupture of membranes >24 hours before delivery
Precipitous labor
Prolonged labor (>24 hours)
Prolonged second stage of labor (>2 hours)
Nonreassuing fetal heart rate patterns
Use of general anesthesia
Uterine tetany
Narcotics administered to mother within 4 hours of delivery
Meconium-stained amniotic fluid
Prolapsed cord
Abruption placentae
Placenta previa
Note: Keep these factors well in mind because they will alert you that depression and possible asphyxia are potential problems.

From Kattwinkel J, editor: *Textbook of neonatal resuscitation,* ed 4, American Academy of Pediatrics and American Heart Association, 2000, with permission.

● BOX 3-2
NEONATAL RESUSCITATION SUPPLIES AND EQUIPMENT

Suction Equipment
Bulb syringe
Mechanical suction and tubing
Suction catheters: 5 Fr or 6 Fr, 8 Fr, 10 Fr or 12 Fr
8-Fr feeding tube and 20-mL syringe
Meconium aspirator

Bag-and-Mask Equipment
Neonatal resuscitation bag with a pressure-release valve or pressure manometer—the bag
   must be capable of delivering 90%–100% oxygen
Face masks: newborn and premature sizes (cushioned rim masks preferred)
Oxygen with flowmeter and tubing

Intubation Equipment
Laryngoscope with straight blades: No. 0 (preterm) and No. 1 (term)
Extra bulbs and batteries for laryngoscope
Endotracheal tubes: 2.5, 3.0, 3.5, 4.0 mm internal diameter (ID)
Stylet (optional)
Scissors
Tape or securing device for endotracheal tube
Alcohol sponges
CO_2 detector (optional)
Laryngeal mask airway (optional)

Medications
Epinephrine 1:10,000: 3-mL or 10-mL ampules
Isotonic crystalloid (normal saline or Ringer's lactate) for volume expansion: 100 or 250 mL
Sodium bicarbonate 4.2% (5 mEq/10 mL): 10-mL ampules
Naloxone hydrochloride: 0.4 mg/mL, 1-mL ampules *or* 1.0 mg/mL, 2-mL ampules
Dextrose 10%: 250 mL
Normal saline for flushes
Feeding tube: 5 ft (optional)
Umbilical vessel catheterization supplies
Syringes: 1, 3, 5, 10, 20, 50 mL
Needles: 25-, 21-, or 18-gauge *or* puncture device for needleless system

Miscellaneous
Sterile gloves and appropriate personal protection
Scalpel or scissors
Povidone-iodine solution
Umbilical tape
Umbilical catheters: 3.5 Fr, 5 Fr
Three-way stopcock
Radiant warmer
Tape: 1/2 or 3/4 inch

From Kattwinkel J, editor: *Textbook of neonatal resuscitation,* ed 4, American Academy of Pediatrics and American Heart Association, 2000, pp 18-19, with permission.

   2. If the answer to all the above questions is "yes," the infant can receive rou-
      tine care (i.e., provide warmth, clear airway, dry).
   3. If the answer to any of the above questions is "no," the infant will need at
      least the initial steps of resuscitation.
B. **Provide the Initial Steps of Resuscitation**
   1. Provide warmth under a radiant heat source.
   2. Clear the airway (as necessary).
      a. Position the infant supine or side-lying with the neck slightly extended
         (Figure 3-1).
      b. If the amniotic fluid is clear, suction the mouth and then the nose to
         clear the airway. The mouth is suctioned first to clear the largest vol-
         ume of secretions; when the nasopharynx is suctioned, a reflex cough,
         sneeze, or cry often results.
         (1) Turn the head to the side to allow secretions to pool in the cheek,
             then remove with a bulb syringe.
         (2) DeLee suction trap or regular suction catheter may be used
             with mechanical suction; suction pressure should not exceed
             80 to 100 mm Hg.
         (3) Deep pharyngeal suction (in a child not requiring positive-pres-
             sure ventilation or intubation) should not be performed during the
             first few minutes after birth to avoid vagal depression.
      c. If the amniotic fluid is meconium-stained, evaluate the need for tracheal
         suctioning (Wiswell 2000).
         (1) Suction the nose, mouth, and posterior pharynx when the head is
             delivered.

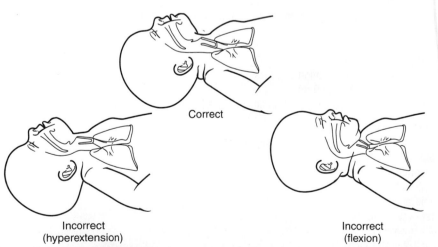

Correct

Incorrect
(hyperextension)

Incorrect
(flexion)

FIGURE 3-1 ● Either hyperextension or underextension of the neck may decrease air entry.
(From Kattwinkel J, editor: *Textbook of neonatal resuscitation*, ed 4, American Academy of
Pediatrics and American Heart Association, 2000, pp 2-6.)

(2) If the infant is vigorous (adequate breathing, good tone, and heart rate >100 bpm), suction the mouth and nose.

(3) If the infant is depressed (inadequate breathing, poor tone, or heart rate <100 bpm), suction the trachea under direct vision using an endotracheal tube, adapter, and mechanical suction (Figure 3-2).

(4) Dry and stimulate the infant and remove wet linen after airway suctioning is complete or positive-pressure ventilation is initiated.

(5) Suction the stomach when airway management is complete and vital signs are stable (usually after 5 minutes).

3. Dry and stimulate; reposition.

a. Dry the infant and remove the wet linen.

b. Provide tactile stimulation.

(1) Slap/flick feet or rub infant's back.

(2) Stimulate once or twice; if the infant remains apneic, immediately begin bag-and-mask ventilation.

(3) Continue gentle rubbing of back, trunk, or extremities to support early respiratory efforts in a depressed infant.

c. If chest wall movement is observed, give oxygen as necessary and proceed to evaluation.

d. If the infant is apneic, begin positive-pressure ventilation.

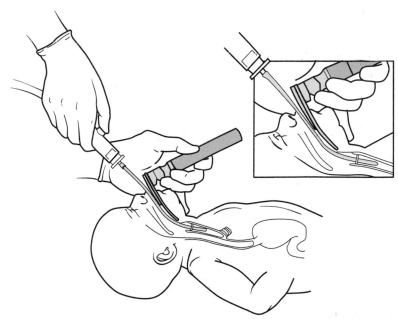

FIGURE 3-2 ● Visualizing the glottis and suctioning meconium from the trachea. Following intubation, the meconium aspirator is connected to the endotracheal tube and suction is applied by occluding the vent with a finger while withdrawing the endotracheal tube. (From Kattwinkel J, editor: *Textbook of neonatal resuscitation,* ed 4, American Academy of Pediatrics and American Heart Association, 2000, pp 2-8.)

4. Provide oxygen (as necessary).
   a. If there is central cyanosis, provide free-flow oxygen.
   b. Acrocyanosis is not an indication for oxygen.
   c. Once the color is pink, oxygen should be gradually withdrawn.

C. **Evaluate the Infant After Each Action for Respirations, Heart Rate, and Color**
   1. If the infant is breathing regularly with heart rate >100 bpm and is centrally pink, continue to observe under guidelines for transition.
   2. If the infant is apneic or gasping, begin positive-pressure ventilation.
   3. If the heart rate is <100, begin positive-pressure ventilation, even though the infant may have spontaneous respirations.
   4. If the infant has central cyanosis (with spontaneous respirations and adequate heart rate), give free-flow oxygen.
      a. Administer by oxygen tubing or mask.
      b. Initially use a high concentration of oxygen: 100% oxygen at 5 L/min provides 80%–100% oxygen with tubing 1/2 inch from nares surrounded by a cupped hand or a mask held firmly on the face.
      c. Once the infant becomes pink, gradually withdraw the oxygen.
      d. If cyanosis persists, reevaluate the quality of respirations and the heart rate; perform a brief physical exam; consider bag-and-mask ventilation or intubation if there is evidence of respiratory distress.
   5. Assign an Apgar score at 1 and 5 minutes (Table 3-1).
      a. The Apgar score is a quantitative description of infant's condition and response to resuscitation: A = appearance (color), P = pulse (heart rate), G = grimace (reflex irritability response to stimulation of sole of foot), A = activity (muscle tone), R = respiration (respiratory effort) (Covey and Butterfield, 1962).
      b. The Apgar score is *not* the basis for resuscitation decisions or prognosis.
      c. A complete description of resuscitative steps is vital to interpret a low Apgar score.
      d. Continue to assign an Apgar score every 5 minutes until the score is ≥7.

● TABLE 3-1
Apgar Score

Sign	0	1	2
Heart rate	Absent	<100 beats/min	≥100 beats/min
Respirations	Absent	Weak cry; hypoventilation	Good, strong cry
Muscle tone	Limp	Some flexion	Active motion
Reflex irritability (response to brisk slap on soles of feet)	No response	Grimace	Cry or active withdrawal
Color	Blue or pale	Body pink; extremities blue	Completely pink

American Academy of Pediatrics and American College of Obstetricians and Gynecologists: Intrapartum care. In Gillstrap LC, Oh W: *Guidelines for perinatal care,* ed 5, Elk Grove Village, IL, 2002, American Academy of Pediatrics, pp 187-198.

RESUSCITATION PROCEDURES

A. Bag-and-Mask Ventilation

    1. Indications for bag-and-mask ventilation

        a. Apnea unresponsive to brief stimulation

        b. Gasping respirations

        c. Heart rate <100 beats/minute

    2. Equipment for bag-and-mask ventilation

        a. Bag choices (Figure 3-3)

            (1) Flow-initiating bag (500–750 mL) with pressure gauge and flow-control valve

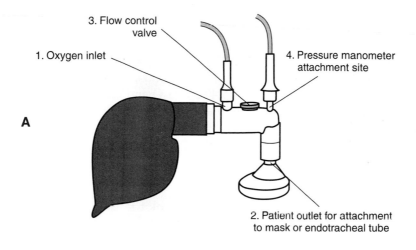

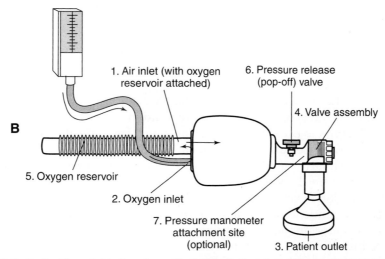

FIGURE 3-3 ● **A,** Flow-initiating bag. **B,** Self-inflating bag. (From Kattwinkel J, editor: *Textbook of neonatal resuscitation,* ed 4, American Academy of Pediatrics and American Heart Association, 2000, pp 3-13.)

        (2) Self-inflating bag (240–750 mL) with oxygen reservoir and pressure-release valve or pressure gauge

    b. Face mask

        (1) Appropriate size (premature, term) to cover chin, mouth, and nose but not eyes

        (2) Preferably cushioned rim

    c. Source of 100% oxygen

    d. Flowmeter to deliver 5–8 L/min,with the capability of increasing to 10–12 L/min

3. Procedure for bag-and-mask ventilation

    a. Test equipment prior to use. **Equipment failure can cause resuscitation failure!**

    b. Position the infant with the neck slightly extended and avoid compression of soft tissues of the neck by holding the mask to the face with fingers resting along the mandible.

    c. If the infant is apneic, give an opening breath with pressure 30–40 cm H_2O and inspiratory time of 1–2 seconds.

    d. Ventilate with pressure 15-40 cm H_2O and rate 40-60 breaths/min.

    e. Observe chest expansion. If adequate:

        (1) Reapply face mask for better seal.

        (2) Reposition the head.

        (3) Suction secretions.

        (4) Open the infant's mouth slightly.

        (5) Increase pressure.

    f. Reevaluate heart rate, respirations, color.

    g. Insert an orogastric catheter (8 Fr feeding tube) after several minutes of bag-and-mask ventilation.

        (1) Measure the insertion depth of the catheter by holding the tip at the bridge of the nose and measuring to the earlobe, then to the xiphoid.

        (2) Insert the catheter through the mouth, not the nose.

        (3) Aspirate gastric contents with a 20-mL syringe and leave the catheter open.

        (4) Tape the catheter to the infant's cheek.

4. Complications of bag-and-mask ventilation

    a. Trauma to eyes or face from improper size or position of mask

    b. Air leak (pneumothorax, subcutaneous air)

    c. Intestinal distention elevating a normal diaphragm or compression lung directly with diaphragmatic hernia

5. Prevention of complications

    a. Use gentle technique and equipment of correct size.

    b. Monitor pressures carefully.

    c. Insert an orogastric tube when indicated.

B. Endotracheal Intubation

1. Indications for intubation

    a. Need for tracheal suctioning

   b. Ineffective bag-and-mask ventilation
   c. Need for prolonged positive-pressure ventilation or surfactant administration
   d. Diaphragmatic hernia
2. Equipment for intubation
   a. Laryngoscope (extra batteries and bulb)
   b. Blades: Miller (straight) size 0 for preterm; size 1 for term
   c. Endotracheal tubes: Internal diameter 2.5, 3.0, 3.5, 4.0 mm
   d. Stylet
   e. Suction
   f. Tape, scissors
   g. Bag and mask, oxygen source
3. Procedure for intubation
   a. Select the correct size endotracheal tube (Table 3-2) and shorten it to 13 cm.
   b. Prepare the laryngoscope, tape, suction, oxygen, bag/mask.
   c. Position the infant with the neck slightly extended.
   d. Provide free-flow oxygen.
   e. Visualize landmarks; identify the epiglottis, vocal cords, and glottis.
   f. Insert the endotracheal tube to the level of the vocal cord guideline near the tip of the tube.
   g. Limit each intubation attempt to 20 seconds.
   h. Confirm endotracheal tube position by:
      (1) Breath sounds (symmetric in axillae)
      (2) Chest wall movement
      (3) Centimeter markings on tube (Table 3-3)
      (4) Chest x-ray
   i. Shorten endotracheal tube to 4 cm beyond lips.
4. Complications of intubation
   a. Hypoxia resulting from prolonged intubation attempts or lack of supplemental oxygen
   b. Apnea/bradycardia resulting from hypoxia or vagal stimulation
   c. Trauma to oropharynx, trachea, vocal cords, esophagus

● TABLE 3-2
● Endotracheal Tube Size

Tube Size (mm) (Inside Diameter)	Weight (g)	Gestational Age (wk)
2.5	Below 1000	Below 28
3.0	1000–2000	28–34
3.5	2000–3000	34–38
3.5–4.0	Above 3000	Above 38

From Kattwinkel J, editor: *Textbook of neonatal resuscitation*, ed 4, American Academy of Pediatrics and American Heart Association, 2000, pp 5-5, with permission.

● TABLE 3-3
Depth of Endotracheal Tube Insertion

Weight (kg)	Depth of Insertion (cm from upper lip)
1*	7
2	8
3	9
4	10

*Babies weighing less than 750 g may require only 6 cm insertion.
From Kattwinkel J, editor: *Textbook of neonatal resuscitation,* ed 4, American Academy of Pediatrics and American Heart Association, 2000, pp 5-19, with permission.

      d. Infection cause by introduction of nosocomial organisms and irritation/obstruction by foreign body
      e. Palatal grooves with prolonged intubation and subglottic stenosis with prolonged, traumatic, or repeated intubation
   5. Prevention of complications
      a. Provide free-flow oxygen during intubation.
      b. Limit intubation attempts to 20 seconds.
      c. Use gentle technique.
      d. Check tube position frequently.
      e. Consider use of palatal stabilizers with prolonged intubation.
C. Chest Compressions
   1. Indications for chest compressions: Heart rate <60 beats/min despite ventilation for 30 seconds with 100% oxygen
   2. Procedure for chest compressions
      a. Position the infant with the neck slightly extended.
      b. Provide firm support for the back.
      c. Perform compressions by two-finger or thumb method (Figure 3-4).
        (1) Position: Lower third of sternum (Orlowski, 1986)
        (2) Rate: 90 times/min
        (3) Depth: One third the anteroposterior diameter of the chest
        (4) Support: Encircling fingers or hand under back
      d. Interpose 30 breaths/min with a 3:1 ratio of compressions to breaths for a total of 120 events/min.
      e. Evaluate the heart rate after 30 seconds.
      f. Continue compressions until the heart rate is >60 beats/min.
   3. Complications of chest compressions
      a. Liver laceration
      b. Rib fractures
      c. Pneumothorax
   4. Prevention of complications
      a. Check position of compressions.

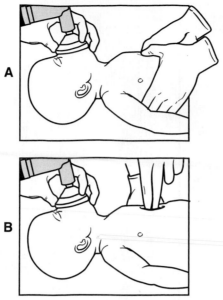

FIGURE 3-4 ● Two techniques for giving chest compressions: thumb (**A**) and two-finger (**B**) methods. (From Kattwinkel J, editor: *Textbook of neonatal resuscitation,* ed 4, American Academy of Pediatrics and American Heart Association, 2000, pp 4-5.)

          b. Maintain contact with the chest during the release portion of the compression cycle.

          c. Avoid excessive force of compressions.

   D. Drugs

     1. Indications for drugs during resuscitation

          a. Epinephrine: heart rate <60 beats/min despite at least 30 seconds of adequate ventilation with 100% oxygen and chest compressions

          b. Sodium bicarbonate

              (1) Documented metabolic acidosis in the presence of adequate ventilation

              (2) Prolonged arrest unresponsive to other therapy including adequate ventilation

          c. Naloxone hydrochloride: severe respiratory depression **and** narcotic administration to the mother in the last 4 hours (*Note*: Naloxone is contraindicated in infants of addicted mothers.)

          d. Volume expanders

              (1) Evidence of acute bleeding and signs of hypovolemia

              (2) Poor response to other resuscitative measures

     2. Procedure for administering drugs (Table 3-4)

          a. Prepare each drug for administration; draw up the appropriate concentration and volume; label.

          b. Calculate the correct dosage of each drug.

● TABLE 3-4
Medications for Neonatal Resuscitation

Medication	Concentration to Administer	Preparation	Dosage/Route	Total Dose/Infant		Rate/Precautions
Epinephrine	1:10,000	1 mL	0.1–0.3 mL/kg IV or ET	**Weight** 1 kg 2 kg 3 kg 4 kg	**Total mL** 0.1–0.3 mL 0.2–0.6 mL 0.3–0.9 mL 0.4–1.2 mL	Give rapidly May dilute with normal saline to 1–2 mL if giving ET
Volume expanders	Whole blood, 5% albumin Normal saline Ringer's lactate	40 mL	10 mL/kg IV	**Weight** 1 kg 2 kg 3 kg 4 kg	**Total mL** 10 mL 20 mL 30 mL 40 mL	Give over 5–10 minutes
Sodium bicarbonate	0.5 mEq/mL (4.2% solution)	20 mL or two 10-mL prefilled syringes	2 mEq/kg IV	**Weight** 1 kg 2 kg 3 kg 4 kg	**Total Dose** 2 mEq 4 mEq 6 mEq 8 mEq **Total mL** 4 mL 8 mL 12 mL 16 mL	Give *slowly*, over at least 2 minutes Give only if infant is being effectively ventilated

				Weight	Total Dose	Total mL	
Naloxone hydrochloride	0.4 mg/mL	1 mL	0.1 mg/kg (0.25 mL/kg) IV, ET IM, SQ	1 kg	0.1 mg	0.25 mL	Give rapidly IV, ET preferred IM, SQ acceptable
				2 kg	0.2 mg	0.50 mL	
				3 kg	0.3 mg	0.75 mL	
				4 kg	0.4 mg	1.00 mL	
	1.0 mg/mL	1 mL	0.1 mL/kg (0.1 mL/kg) IV, ET IM, SQ	1 kg	0.1 mg	0.1 mL	
				2 kg	0.2 mg	0.2 mL	
				3 kg	0.3 mg	0.3 mL	
				4 kg	0.4 mg	0.4 mL	
				Weight	Total µg/min		
Dopamine			Begin at 5 µg/kg/min (may increase to 20 µg/kg/min if necessary) IV	1 kg	5–20 µg/min		Give as a continuous infusion using an infusion pump Monitor heart rate and blood pressure closely Seek consultation
				2 kg	10–40 µg/min		
				3 kg	15–60 µg/min		
				4 kg	20–80 µg/min		

$$\frac{\text{Weight (kg)} \times \text{Desired dose (µg/kg/min)} \times 6}{\text{Desired fluid (mL/h)}} = \text{mg of dopamine per 100 mL of solution}$$

IM, intramuscular; *ET*, endotracheal; *IV*, intravenous; *SQ*, subcutaneous.
From Bloom RS, Cropley C, and the AHA/AAP Neonatal Resuscitation Program Steering Committee: *Textbook of neonatal resuscitation*, Dallas, TX, 1994, American Academy of Pediatrics and American Heart Association, pp 6-51, with permission.

    c. Administer drug by the correct route and at proper rate (Hagasawa, 1986).

    d. Reevaluate for desired effect and take follow-up action.

3. Complications of drug administration

    a. Extravasation with intravascular administration

    b. Hepatic injury with low umbilical venous catheters

    c. Unpredictable absorption with endotracheal and intramuscular administration

    d. Adverse pharmacologic effects

      (1) Epinephrine: Risk for significant hypertension, germinal matrix hemorrhage, and cardiac injury with higher doses (Burchfield et al., 1993)

      (2) Sodium bicarbonate: Worsened acidosis with impaired ventilation, worsened intracellular acidosis, hyperosmolar load, high sodium load, decreased myocardial performance (Hein, 1993; Howell, 1987)

    e. Volume overload

4. Prevention of complications

    a. Choose correct route of administration.

    b. Position umbilical lines correctly.

    c. Evaluate for adverse effects after each dose.

    d. Avoid calcium and atropine in delivery room settings.

      (1) Calcium is indicated for hypocalcemia or hyperkalemia; these are infrequent problems in the delivery room.

      (2) Atropine may mask hypoxia-related bradycardia (Sims et al., 1994).

REFERENCES

American Academy of Pediatrics and American College of Obstetricians and Gynecologists: Intrapartum care. In Gillstrap LC, Oh W: *Guidelines for perinatal care,* ed 5, Elk Grove Village, IL, 2002, American Academy of Pediatrics, pp 187-198.

Burchfield DJ, Berkowitz ID, Berg RA, Goldberg RN: Medications in neonatal resuscitation, *Ann Emerg Med* 22:435-439, 1993.

Covey MJ, Butterfield LJ: Practical epigram of the Apgar score, *JAMA* 181:353, 1962.

Emergency Cardiovascular Care Committee and Subcommittees, AHA; International guidelines for neonatal resuscitation: an excerpt from the Guidelines 2000 for Cardiopulmonary Resuscitation and Emergency Cardiovascular Care, *International Consensus on Science Circulation* 102(Suppl I):I-543-T-357, 2000.

Hasagawa EA: The endotracheal use of emergency drugs, *Heart Lung* 15:60-63, 1986.

Hein HA: The use of sodium bicarbonate in neonatal resuscitation: help or harm? *Pediatrics* 91:496-497, 1993.

Howell JH: Sodium bicarbonate in the perinatal setting—revisited, *Clin Perinatol* 14:807-816, 1987.

Kattwinkel J, editor: *Textbook of neonatal resuscitation,* ed 4, American Academy of Pediatrics and American Heart Association, 2000.

Orlowski JP: Optimum position for external cardiac compression in infants and young children, *Ann Emerg Med* 15:667-673, 1986.

Sims DG, Heal CA, Bartle SM: Use of adrenaline and atropine in neonatal resuscitation, *Arch Dis Child* 70:F3-F10, 1994.

Wiswell T and the Meconium in the Delivery Room Trial Group: Delivery room management of the apparently vigorous meconium-stained neonate: results of the multicenter collaborative trial, *Pediatrics* 105:1-7, 2000.

4 Recognition and Management of Neonatal Emergencies

Susan Niermeyer, MD ■ *Anne Gross*, RNC, MS, NNP

EMERGENCIES

A. Airway Obstruction/Anomalies

1. Physical examination
   a. Choanal atresia/stenosis: Noisy respirations; pink when crying, cyanotic when quiet; inability to pass suction catheter per nares
   b. Laryngeal/tracheal obstruction: Mass (internal or external), trauma (perforation), atresia/stenosis
   c. Pneumothorax, cystic adenomatoid malformation: Unequal breath sounds

2. Stabilization
   a. Provide supplemental oxygen as needed.
   b. Attempt to bypass the level of obstruction: An oral airway and prone positioning may decrease upper airway obstruction; lower airway obstruction requires intubation or emergency tracheostomy.
   c. Transilluminate to detect a pneumothorax or obtain a chest radiograph to detect other parenchymal anomalies; perform needle thoracentesis or insert a chest tube to relieve a symptomatic pneumothorax (see "Procedures" below).

B. Severe Asphyxia or Hypovolemia

1. Physical examination: Hypotonia, seizures, pallor, poor perfusion, absence of spontaneous respirations

2. Stabilization
   a. Place an endotracheal tube for prolonged apnea or hypoxemia.
   b. Insert umbilical lines (see "Procedures" below).
   c. Give volume support and/or pressors for shock.
   d. Monitor hematocrit, urine output, neurologic status carefully.

C. Sepsis

1. Physical examination
   a. Congenital infection: Hepatomegaly, cutaneous lesions, pallor, external or internal ocular abnormalities
   b. Perinatal infection: Hypotonia, poor perfusion, poorly compliant lungs (pneumonia), foul odor.

   2. Stabilization
      a. Place an endotracheal tube for severe respiratory distress.
      b. Insert umbilical lines (see "Procedures" below).
      c. Obtain blood culture and administer antibiotics.
      d. Give volume support and pressors for shock.

   D. **Congenital Diaphragmatic Hernia**
      1. Physical examination: Barrel chest and scaphoid abdomen, cardiac point of maximum intensity (PMI) shifted toward side opposite hernia (usually toward the right chest), asymmetric breath sounds, worsening respiratory distress with bag-mask ventilation
      2. Stabilization
         a. Immediately place endotracheal tube.
         b. Decompress the bowel with an orogastric sump tube attached to low intermittent suction.
         c. Insert umbilical lines (see "Procedures" below).
         d. Arrange emergency transport to a facility with pediatric surgery, availability of nitric oxide, and extracorporeal membrane oxygenation (ECMO).

   E. **Pulmonary Hypoplasia/Oligohydramnios Sequence**
      1. Physical examination: Flattened, deviated nose; infraorbital creases; low-set, crumpled ears; small chin; positional deformities of the extremities
      2. Stabilization
         a. Place an endotracheal tube (see Chapter 3) and umbilical lines (see "Procedures" below).
         b. Ventilate with pressure/rate necessary to normalize arterial blood gases.
         c. Monitor closely for pulmonary air leak.
         d. Arrange emergency transport to a facility with high-frequency ventilation, nitric oxide capability.

   F. **Hydrops Fetalis**
      1. Physical examination: Body wall edema, ascites, pallor, poor perfusion, poorly compliant lungs (pleural effusion), unequal breath sounds (pneumothorax), distant heart sounds (pericardial effusion)
      2. Stabilization
         a. Place an endotracheal tube.
         b. Perform posterolateral needle thoracentesis bilaterally if unable to ventilate. Consider paracentesis if ascites compromises lung expansion.
         c. Place chest tube for pneumothorax (see "Procedures" below).
         d. Insert umbilical lines (see "Procedures" below).
         e. Monitor hematocrit, blood pressure, urine output closely.
         f. Initiate diagnostic studies to determine cause of hydrops.

   G. **Abdominal Wall Defect**
      1. Physical examination: Midline abdominal wall defect at base of umbilical cord (omphalocele) or lateral to cord insertion (gastroschisis); herniation may involve stomach, intestines, liver, ovaries/fallopian tubes
      2. Stabilization

  a. Protect exposed tissue with gauze soaked in warmed saline and cover with an evaporative barrier.

  b. Begin parenteral fluids promptly at 1.5 times maintenance rate.

  c. Position the infant side-lying, support the exposed organs, and monitor perfusion of herniated intestines.

  d. Place orogastric tube and attach to low intermittent suction.

  e. Monitor temperature and urine output closely.

  f. Examine carefully for other anomalies.

  g. Arrange prompt transport to a center with appropriate specialists in pediatric surgery.

H. Neural Tube Defect

 1. Physical examination: Open spinal defect (myelomeningocele), cranial defect with out-pouching brain tissue (occipital or frontal encephalocele), failure of formation of skull and brain (anencephaly)

 2. Stabilization

  a. Provide supportive care unless prenatal diagnosis of a lethal anomaly has allowed parents and professionals to formulate a plan for limited resuscitation/support.

  b. Protect exposed tissue with gauze soaked in warmed saline and cover with an evaporative barrier.

  c. Monitor temperature and cardiorespiratory status closely.

  d. Arrange prompt transport to a center with appropriate specialists in pediatric neurosurgery, genetics, orthopedics, urology, and rehabilitation.

I. Extremely Low-Birth-Weight Infant

 1. Physical examination: Birth weight <1000 g; thin, translucent skin; respiratory distress with grunting, flaring, retractions

 2. Stabilization

  a. Provide supportive care unless prenatal diagnosis of extreme prematurity (<26 weeks) has allowed parents and professionals to formulate a plan for limited resuscitation/support.

  b. Intubate for respiratory distress.

  c. Evaluate for use of artificial surfactant.

  d. Place umbilical lines (see "Procedures" below).

  e. Monitor temperature, cardiorespiratory status (including blood pressure), glucose, and urine output closely.

  f. Obtain blood culture and begin antibiotics in the setting of possible perinatal infection.

  g. Consider transport to a center with neonatology specialists.

PROCEDURES

A. Thoracentesis/Chest Tube Placement

 1. Recognition of pneumothorax

  a. Risk factors

   (1) Respiratory distress syndrome (5%–10% incidence)

   (2) Aspiration syndrome

      (3) Assisted ventilation (10%–15% with continuous positive airway pressure; 20%–40% with intermittent mandatory ventilation)

      (4) Spontaneous breaths in healthy newborns (1%–2%)

   b. Clinical signs

      (1) Sudden cyanosis

      (2) Tachypnea and increased work of breathing

      (3) Asymmetric chest

      (4) Shift in PMI

      (5) Asymmetric breath sounds

      (6) Abdominal distention

      (7) Hypotension

      (8) Mottling/poor perfusion

   c. Diagnostic techniques

      (1) Transillumination

      (2) Chest x-ray (anteroposterior [AP] and cross-table lateral) showing hyperlucent rim of air or hyperlucent lung field, downward displacement of the diaphragm, midline shift

      (3) Arterial blood gases: hypoxia, hypercarbia, acidosis

2. Management of pneumothorax

   a. Nontension pneumothorax

      (1) Observation

      (2) Nitrogen washout in term newborn: 100% oxygen by hood for several hours to replace trapped nitrogen in pneumothorax with more readily absorbed oxygen

   b. Tension pneumothorax

      (1) Needle aspiration

      (2) Tube thoracostomy

3. Procedure for needle aspiration (Figure 4-1)

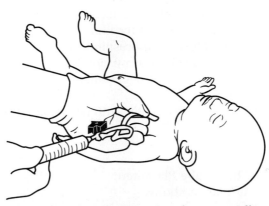

FIGURE 4-1 ● Aspiration of a pneumothorax with scalp vein needle, stopcock, and syringe. (From Schreiner RL, Bradburn NC: *Care of the newborn*, ed 2, New York, 1988, Raven Press, with permission.)

      a. Assemble 23-gauge butterfly needle, three-way stopcock, 60-mL syringe.

      b. Restrain the infant and prep the third intercostal space, midclavicular line.

      c. Insert the needle perpendicularly just above the fourth rib.

      d. Pull back on the syringe as soon as the needle enters the skin; stop advancing the needle when air is obtained.

      e. Aspirate the air collection; empty the syringe by closing stopcock to needle.

      f. Withdraw needle when air no longer aspirates easily.

      g. Reassess condition; consider chest tube placement.

4. Procedure for chest tube placement

      a. Assemble equipment.

          (1) 1% lidocaine

          (2) Syringe with 25-gauge needle

          (3) Mask, gown, sterile gloves

          (4) Povidone-iodine, alcohol

          (5) No. 15 scalpel

          (6) Small curved hemostat

          (7) Chest tube (8, 10, 12 Fr)

          (8) 3-0 suture and needle holder

          (9) Tape

          (10) Suction adaptor, suction apparatus, wall suction

      b. Prepare the suction apparatus (10 cm H_2O suction).

      c. Position the infant with affected side at 60-degree angle upward and supported; extend arm over head.

      d. Monitor the infant with cardiorespiratory monitor and pulse oximetry.

      e. Prep and anesthetize over fourth–sixth rib and midaxillary line.

      f. Make a 3- to 4-mm incision over the sixth rib.

      g. Tunnel with hemostat to above fifth rib, slide over the rib, and pop through the parietal pleura (Figure 4-2, *A*).

      h. Insert chest tube through opened hemostat (Figure 4-2, *B*); remove hemostat.

      i. Connect chest tube to suction; observe for condensation in the tube and bubbling in the suction apparatus when connected.

      j. Suture the chest tube in place and tape (Figure 4-2, *C*).

      k. Obtain AP and lateral chest x-ray for placement.

5. Complications of chest tube insertion

      a. Bleeding from intercostal vessels, internal mammary artery, mediastinal vessels, heart (Quak et al., 1993)

      b. Lung perforation

      c. Phrenic nerve injury (Arya et al., 1991)

      d. Cutaneous scars

6. Prevention of complications

      a. Insert chest tube over a rib.

      b. Avoid second chest tube on the same side.

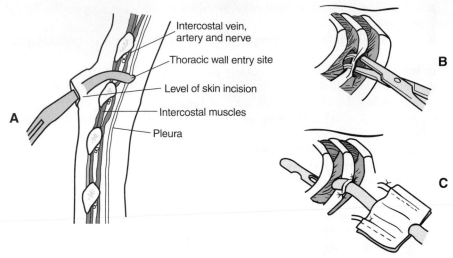

A

Intercostal vein,
artery and nerve

Thoracic wall entry site

Level of skin incision

Intercostal muscles

Pleura

B

C

FIGURE 4-2 ● Procedures of chest tube insertion. **A,** Level of skin incision and thoracic wall entry site in relation to the rib and neurovascular bundle. **B,** Opened hemostat through which chest tube is inserted. **C,** Chest tube secured to skin with silk sutures. (From Gomella TL, editor: *Neonatology,* New York, 1999, Appleton & Lange, p 16, with permission.)

     c. Place incision away from breast tissue, behind pectoralis muscle (Rainer et al., 2003).
B. Umbilical Vessel Catheterization
    1. Indications for use of umbilical vessel catheters
       a. Arterial
         (1) Blood gas analysis
         (2) Frequent blood sampling for other analyses
         (3) Central arterial blood pressure monitoring
       b. Venous
         (1) Emergency administration of drugs
         (2) Emergency measurement of Pco_2 and pH
         (3) Fluid administration (hypertonic solutions or inadequate peripheral access)
         (4) Central venous pressure monitoring
         (5) Exchange transfusions
    2. Equipment for umbilical vessel catheterization
       a. Overhead radiant warmer, cardiac monitor
       b. Restraints (four-point)
       c. Instrument tray
         (1) Curved iris forceps
         (2) Straight iris forceps
         (3) Scissors
         (4) Needle holder
         (5) Curved mosquito clamp (2)

      (6) Straight mosquito clamps (2)

      (7) Knife handle and blade

      (8) 3-0 silk suture

      (9) Umbilical tape

     (10) Three-way stopcock (Luer lock)

        (a) Catheters

          (i) Arterial: 3.5 or 5.0 Fr, polyvinyl chloride (PVC) or Silastic

          (ii) Integral connector or blunt needle adapter

        (b) Venous

          (i) 5.0 Fr for emergency drugs, fluids

          (ii) 8.0 Fr for exchange transfusion in large babies (side-hole catheter for exchange)

3. Procedure for umbilical artery catheterization (for alternative side-entry method, see Squire et al. 1990)

    a. Measure the baby to estimate depth of insertion (Figure 4-3); add 2 cm to estimate depth per nomogram (Greenough 1993; Shukla and Ferrara, 1986).

    b. Prepare the catheter with stopcock and flush.

    c. Prep and drape the umbilicus.

    d. Encircle the cord with umbilical tape and cut the cord, leaving a 2- to 3-cm stump (Figure 4-4, *A*).

    e. Place upward traction on the cord and identify the muscular umbilical arteries (Figure 4-4, *B*).

    f. Dilate an artery with curved iris forceps by inserting first one tip, then both tips, and then using a gentle spreading motion (Figure 4-4, *C*).

    g. Insert the catheter while maintaining traction on the cord upward and toward the head.

    h. If resistance is met, maintain steady pressure.

    i. Aspirate blood into the syringe; clear air bubbles; flush heparinized fluids through the catheter.

    j. Secure the catheter with purse-string suture and tape (Figure 4-5, *A*).

    k. Check placement with x-ray (tip at L3–L4 interspace).

    l. Reposition if necessary and recheck x-ray.

    m. Stop umbilical arterial bleeding by tightly grasping the umbilicus and skin below for 5 minutes.

4. Procedure for umbilical vein catheterization

    a. Emergency placement (low)

      (1) Encircle the cord with umbilical tape and cut the cord.

      (2) Identify the vein and insert catheter 2–3 cm.

      (3) Aspirate blood into the syringe; clear air from the line.

      (4) Remove catheter prior to moving infant.

      (5) Stop umbilical venous bleeding by pressure on the abdomen above the umbilicus.

    b. Indwelling venous central line (high).

      (1) Measure the baby to estimate depth of insertion (see Figure 4-3) (Shukla and Ferrara, 1986).

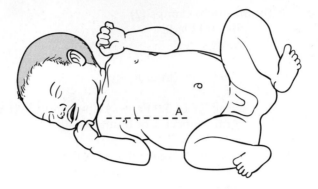

To determine shoulder-umbilicus length, measure along line A.

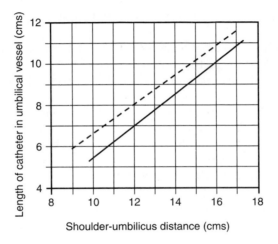

Shoulder-umbilicus distance (cms)

– – · Umbilical vein to junction of inferior vena cava and right atrium

——— Umbilical artery to bifurcation of aorta

FIGURE 4-3 ● Umbilical vein catheterization. Nomogram for insertion depth of umbilical artery and vein catheters. (From Klaus MH, Fanaroff AA: *Care of the high-risk neonate*, ed 5, Philadelphia, 2001, WB Saunders, p 501, with permission. Nomogram adapted from Dunn P: Localization of the umbilical catheter by post-mortem measurement, *Arch Dis Child* 41:69, 1966.)

(2) Prepare cord as for artery and identify the thin-walled vein.

(3) Grasp the edge of the vein and side of the cord with forceps (Figure 4-5, *B*).

(4) Insert the catheter while maintaining traction on the cord toward the left foot (Figure 4-5, *C*).

(5) If resistance is met, withdraw the catheter to 2–3 cm, twist, and reinsert.

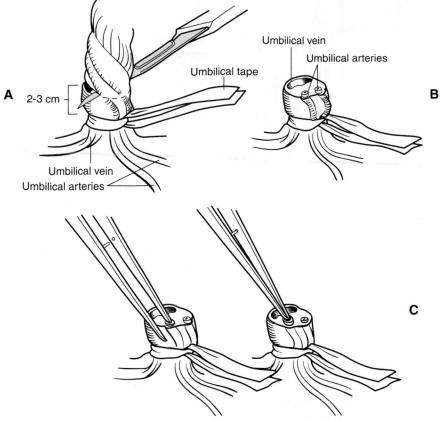

FIGURE 4-4 ● Umbilical artery catheterization. **A,** Umbilical cord is cut, leaving a 2- to 3-cm stump. **B,** Identification of umbilical vessels. **C,** Umbilical artery is dilated gently with forceps. (From Gomella TL, editor: *Neonatology*, ed 4, New York, 1999, Appleton & Lange, p 152, with permission.)

(6) Connect, secure, and confirm/adjust/confirm position at or just above the diaphragm.

5. Complications of umbilical vessel catheterization
   a. Arterial
      (1) Rapid blood loss
      (2) Vasospasm, arterial disruption, and occlusion (Schneider et al., 1989)
      (3) Thrombi or emboli resulting in late hypertension, leg growth abnormalities (Kempley et al., 1993; Seibert et al., 1991; Boo et al., 1999)
      (4) Hypoglycemia with high catheters
      (5) Sepsis
   b. Venous
      (1) Blood loss

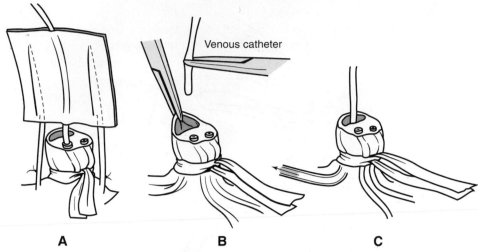

A   **B**   **C**

FIGURE 4-5 ● **A,** Umbilical artery catheter is secured with silk tape, which is attached to base of umbilicus with 3-0 silk sutures. **B,** Umbilical stump is held upright before catheter is inserted. **C,** Catheter is passed into umbilical vein. (From Gomella TL, editor: *Neonatology,* ed 4, New York, 1999, Appleton & Lange, pp 154, 187, with permission.)

(2) Hepatic damage
(3) Venous perforation
(4) Thrombosis
(5) Air embolus
(6) Sepsis
6. Prevention of complications
   a. Insert catheters gently—never force!
   b. Aspirate clots immediately after catheter insertion.
   c. Confirm correct position by x-ray.
   d. Use pressure transducer monitoring to detect line disconnection.
   e. Use meticulous sampling technique; always draw out before flushing and flush slowly while observing catheter and baby.
   f. Add heparin to infusion solutions.
   g. Remove catheter promptly when no longer needed or if complications arise.
C. Percutaneous Venous Catheterization
   1. Indications
      a. Administration of IV medications
      b. Administration of IV fluids
      c. Administration of parenteral nutrition
   2. Materials required
      a. Arm board
      b. Tape
      c. Betadine and alcohol swabs

    d. Tourniquet or rubber band

    e. Normal saline or flush solution in a 1- or 3-mL syringe

    f. 23- or 25-gauge scalp vein needle or 24- to 22-gauge angiocath (catheter-over-needle)

3. Procedure

    a. Scalp vein

        (1) Select vein to use (Figure 4-6).

        (2) Apply arm board or have assistant hold extremity or head.

        (3) Apply tourniquet proximal to puncture site.

        (4) Prepare site of puncture with Betadine swab, followed by saline swab when dry.

        (5) Fill tubing with flush and detatch syringe.

        (6) Grasp the plastic wings with needle bevel up.

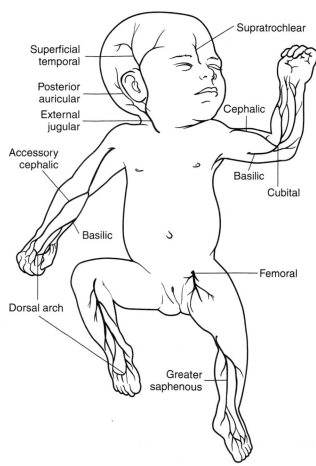

FIGURE 4-6 ● Sites for venous access frequently used in the neonate. (From Gomella TL, editor: *Neonatology*, ed 4, New York, 1999, Appleton & Lange, p 180, with permission.)

(7) With the thumb or index finger of the free hand, apply downward traction to stabilize the vein.

(8) At a point 0.5 cm distal to the anticipated site of vessel puncture, insert the needle point, bevel up.

(9) Advance needle until blood appears in the tubing.

(10) Remove the tourniquet and inject some of the flush solution gently to ensure patency of the needle and correct position within the vein.

(11) Tape the needle in position and connect IV tubing and fluid to needle (Figure 4-7).

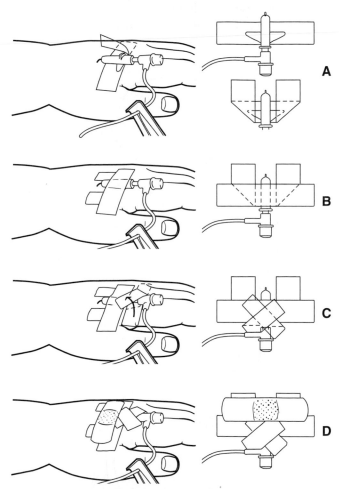

FIGURE 4-7 ● Securing venous catheter. **A,** Diagonally fold tape over catheter wings and back on itself. **B,** Place next strip of tape over wings of catheter and over first piece of tape. **C,** Apply third piece of tape, folding chevron style. **D,** Apply adhesive bandage over insertion site. (From Taeusch H, Christiansen RO, Buescher ES: *Pediatric and neonatal tests and procedures,* Philadelphia, 1996, WB Saunders.)

  b. Catheter-over-needle
    (1) Follow steps 1 through 4 above for scalp vein needle procedure.
    (2) Apply traction on skin to stabilize the vein.
    (3) Enter the skin 0.5 cm distal to anticipated vessel entrance site with bevel up; then enter vessel itself in separate motion.
    (4) Carefully advance needle until blood appears in the hub.
    (5) Withdraw the inner needle while advancing the catheter.
    (6) Remove tourniquet and gently inject flush solution into catheter to ensure patency.
    (7) Connect IV tubing and fluid and tape in position (see Figure 4-7).
  c. Complications
    (1) Infection
    (2) Hematoma
    (3) Infiltration
    (4) Phlebitis
    (5) Air embolism or clot
    (6) Vasospasm
D. **Venipuncture**
  1. Indications
    a. To obtain a blood sample for culture or analysis
    b. To administer IV medications
  2. Materials required
    a. 25- or 23-gauge scalp vein needle
    b. Povidone-iodine and saline swabs
    c. Rubber band or tourniquet
    d. Syringe
    e. Specimen container(s)
    f. Cotton balls or sterile gauze pad
  3. Procedure
    a. Choose vein to be used (see Figure 4-6).
    b. If needed, have assistant restrain the infant.
    c. Occlude the vein with tourniquet or rubber band, or have assistant encircle area with hand.
    d. Prepare site with povidone-iodine swab, allow to dry, then swab with saline swab.
    e. Puncture skin with needle bevel up, then direct needle into vein at 45-degree angle.
    f. As blood enters the tubing, attach syringe and collect blood slowly (or administer medication).
    g. Remove tourniquet.
    h. Remove needle and apply gentle pressure on the area until bleeding has stopped.
    i. If blood has been collected, place in proper containers and send to laboratory.
  4. Complications
    a. Infection

   b. Hematoma or hemorrhage
   c. Venous thrombosis
E. Arterial Puncture (Radial Artery Puncture)
   1. Indications
      a. To obtain blood for blood gas analysis
      b. When blood gas sample is needed and venous or capillary blood samples cannot be obtained
   2. Materials needed
      a. 25- or 23-gauge scalp needle or 25-gauge needle attached to a syringe
      b. Betadine and saline swabs
      c. 1- or 3-mL syringe
      d. 1:1000 heparin
      e. Gauze pad
   3. Procedure (Figure 4-8)
      a. If drawing a blood gas sample, obtain heparinized 1- or 3-mL syringe. If not available, draw up a small amount of 1:1000 heparin (approximately 0.2 mL) and then discard from syringe.
      b. Place patient's hand in your left hand (if right-handed) and extend wrist. Palpate radial artery with the left index finger.
      c. Prepare site with povidone-iodine swab, allow to dry, then swab with saline swab.
      d. Puncture the skin at approximately a 10- to 30-degree angle, bevel up, over the artery; slowly advance the needle while applying a small amount of negative pressure to the syringe. Advance the needle until blood appears in the tubing.
      e. Collect blood needed by slowly withdrawing on syringe.
      f. Withdraw needle and immediately apply firm, but not occlusive, pressure at the puncture site for at least 5 minutes with gauze pad.

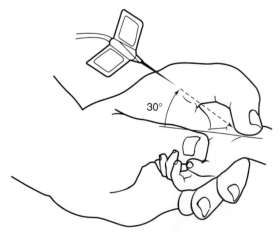

FIGURE 4-8 ● Technique of arterial puncture in the neonate. (From Gomella TL, editor: *Neonatology*, ed 4, New York, 1999, Appleton & Lange, p 149, with permission.)

      g. Remove air bubbles from blood sample before sending to laboratory.

      h. Tightly cap syringe, place on ice, and take to laboratory.

    4. Complications

      a. Arteriospasm

      b. Hematoma

      c. Thrombosis, embolism

      d. Infection

      e. Inaccuracy of blood gas results secondary to excess heparin or air bubbles

F. Lumbar Puncture (Spinal Tap)

    1. Indications

      a. To obtain cerebrospinal fluid (CSF) for diagnosis of disorders such as meningitis or subarachnoid hemorrhage

      b. To drain CFS in communicating hydrocephalus in association with intraventricular hemorrhage

      c. Administration of intrathecal medications

    2. Materials and equipment for lumbar puncture (lumbar puncture tray)

      a. Three sterile specimen tubes

      b. Sterile 22-gauge spinal needle with stylet

      c. Sterile drapes

      d. 1% lidocaine

      e. Betadine solution

      f. Sterile sponges for back preparation

      g. Adhesive bandage

      h. Alcohol swab

      i. Sterile gauze

      j. Sterile gloves

    3. Procedure

      a. An assistant must restrain the infant in a sitting or lateral decubitus position. If the infant is intubated, the lateral decubitus position should be used (Figure 4-9).

      b. Once infant is positioned, palpate the iliac crest and slide finger down to L4–L5 interspace. This is the site for lumbar puncture.

      c. Prepare equipment by opening sterile containers and pouring Betadine in well of lumbar puncture tray.

      d. Put on gloves and prep lumbar area with Betadine, starting with the chosen interspace. Prep in a widening circle, from this interspace up and over the iliac crest

      e. Remove Betadine from specified insertion site with alcohol after allowing Betadine to dry.

      f. Place one sterile drape under infant and one over infant, exposing only the insertion site.

      g. Inject 0.1 to 0.2 mL of 1% lidocaine subcutaneously at the insertion site for pain relief.

      h. After 1 to 2 minutes, insert the spinal needle with stylet in place, midline, with steady force aimed toward the umbilicus.

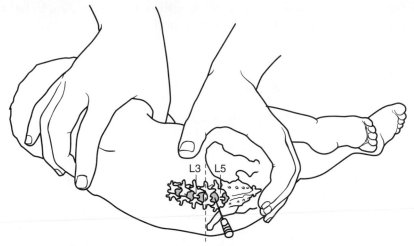

FIGURE 4-9 ● Positioning and landmarks used for lumbar puncture. The iliac crest *(dotted line)* marks the approximate level of L4. (From Gomella TL, editor: *Neonatology*, ed 4, New York, 1999, Appleton & Lange, p 173, with permission.)

    i. Advance the needle slowly and then remove the stylet to check for the appearance of spinal fluid. If no fluid is obtained, replace the stylet and advance needle again slowly. It may be necessary to remove the stylet frequently to keep from going too far and obtaining a bloody specimen.

    j. Obtain 1 mL of fluid in each of the three specimen tubes by allowing the fluid to drip into the tubes. Viral or other special studies may require additional volume

    k. When fluid has been obtained, replace the stylet and withdraw the needle in a single motion.

    l. Maintain pressure over the puncture site and remove excess Betadine with alcohol swabs.

    m. Place adhesive bandage over insertion site.

    n. Send specimen tubes to the laboratory.
        (1) Tube 1: For Gram stain, culture, and sensitivity
        (2) Tube 2: For glucose, protein levels
        (3) Tube 3: For cell count and differential

  4. Complications
    a. Apnea and bradycardia
    b. Hypoxia
    c. Infection
    d. Bleeding
    e. Spinal cord and nerve damage
    f. Herniation of cerebral tissue through foramen magnum

G. Nasogastric Tube Placement
  1. Indications
    a. Enteric feedings

        b. Gastric decompression

        c. Administration of medications

        d. Analysis of gastric contents

    2. Equipment for nasogastric tube placement

        a. For enteric feeding, infant feeding tube, 5 or 8 Fr

        b. For gastric decompression, Salem sump or Replogel tube, 8 or 10 Fr

        c. Stethoscope

        d. Sterile water

        e. 5- or 10-mL syringe

        f. Tape

        g. Suction equipment

    3. Procedure

        a. Check tube for defects such as cracks and/or occlusions. If tube has a guidewire, remove and reinsert wire to ensure that it can easily be removed once placed in the patient.

        b. Monitor heart rate and respirations during insertion of tube.

        c. Place infant in supine position.

        d. Measure for tube length and proper placement. This is done by placing the distal opening at the end of the nose. Then extend tubing to ear lobe and down to a point midway between the xiphoid process and umbilicus (Ziemer and Carroll, 1978).

        e. Place a piece of tape on tube to mark this distance.

        f. The tube may be inserted orally (Figure 4-10, *A*) or nasally (Figure 4-10, *B*).

            (1) Nasal insertion: Flex the neck, direct nose upward, insert tube straight back, and advance to determined length.

            (2) Oral insertion: With tongue down, pass tube into oropharynx and then advance slowly to determined length.

        g. Observe for apnea, respiratory distress, and bradycardia during procedure.

        h. Remove guidewire from enteric feeding tube. Never reinsert wire while tube is in patient because wire may exit through feeding port and cause trauma or perforation of stomach.

        i. Determine location of tube

            (1) Inject 5 mL of air into tube and listen with stethoscope over stomach for rush of air.

            (2) Palpate tube in the abdomen.

            (3) Aspirate stomach contents and test with pH paper.

            (4) If tube placement still cannot be determined, obtain x-ray.

        j. Tape tube in place securely to face (Figure 4-10, *B*).

    4. Complications

        a. Apnea and bradycardia

        b. Hypoxia

        c. Aspiration

        d. Perforation of esophagus, posterior pharynx, stomach, or duodenum

H. Bladder Aspiration (Suprapubic Urine Collection)

    1. Indication: To obtain urine culture when less invasive technique is not possible

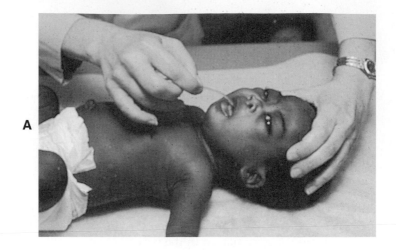

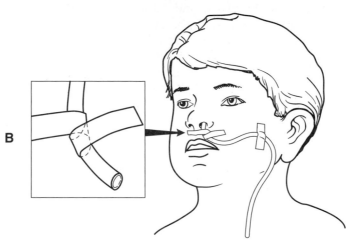

FIGURE 4-10 ● Insertion of nasogastric tube. **A,** Oral placement. **B,** Nasal placement. Position of tube is secured by crossover method. (**A,** From Wong DL et al.: *Wong's Essentials of pediatric nursing,* ed 6, St Louis, 2001, Mosby, p 814. **B,** From Taeusch H, Christiansen RO, Buescher ES: *Pediatric and neonatal tests and procedures,* Philadelphia, 1996, WB Saunders.)

2. Materials and equipment
   a. Povidone-iodine solution
   b. Sterile gloves
   c. Sterile container for urine
   d. Gauze pads
   e. 23- or 25-gauge 1-inch needle attached to a 3-mL syringe
3. Procedure
   a. Be certain that there is adequate urine in the bladder to collect a sample. There is usually adequate urine in the bladder if the infant has not voided in the previous 1 to 2 hours.

    b. Have an assistant hold the infant's legs in a frog-leg position.

    c. Determine site of bladder puncture (0.5–1 cm above the pubic symphysis and midline in the lower abdomen).

    d. Put on sterile gloves and prepare site with povidone-iodine.

    e. Palpate the pubic symphysis. Puncture the needle through the skin approximately 0.5–1 cm above the pubic symphysis at a 90-degree angle (Figure 4-11).

    f. Aspirate while advancing the needle. Do not advance the needle once urine is obtained.

    g. Withdraw needle while placing pressure over the puncture site.

    h. Transfer urine to sterile container or cap tightly and send to laboratory.

  4. Complications

    a. Perforation of bowel

    b. Bleeding

    c. Infection

I. Bladder Catheterization

  1. Indications

    a. To obtain urine specimen when clean-catch specimen or suprapubic aspiration cannot be obtained

    b. To monitor urinary output

    c. To relieve urinary retention

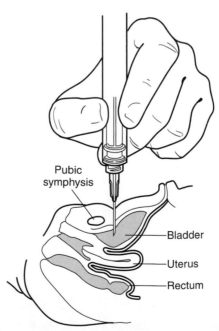

FIGURE 4-11 ● Technique of suprapubic bladder aspiration. (From Gomella TL, editor: *Neonatology*, ed 4, New York, 1999, Appleton & Lange, p 156, with permission.)

d. During genitourinary testing, such as cystogram or voiding cystourethrogram

2. Equipment and materials
   a. Urethral catheters
      (1) 3.5 Fr umbilical artery catheter for infants <1000 g
      (2) 6 Fr Foley catheter or 5 Fr feeding tube for infants 1000–1800 g
      (3) 8 Fr feeding tube or Foley catheter for infants >1800 g
   b. Urinary catheter tray
      (1) Sterile gloves
      (2) Cotton balls
      (3) Povidone-iodine solution
      (4) Sterile drapes
      (5) Sterile lubricant
      (6) Sterile specimen container

3. Procedure
   a. Male catheterization (Figure 4-12, *A*)
      (1) Place infant on back and restrain legs or have assistant hold legs.
      (2) Clean penis with povidone-iodine solution, starting at meatus and moving down the penis.
      (3) Put on sterile gloves and drape area with sterile towels.
      (4) Apply sterile lubricant to catheter tip.
      (5) Hold the penis perpendicular to the body. Place the catheter in the urethra and advance until urine appears in the catheter. Slight resistance may be felt as the catheter passes through the external sphincter. Steady, gentle pressure is usually needed to pass beyond this area; never force the catheter.

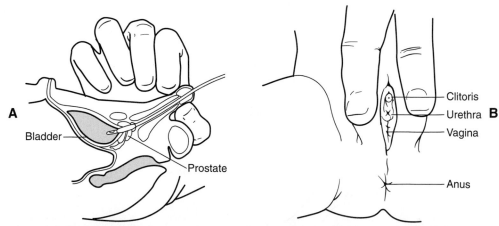

FIGURE 4-12 ● **A,** Bladder catheterization of male infant. **B,** Landmarks used for bladder catheterization of female infant. (From Gomella TL, editor: *Neonatology,* ed 4, New York, 1999, Appleton & Lange, pp 158-159, with permission.)

(6) Collect the urine specimen in the sterile container and send to the laboratory.

(7) If a Foley catheter is used, inflate the balloon with 2–5 mL sterile water, depending on balloon size.

(8) If catheter is to remain in place, tape securely to the lower abdomen.

   b. Female catheterization (Figure 4-12, *B*)

(1) Place infant on back and secure legs in frog-leg position. Secure with restraints or have an assistant hold the legs.

(2) Separate the labia and clean the area around the meatus with povidone-iodine solution using front-to-back strokes.

(3) Put on sterile gloves and apply sterile drapes around the labia.

(4) Spread the labia and identify the urethra.

(5) Apply sterile lubricant to the tip of the catheter.

(6) Insert the catheter in the urethra and advance until urine appears.

(7) Inflate bulb of Foley catheter, if applicable, and tape catheter to leg.

  4. Complications

   a. Infection

   b. Hematuria

   c. Trauma to urethra

   d. Stricture

J. Electrocardiogram Lead Placement

  1. Indication: To monitor infant who has evidence of respiratory or cardiovascular instability

  2. Lead placement

   a. It is important that electrodes make good skin contact. This means that the area used for electrodes must be clean and dry. The skin should be free of blood, vernix, and amniotic fluid.

   b. Electrodes should be placed at the periphery of the anterior chest. This facilitates auscultation of the heart and lungs. It also avoids interference with chest compressions and x-ray artifact.

   c. Electrodes are typically placed on shoulders or lateral chest surfaces, and the ground electrode is placed on the abdomen or thigh.

K. Venous Pool Puncture

  1. Indications

   a. To obtain blood when superficial veins are unavailable

   b. To obtain blood when capillary sample is unavailable

  2. Equipment and materials

   a. 25- or 23-gauge scalp vein needle or 25-gauge needle attached to syringe

   b. Povidone-iodine and alcohol swabs

   c. Gauze pad

   d. Appropriate specimen containers

  3. Procedure (University Hospital, 1993)

   a. Locate venous pool site on the anterior forearm below the cubital fossa (inside of the elbow) (Figure 4-13). This area is specifically defined as the area where the flexor carpi radialis, palmaris longus, flexor carpi ulnaris, and brachioradialis muscles (the superficial forearm muscles) meet.

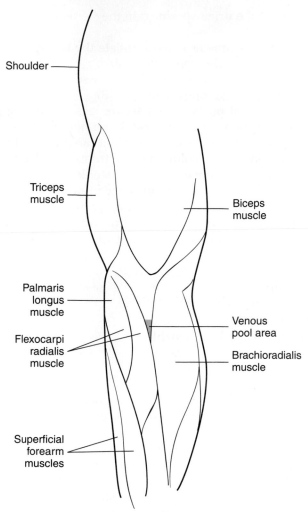

Shoulder

Triceps muscle

Biceps muscle

Palmaris longus muscle

Venous pool area

Flexocarpi radialis muscle

Brachioradialis muscle

Superficial forearm muscles

FIGURE 4-13 ● Location of venous pool site. (From University Hospital: *Venipuncture for obtaining blood sample in neonate* [policy number V-1-NN], Denver, 1993, University of Colorado Health Sciences Center, University Hospital, p 3.)

b. Clean area with povidone-iodine; allow to dry; then swab with alcohol.
c. Insert scalp vein needle or needle attached to syringe, at no more than a 30-degree angle, into the venous pool.
d. When blood appears in the tubing or hub, withdraw needed amount of blood.
e. Withdraw needle and apply gentle pressure with gauze pad.
f. Transfer blood to proper specimen container and take to laboratory.

4. Complications
   a. Hematoma
   b. Injury to brachial artery with insertion angle >30 degrees
   c. Infection

REFERENCES

Arya H, Williams J, Ponsford SN, Bissenden JG: Neonatal diaphragmatic paralysis caused by chest drains, *Arch Dis Child* 66:441-442, 1991.

Boo NY, Wong NC, Zulkifli SZ, Lye NS: Risk factors associated with umbilical vascular catheter-associated thrombosis in newborn infants, *J Pediatr Child Health* 35:460-465, 1999.

Gomella T, editor: *Neonatology,* New York, 1999, Appleton & Lange.

Greenough A: Where should the umbilical catheter go? *Lancet* 341:1186-1187, 1993.

Hazinski M, editor: *Pediatric advanced life support,* Dallas, TX, 1994, American Heart Association.

Kattwinkel J, Cook LJ, Hurt H, et al: *Perinatal continuing education program. Book II. Newborn care: concepts and procedures,* Charlottesville, VA, 1995, University of Virginia Health Sciences Center, Division of Neonatal Medicine.

Kempley ST, Bennett S, Loftus BG, et al: Randomized trial of umbilical arterial catheter position: clinical outcome, *Acta Paediatr* 82:173-176, 1993.

Quak JM, Szatmari A, van den Anker JN: Cardiac tamponade in a preterm neonate secondary to a chest tube, *Acta Paediatr* 82:490-491, 1993.

Rainer C, Gardetto A, Fruhwirth M, et al: Breast deformity in adolescence as a result of pneumothorax drainage during neonatal intensive care, *Pediatrics* 3:80-86, 2003.

Schneider K, Hartl M, Fendel H: Umbilical and portal vein calcification following umbilical vein catheterization, *Pediatr Radiol* 19:468-470, 1989.

Seibert JJ, Northington FJ, Miers JF, Taylor BJ: Aortic thrombosis after umbilical artery catheterization in neonates: prevalance of complications on long-term follow-up, *Am J Roentgenol* 156:567-569, 1991.

Shukla H, Ferrara A: Rapid estimation of insertional length of umbilical catheters in newborns, *Am J Dis Child* 140:786-788, 1986.

Squire SJ, Hornung TL, Kirchhoff KT: Comparing two methods of umbilical artery catheter placement, *Am J Perinatol* 7:8-12, 1990.

Taeusch HW, Christiansen RO, Buescher ES: *Pediatric and neonatal tests and procedures,* Philadelphia, 1996, WB Saunders.

University Hospital: *Venipuncture for obtaining blood sample in neonate* (policy number V-1-NN), Denver, 1993, University of Colorado Health Sciences Center, University Hospital.

Ziemer M, Carroll JS: Infant gavage reconsidered, *Am J Nurs* 78:1543-1544, 1978.

Evaluation and Care of the Newborn Infant During the Transitional Period and Beyond

The initial evaluation, assessment, and management of the newly born must be directed to promote and facilitate normal adaptation to extrauterine life and to provide early detection of significant medical problems so that they can be evaluated and treated appropriately.

Birth is an obligatory change of environments. In adjusting to extrauterine life, the newly born infant experiences a complex series of biologic, physiologic, and metabolic changes. These changes are evoked by a variety of processes, including perinatal surges in hormones, labor, delivery, gaseous ventilation and oxygenation of the lung, umbilical cord occlusion, decreased environmental temperature, and activation of the sympathoadrenal system.

These complex changes are essential for survival. Every infant must successfully complete this process of transition in order to survive in the extrauterine environment. For a small percentage of infants, transition is never achieved; for a slightly larger number, transition is delayed or complicated; however, for most infants, transition is so smooth it appears uneventful.

5 Adaptation to Extrauterine Life and Management During Normal and Abnormal Transition

Jacinto A. Hernandez, MD, MHA ■ *Lucy Fashaw,* RNC, BSN ■ *Ruth Evans,* RNC, MS, NNP

The transition from fetal to newborn life is a highly vulnerable time for the infant. The high neonatal morbidity and mortality rates during this remarkable sequence of adaptive events attest to the fragility of life in this period of transition. Consequently, the optimum care of the neonatal patient during this period is prospective and anticipatory. The focus should be on early recognition of those perinatal factors adversely affecting the normal transition and the detection of those infants whose transition is in jeopardy.

CARDIOPULMONARY CHARACTERISTICS OF THE FETUS

A. **Placental-Fetal Circulation**
   1. Placenta
      a. Responsible for blood oxygenation and elimination of waste products of metabolism; transfer of O_2 and CO_2 across the placenta is by simple diffusion.
      b. High rate of metabolism; uses one third of all the oxygen and glucose supplied by the maternal circulation for its own metabolic needs.
      c. Low-resistance circuit; receives approximately 50% of fetal cardiac output.
      d. Uterine venous blood entering the intervillous space has a PaO_2 of 40–50 mm Hg and a pH of 7.36.
   2. Fetal shunts and blood flow (Figure 5-1)
      a. Umbilical vein (PaO_2 = 35 mm Hg) carries oxygenated blood from the placenta to the fetus.
      b. Ductus venosus: One half of the umbilical venous blood bypasses the liver through the ductus venosus to the inferior vena cava, while the

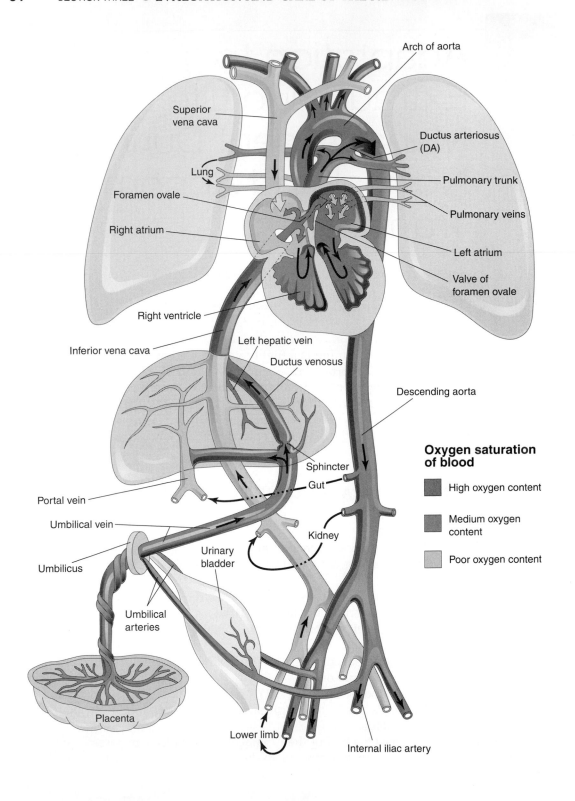

other half passes through the liver and enters the inferior vena cava via the hepatic veins. This mixing of blood slightly lowers the PaO_2.

c. Inferior vena cava blood (PaO_2 = 25–28 mm Hg) is largely deflected across the right atrium through the foramen ovale into the left atrium.

d. Left atrium: Receives the blood from the right atrium and mixes it with a small amount of blood returning from the lungs via the pulmonary veins.

e. Left ventricular blood (PaO_2 = 25–28 mm Hg) is virtually all from the inferior vena cava by way of the right atrium–foramen ovale–left atrium pathway. Left ventricular blood is pumped through the aorta to the brain from the upper part of the aortic arch. Approximately two thirds of the blood from the ascending aorta flows to the brain and upper extremities.

f. Superior vena cava receives deoxygenated blood returning from the brain and upper extremities. Of this blood, 97% enters the right atrium and flows to the right ventricle; only 3% goes to the left atrium via the foramen ovale.

g. Right atrium: Some mixing occurs here between the deoxygenated superior vena caval blood and the portion of the oxygenated inferior vena caval blood not shunted directly into the left atrium via the foramen ovale.

h. Right ventricle: This is the dominant ventricle (PaO_2 = 19–22 mm Hg), ejecting about two thirds of the total cardiac output. Most of the blood is directed away from the lungs through the ductus arteriosus to the descending aorta and subsequently to the placenta through the umbilical arteries.

i. Ductus arteriosus: Equal in size to the aorta; connects the pulmonary artery to the descending aorta. The blood flows right to left (pulmonary artery to aorta) across the ductus arteriosus because of high pulmonary vascular resistance and low placental resistance.

j. Low pulmonary blood flow (only 8%–10% of right ventricular output) results from high pulmonary vascular resistance.

k. Descending aorta supplies kidneys and intestines, divides into two arteries, and returns blood to the placenta for oxygenation.

B. **The Fetal Lung**
   1. Decreased blood flow compared with extrauterine life, due in part to the compression of the pulmonary capillaries by the fetal lung fluid.
   2. The small pulmonary arteries of the fetus have a thick muscular medial layer. Pulmonary vascular resistance increases throughout fetal life. The low

FIGURE 5-1 ● Simplified scheme of fetal circulation. *Shaded areas* indicate oxygen saturation of the blood, and *arrows* show the course of fetal circulation. Organs are not drawn to scale. (From Moore KL, Persaud TVN: *The developing human: clinically oriented embryology,* ed 7, Philadelphia, 2003, WB Saunders.)

fetal oxygen tension in fetal life also contributes to the high pulmonary vascular resistance, and even very early in gestation the pulmonary vessels are quite sensitive to hypoxia and other stimuli.

3. There is active secretion of fluid by the lungs with decreased secretion of lung fluid toward term. At term the lung contains approximately 30 mL/kg body weight of a plasma ultrafiltrate, comparable to the normal postnatal thoracic gas volume of 25 mL/kg; an adequate fluid volume is necessary for lung development. Net flux of fluid is out through the trachea.

4. In utero, fetal breathing movements are present and have been detected as early as 11 weeks gestation. This breathing movement contributes to lung development.

5. Surfactant is secreted into the amniotic fluid by the fetal lung beginning prior to 20 weeks gestation. The absolute quantity of surfactant increases throughout gestation in both lung and amniotic fluid, being of sufficient quantity to support extrauterine respiration at an average of 34 weeks gestation.

PHYSIOLOGIC CHANGES AT BIRTH

A. **Circulatory Adjustments to Postnatal Life** (Figure 5-2): Dramatic changes occur in the cardiovascular system at birth. The circulation changes from one characterized by the presence of central shunts, a relatively low combined ventricular output, right ventricular dominance, and pulmonary vasoconstriction to a circulation in series with a high cardiac output equally divided between the two ventricles, and a greatly dilated pulmonary vascular bed.

1. When the umbilical cord is clamped, the following occurs:
   a. The placenta is separated from the circulation, and the umbilical arteries and veins constrict.
   b. As the low-resistance placental circuit is removed, there is a resultant increase in systemic blood pressure; the systemic vascular resistance then exceeds the pulmonary vascular resistance.

2. The three major fetal shunts (ductus venosus, foramen ovale, and ductus arteriosus) functionally close during transition.
   a. Ductus arteriosus: The lungs now provide more efficient oxygenation of the blood, and the arterial tension rises. This rise in the PaO_2 is the most potent stimulus to constriction of the ductus arteriosus, with circulating prostaglandins also contributing to ductal closure.
   b. Foramen ovale: The fall in pulmonary vascular resistance results in a drop in right ventricular and right atrial pressure, and the increased

FIGURE 5-2 ● Simplified representation of the circulation after birth. Adult derivatives of fetal vessels and structures that become nonfunctional at birth are also shown. *Arrows* indicate the course of neonatal circulation. Organs are not drawn to scale. (From Moore KL, Persaud TVN: *The developing human: clinically oriented embryology,* ed 7, Philadelphia, 2003, WB Saunders.)

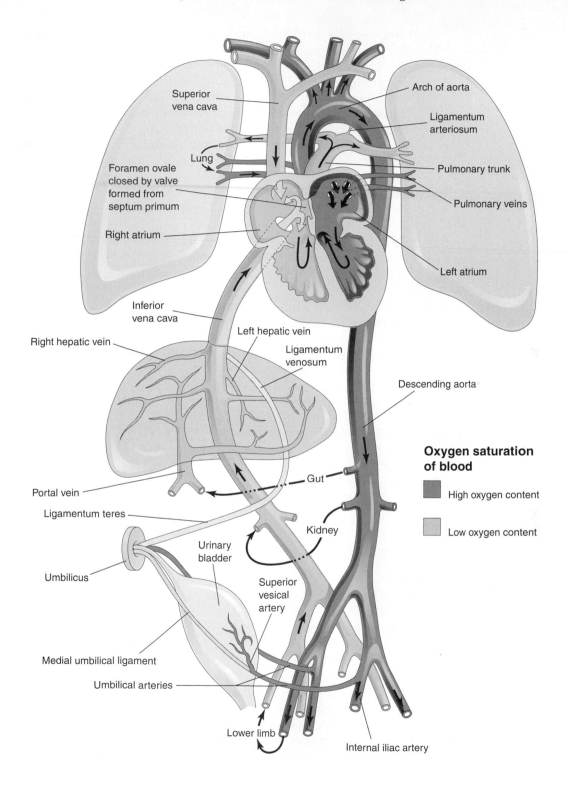

systemic vascular resistance results in an increase in left atrial and ventricular pressures, causing the foramen ovale to close.

(1) The foramen ovale becomes sealed by the deposition of fibrin and cell products during the first month of life.

(2) Until the foramen ovale is anatomically sealed, anything that produces a significant increase in right atrial pressure can reopen the foramen ovale and allow a right-to-left shunt.

    c. Ductus venosus: Absent umbilical venous return leads to closure of the ductus venosus. Functionally closes within 2-3 days; becomes the ligamentum venosum.

  3. The postnatal circulation

    a. Systemic venous blood enters the right atrium from the superior vena cava and the inferior vena cava.

    b. Poorly oxygenated blood enters the right ventricle and passes through the pulmonary artery into the pulmonary circulation for oxygenation.

    c. The oxygenated blood returns to the left atrium through the pulmonary veins.

    d. This blood passes through the left ventricle and into the aorta to supply the systemic circulation.

B. Pulmonary Adaptation at Birth

  1. With delivery of the infant and the onset of respiration, the lungs become the organ of gas exchange. It is now well established that breathing does not start at birth but occurs intermittently long before in utero. Breathing is a continuation of movements and reflexes that have been established and "exercised" for a long time in utero.

  2. Many factors are responsible for the onset of postnatal breathing: sensory stimuli such as cold, light, noise, and pain; chemical stimuli such as hypoxemia, hypercarbia, and acidosis; and mechanical gasp reflexes caused by the elastic recoil of the thorax after delivery.

  3. The initial lung inflation may require negative intrathoracic pressures of 30–40 cm H_2O, but pressures as high as 60–70 cm H_2O are not uncommon. Subsequent breaths in the normal newborn require 15–20 cm H_2O pressure.

  4. As much as two thirds of the fetal lung fluid is removed during labor and during the passage through the birth canal as the result of a "physiologic squeeze." With the first breath, air enters the lungs.

    a. Aeration of the lung drives fluid into the interstitium and stimulates increased blood flow and resorption of this fluid by the circulation and by lymphatics. The rate at which this occurs is variable; it is not unusual to hear fine crackling rales throughout the lungs before this process is completed.

    b. The pulmonary vessels respond to the increase in Po_2 with vasodilation. Pulmonary vascular resistance progressively decreases until adult levels are reached at 2–3 weeks of age.

  5. The work of inspiration is mainly (80%) devoted to overcoming the surface tension of the walls of the terminal lung units at the gas-tissue interface. On expiration, the ability to retain air depends on surfactant.

     a. Surfactant is a lipoprotein produced by type II alveolar pneumocytes; surfactant release increases in response to increased catecholamine at birth.

     b. Surfactant has the ability to lower surface tension at an air-liquid interface.

     c. As surfactant lowers surface tension in the alveolus at end-expiration, it stabilizes the alveoli and prevents collapse.

  6. There is an increased functional residual capacity with each breath; thus less inspiratory pressure is required for subsequent breaths.

  7. Lung compliance improves in the hours following delivery, secondary to circulating catecholamine. The increased levels of catecholamine (especially epinephrine) also clear the lungs by decreasing secretion of lung fluids and increasing their absorption through the lymphatic system.

THE NORMAL TRANSITIONAL PERIOD

  A. The First Few Hours of Life: During the first few hours after birth, the normal infant progresses through a fairly predictable sequence of events, recovering from the stress of delivery and adapting to extrauterine life. This is referred to as "transition." Both the intrapartum and the immediate neonatal events result in sympathetic discharges that are reflected in changes in heart rate, color, respiration, motor activity, gastrointestinal function, and body temperature of the infant. Figure 5-3 shows Desmond's classical description of the transitional period, which includes the following three stages:

    1. First stage (0–30 minutes) = "first period of reactivity." Changes are predominantly sympathetic. During this period:

     a. There is a rapid increase in the heart rate to the range of 160 to 180 beats per minute. This range lasts 10–15 minutes, with a gradual fall over 30 minutes to a baseline rate between 100 and 120 beats per minute.

     b. Respirations are irregular during the first 15 minutes, with peak respiratory rates between 60 and 80 breaths per minute.

     c. Rales are present on auscultation. Grunting, flaring and retractions also may be noted, and there may be brief periods of apnea (<10 seconds in duration).

     d. The infant is alert, and behavior is marked by spontaneous startle reactions, gustatory movements, tremors, crying, and side-to-side head movements.

     e. There is a decrease in body temperature and a generalized increase in motor activity with increased muscle tone.

     f. Bowel sounds are absent, and the production of saliva is minimal.

    2. Second stage (30 minutes to 2 hours) = "period of decreased responsiveness."

     a. The infant either sleeps or has a marked decrease in motor activity. Muscle tone returns to normal, and responsiveness is diminished.

     b. Fast, shallow, synchronous breathing (up to 60 breaths per minute) without dyspnea should not be alarming at this time. Color should be excellent. An increase in the anterior-posterior diameter (barreling) of the chest may be present.

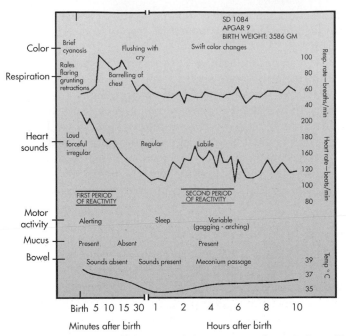

FIGURE 5-3 ● Clinical transitional behavior of the term newborn infant. (From Desmond MM, Rudolph AJ, Philtaksphraiwan P: The transitional care nursery: a mechanism for preventive medicine in the newborn, *Pediatr Clin North Am* 13:656, 1966, with permission.)

    c. The heart rate falls into the range of 100–120 beats per minute and is relatively less responsive.

    d. The abdomen should be rounded and bowel sounds audible. Peristaltic waves may occasionally be visible. Oral mucus is absent.

    e. Spontaneous jerks and twitches are common, but the infant quickly returns to rest.

  3. Third stage (2–8 hours) = "second period of reactivity." During this period, responsiveness returns and may become exaggerated.

    a. The infant again exhibits tachycardia, brief periods of rapid respiration, and abrupt changes in tone, color, and bowel sounds.

    b. Oral mucus again may become prominent, and gagging and vomiting are not unusual. The bowel may be cleared of meconium.

    c. The infant becomes more responsive to exogenous and endogenous stimuli, and heart rate becomes labile.

    d. The second period of reactivity may be brief or last several hours. As it diminishes, the infant appears to be relatively stable and ready for feedings.

The sequence of clinical behavior just described is common to all well newborns after birth regardless of gestational age or route of delivery. Knowledge of the normal changes occurring during the transitional period allows early recognition of the infant who is not making a normal extrauterine adaptation.

MANAGEMENT OF THE NEWBORN DURING TRANSITION

Traditionally, nursery care was based on the optimistic assumption that the majority of babies will have no transitional difficulty after delivery and that the term infant in particular will do exceedingly well. Nursery care was geared for the 85%–90% of newborns who do well rather than for the 10%–15% with transitional complications. The present approach to postdelivery care of newborn infants recognizes the awesome complexity of the transition process.

A. **The Newborn as a Recovery Patient**
   1. The "intensive care" concept: This concept, proven to be successful in the immediate postsurgical period for all patients, has been introduced to the care provided in the immediate neonatal period. All newborns are to be regarded as recovering patients until they have demonstrated evidence of smooth transition.
   2. Who should provide the care? Present standards of care have created a need for skilled personnel to care for infants in the delivery room during the first minutes after birth and in the nursery thereafter. This type of personnel must be available 24 hours a day in every delivery service. It is imperative that all nursery caregivers become familiar with the transitional changes occurring after birth. It is clear that optimal outcomes are basically dependent on constant scrutiny of infants by qualified personnel rather than by monitors.
   3. The role of the neonatal nurse: Primary evaluation and care of infants at birth following a normal or low-risk pregnancy should be delegated to an appropriately trained neonatal nurse who can consult a qualified physician when the need arises. For intermediate or high-risk pregnancies, the presence of a qualified physician and/or experienced neonatal nurse practitioner at the delivery is imperative.

B. **Physiologic Monitoring and Stabilization During Transition**
   1. Body temperature and neutral thermal environment: The newborn is likely to lose a great deal of body heat after birth. If measures are not taken to prevent heat loss, body temperature can fall precipitously.
      a. Neutral thermal environment (NTE): In the transition nursery, an infant who needs frequent or continuous observation can be nursed unclothed in an incubator or under a radiant warmer set to maintain an NTE.
         (1) NTE is the range of ambient temperature and humidity at which heat loss is minimal and metabolic demands and oxygen consumption are the lowest. For an undressed, normal-term newborn, this is in the range of 31°–34° C at 50% humidity.
         (2) Under these conditions the normal range of body temperature in a healthy newborn is 36.5°–37.0° C by axillary temperature or 36.0°–36.5° C by skin temperature. This range varies with weight, gestational age, and chronologic age.

(3) Once the term newborn is maintaining a stable temperature, the infant can be cared for in an open crib if clothed and wrapped in a blanket. A draft-free room of 24°–26° C should provide an adequate thermal-neutral condition.

b. Temperature care considerations

(1) Check axillary temperature every 30–60 minutes during transition when the child is under a radiant warmer. Avoid hyperthermia (skin temperature >37.0° C or axillary temperature >37.5° C). Monitoring the axillary temperature allows time for successful intervention before a fall in core temperature indicates failure of the body's compensatory heat regulation mechanisms.

(2) For infants in an incubator or under a radiant warmer, record the environmental temperature simultaneously with the infant's temperature assessments to monitor the infant's environmental temperature requirements. These requirements can be checked against published normal ranges of neutral thermal environmental temperatures as a tool in evaluating an infant; if too much or too little external heat is required to maintain a normal infant temperature, it may be a sign of infection or other problem.

(3) First bath should be delayed until body temperature has stabilized at 36.5°–37.0° C. Check temperature 30 minutes after the bath and 1 hour after transfer to open crib (Behring et al., 2003).

(4) Thereafter, check temperature at least every 2 to 4 hours until infant is stable, then every 8 hours until discharge.

2. Cardiopulmonary function: The heart rate, respiratory rate, quality of respirations, blood pressure, and color of skin and mucous membranes should be checked frequently during the first 6 hours after birth and the findings recorded. Routine blood pressure monitoring is not specifically recommended by the American Academy of Pediatrics (AAP) but should be obtained in any infant who has other abnormal vital signs or is experiencing abnormal transition (AAP, 1993). This is the period when the majority of threatening cardiopulmonary disease may appear.

a. Heart rate: In the first 15 minutes after birth, the average heart rate is 160 bpm, but it varies from 120 to 190. Thereafter, the average is 120–140 bpm (range 90–175). Consistently low or high heart rates suggest a pathologic condition.

b. Respirations: The pattern of respirations should be checked frequently for evidence of respiratory distress and the findings recorded. Table 5-1 shows a useful scoring system for this purpose. A score <2 in the first hour of life is within normal limits. Further investigation is warranted for a score >4 in the immediate newborn period or for any abnormalities after the first hour of life.

c. Brief episodes of apnea: During sleep, newborn infants normally have brief pauses in respiration. These are usually 5 seconds or less in duration, but occasionally as long as 9 seconds. Prolonged apnea or apnea with associated bradycardia is abnormal and requires investigation.

● TABLE 5-1
Clinical Respiratory Distress Scoring System*

Score	0	1	2
Respiratory rate (breaths/min)	60	60–80	>80 or apneic episode
Cyanosis	None	In room air	In 40% F_{IO_2}
Retractions	None	Mild	Moderate to severe
Grunting	None	Audible with stethoscope	Audible without stethoscope
Air entry†	Clear	Delayed or decreased	Barely audible

*The RDS score is the sum of the individual scores for each of the five observations.
†Air entry represents the quality of the inspiratory breath sounds as heard in the midaxillary line.
From Downes JJ, Vidyasager D, Boggs TR Jr, Morrow GM 3d: Respiratory distress syndrome in newborn infants.
I. New clinical scoring system (RDS score) with acid-base and blood-gas correlates, *Clin Pediatr* 9:325-331, 1970, with permission.

  d. Blood pressure: The normal range for indirectly measured blood pressure is 65–95 mm Hg systolic and 30–60 mm Hg diastolic in term infants. Pressure varies with birth weight, tending to be lower in smaller babies (Figure 5-4). The average mean blood pressure is 50–55 mm Hg in infants over 3 kg during the first 12 hours of life.

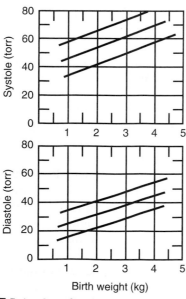
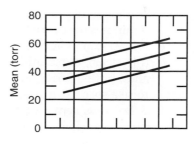

FIGURE 5-4 ● Systolic, diastolic, and mean aortic blood pressure as a function of birth weight. (From Versmold HT, Kitterman JA, Phibbs RH, et al: Aortic blood pressure during the first 12 hours of life in infants with birth weight 610 to 4220 grams, *Pediatrics* 67:607, 1981.)

3. Gastrointestinal function
   a. Passage of meconium (Clark, 1977): Approximately 70% of normal newborns pass meconium during the first 12 hours, 25% between 12 and 24 hours, and the remaining 5% by approximately 48 hours. Failure to stool by 36 hours should be investigated for obstruction. The time of initial stooling should be recorded.
   b. Response to first feeding: The first feeding must be observed carefully; anomalies such as esophageal atresia/tracheoesophageal fistula may become evident.
4. Urinary function
   a. Passage of urine (Clark, 1977): Approximately 68% of newborns urinate within 12 hours of birth, 93% by 24 hours, and 100% by 48 hours. The time of initial urination should be recorded.
   b. Failure to pass urine by 24 hours requires investigation. It may be due to prerenal causes or obstruction to urinary outflow.
C. **Routine Care of the Newborn in Transition**: Delivery room and nursery routines should be developed to meet the demand for careful monitoring in the transitional period and promotion and facilitation of maternal-infant interaction.
   1. Assessment and care in the delivery room
      a. Newborn infants should be regarded as recovering patients and kept under close surveillance during the first few hours after birth.
      b. Assign a qualified person (physician or nurse) to each delivery. This person is responsible for obtaining a pertinent history of pregnancy, labor, and delivery.
      c. Upon delivery, place the infant in a prewarmed incubator or infant warmer. The infant should be dried immediately in a towel and the mouth and nose should be gently suctioned.
      d. Assessment of heart rate, respirations, and color are used to guide any further resuscitation efforts, and Apgar scores are assigned at 1 and 5 minutes (or every 5 minutes until 20 minutes or until score >7).
      e. A brief examination should be performed by the clinician in attendance (physician, nurse midwife, neonatal nurse) to detect significant anomalies, birth injuries, and cardiorespiratory disorders that may compromise a successful adaptation to extrauterine life.
      f. If the assessment is normal, the infant may remain with the mother in the labor and delivery room or be transferred to the transitional care nursery. In either case, trained personnel aware of the changes to be expected during the transitional period should observe the infant frequently and intensively until the infant has achieved a smooth transition.
      g. Maternal-infant interaction
         (1) Every attempt should be made to facilitate and encourage maternal-infant contact.
         (2) If the infant is generally stable, with pink color and 5-minute Apgar score >7, the baby is rewrapped in warm, dry blankets and given to the parents for holding.

(3) At 15 minutes of age the infant must be assessed for general condition, respiratory activity, color, muscle tone, and temperature. This assessment must be documented on the progress note.

(4) Regardless of where the infant is being cared for, by 30 minutes of age all infants must be examined by a neonatal nurse.

2. Assessment and care in the transition nursery

   a. Vital signs and anthropometric measurements: On admission, heart rate, respiratory rate, axillary temperature, blood pressure, head circumference, length, and weight are recorded.

   b. Glucose screening (Cornblath et al., 2000)

   (1) Perform by a reliable method such as Chemstrip bG reagent strips, One Touch II, or AccuCheck on capillary whole blood; should be performed by 30–60 minutes of age on infants with the following risk factors:

   (a) Asphyxia, cold stress, increased work of breathing, possible sepsis (hypoglycemia secondary to increased metabolic response with increased use of glucose).

   (b) Mothers who have been administered excess intrapartum glucose or those receiving drug therapy including terbutaline, ritodrine, propranolol, and oral hypoglycemic agents.

   (c) Premature and postmature infants, infants with evidence of IUGR, or discordant twins.

   (d) Infants with diabetic mothers or large-for-gestational age infants (hyperinsulinemia resulting in rapid removal of glucose from the circulation).

   (e) Any infant with symptoms that could be secondary to hypoglycemia (i.e., jitteriness, hypothermia, apnea, tremor, hypotonia, cyanotic spells).

   (2) Some nurseries perform one glucose screen on all infants.

   (3) Abnormal screen is usually considered to be glucose <45 mg/dL.

   (a) See Figure 16-1 for further evaluation of an abnormal screen.

   (b) Abnormal screening values need to be investigated to determine the etiology of the abnormal screen.

   c. Eye care

   (1) Application may be delayed up to 1 hour after birth and can be delayed until after the first breastfeeding.

   (2) Prophylactic agents: 1% silver nitrate solution, 0.5% erythromycin ophthalmic ointment, 1% tetracycline ophthalmic ointment, or 2.5% povidone-iodone ophthalmic solution for prophylaxis of ophthalmia neonatorum due to *Neisseria gonorrhoeae* (AAP/ACOG, 2002).

   (3) Technique: Instill into conjunctival sac within 1 hour of birth. A new tube should be used for each infant. Medication should not be flushed from the eye following application.

   (4) Side effects include sensitivity reaction: Chemical conjunctivitis can be observed following silver nitrate instillation.

     d. Vitamin K (AquaMEPHYTON, phytonadione)

       (1) Given within 1 hour of birth

       (2) Dosage (AAP/ACOG, 2002)

         (a) Infant weight <1.5 kg: 0.5 mg IM as a single dose.

         (b) Infant weight >1.5 kg: 1.0 mg IM as a single dose.

         (c) Oral vitamin K not yet recommended by the American Academy of Pediatrics (AAP/ACOG, 2002).

       (3) Rationale for use

         (a) Vitamin K is needed to promote the hepatic biosynthesis of vitamin K–dependent clotting factors.

         (b) Newborns are predisposed to vitamin K hepatic deficiency secondary to immaturity, reduced liver stores of vitamin K, and absence of intestinal flora (major source of vitamin K production).

     e. Hepatitis B vaccine: Universal immunization of all newborns recommended by the Centers for Disease Control and Prevention and the AAP (see Chapter 12; AAP/ACOG, 2002).

  3. Physical examination in the transition nursery (see Chapter 7)

     a. During the first hours of life newborns follow the sequence of clinical behavior as previously described.

     b. A head-to-toe physical examination is performed (see Chapter 7). The following findings seen during transition are within normal limits:

       (1) Respirations and breath sounds

         (a) Initially coarse rales and moist tubular breath sounds are present until clearing of lung fluid is complete.

         (b) Prolonged expiratory phase.

         (c) Respiratory rate 30–60 breaths/minute.

         (d) Grunting and retracting (intercostal, substernal) may be present during the first hours of life as lung fluid is cleared.

       (2) Heart and heart sounds

         (a) Normal rate is 120–160 bpm; may range initially from 80 during sleep to 180 bpm when active and crying.

         (b) Loud second heart sound during first few hours to days of life secondary to slight pulmonary hypertension; splitting of the first heart sound is rare, but there is often narrow splitting of the second heart sound, which may be difficult to detect.

         (c) Murmur: Soft grade II/VI systolic murmur may be present and represents a left-to-right shunt across the ductus arteriosus prior to its closure.

       (3) Falling body temperatures: Mean low temperature is 35.6° C with lowest temperature reached at a mean age of 75 minutes after delivery (Desmond et al., 1966).

       (4) Acrocyanosis: Vasoconstriction of peripheral vessels resulting in a mottled appearance.

       (5) Petechiae of the face and facial bruising may be seen in the infant born vertex after a rapid second stage or after a tight nuchal cord.

      (6) Considerable overriding of the skull bones may take place to facilitate passage through the birth canal. This is commonly referred to as molding and resolves over the first few hours to days.

      (7) Gastrointestinal tract:

        (a) Absent bowel sounds initially.

        (b) As the bowel begins to fill with air, motility and bowel sounds are generally present within 15 minutes.

        (c) Anus patency.

      (8) Extremities: Findings may include deformities secondary to intrauterine positioning or fracture secondary to traumatic delivery.

  4. Feeding during transition (see also Chapter 8)

    a. Most infants are ready to be fed upon completion of the adaptation period; however, an infant can begin feeding at any stage of transition if evaluation is within normal limits.

    b. Evaluation of an infant prior to feeding must reveal:

      (1) Normal suck

      (2) Swallowing mucus without excessive accumulation in oropharynx

      (3) Absence of emesis

      (4) Respiratory rate <70 breaths/minute, patent nares, and normal breathing pattern

      (5) Normal color and perfusion

      (6) Bowel sounds present, no abdominal distension, and patent anus

  5. Identification of abnormal transition or illness

    a. Observe for abnormal symptoms or signs that may suggest developing problems. A checklist of the significant observations during transitional care must be made available to the caregivers; findings that are unimpressive by themselves may acquire significance if observed and recorded objectively (Figure 5-5). Infants who remain with their mothers must be returned to the nursery any time their condition become unstable.

    b. If transition is complicated, it is recommended that the infant be transferred to the neonatal intensive care unit.

ABNORMAL TRANSITION

  A. Normal Adaptive Changes Versus Abnormal Transition

    1. Normal adaptation: After birth, the sequence of clinical behavior just described is common to all newborns regardless of gestational age, route of delivery, or presence of disease. Advance knowledge of these anticipated changes allows early identification of those infants who are not making a normal extrauterine adaptation.

    2. Risk factors for altered normal transition or abnormal transition: Significant deviation from the normal sequence of events during transition may result from a variety of influences. Box 5-1 indicates factors and conditions that may alter the pattern and/or sequence of changes expected to occur after birth and that can result either in a healthy infant or one with significant illness. It is important to consider these factors

DATE: _____

TIME: _____

ACTIVITY	√	ACTIVE				
	+	Activity decreased				
	+	Tires easily				
	+	Lethargic				
	+	Floppy				
	+	Irritable				
	+	Pacifier required				
	+	Frantic				
	+	Swaddled				
	+	Tremors				
	+	Rigid				
	+	Opisthotonos				
	+	Moro poor or absent				
APPEARANCE	√	COLOR STABLE				
	+	Pallor				
	+	Plethora				
	+	Mottled				
	+	Harlequin syndrome				
	+	Jaundice				
	+	Dusky				
	+	Cyanosis: Generalized				
	+	Circumoral				
	+	Circumocular				
	+	Extremities				
	+	Tearing				
	+	Eye discharge				
FEEDINGS (GASTROINTESTINAL)	√	HUNGRY				
	√	DEMANDING				
	√	SUCKS WELL				
	+	Sucks poorly				
	√	GAVAGED WELL				
	√	Gavaged well/slowly				
	+	Gavage poorly				
	+	Gavage resisted				
	+	Mucus on tube				
	+	Mucus, other				
	+	Drooled				
	+	Gagged				
	+	Regurgitated				
	+	Vomited				
	+	Abdomen distended				
	cm	Abdomen, circumference				
	+	Hiccoughs				
	+	Sore buttocks				

DATE: _____

TIME: _____

RESPIRATIONS	√	CRY GOOD				
	+	Cry high-pitched				
	+	Cry weak				
	+	Sneezes				
	+	Stuffy Nose				
	+	Yawning				
	+	Hoarseness				
	+	Stridor				
	√	RESPIRATIONS: Regular				
	+	Shallow				
	+	Labored				
	+	Deep				
	+	Irregular				
	+	See saw				
	+	Periodic Breathing				
	+	Rest Periods 10 sec				
	+	10—30 sec				
	+	Apnea 30 sec				
	+	Alae nasi dilated				
	+	Cough				
	+	Grunting				
	+	Retraction				
SKIN	√	SKIN NORMAL				
	+	Dry and peeling				
	+	Irritated				
	+	Petechiae (area)				
	+	Ecchymosis (area)				
	+	Bleeding (area)				
	+	Dehydrated				
	+	Edema				
	+	Pustular rash				
	+	Erythema toxicum				
	+	Other rash (specify)				
	+	Abscess (area)				
	+	Sclerema				
	+	Umbilical redness				
	+	Umbilical oozing				

Completed by the nurse, this checklist indicates the presence of findings (√), severity (+, ++, +++), timing (ac, pc) etc. Capitalized items indicate normal findings. Each column signifies a period of observations. Significant additional data are recorded in the progress notes.

FIGURE 5-5 ● Checklist of significant observations in newborns. (From Lubchenco LO: *Pediatr Clin North Am* 8:471, 1961.)

when caring for an infant experiencing a delayed or altered period of transition (see below).

3. Abnormal transition: Although the pattern and time sequence of normal transition events may be altered by the risk factors noted above, those events still occur. The challenge for the caregiver is to be able to discriminate the signs of disease that produce an ill infant from the dynamic, rapidly changing features that accompany the physiologic adjustments of normal or altered transition but that still result in a healthy infant (Desmond et al., 1966; Gritton, 1998).

B. **Risk Factors for Abnormal Transition**: Box 5-1 identifies risk factors that may precipitate abnormal transition. Details for some of these conditions are provided in this section (Padbury, 1988; Siassi, 1988).

● BOX 5-1

MATERNAL, OBSTETRIC, AND NEONATAL CONDITIONS THAT INCREASE THE RISK FOR ABNORMAL TRANSITION

Maternal factors	Chronic hypertension
	Pregnancy-induced hypertension
	Diabetes mellitus
	Renal disease
	Infection
	Abuse of tobacco, alcohol, or illicit drugs
	Collagen vascular diseases
	Homozygous hemoglobinopathies
	Certain maternal medications
	Rh or other isoimmunization
Obstetric factors	Fetal growth retardation
	Decreased fetal movements
	Multiple gestation
	Oligohydramnios or polyhydramnios
	Premature rupture of membranes
	Third trimester bleeding
	Delivery by cesarean section
Neonatal factors	Prematurity (<37 weeks)
	Postmaturity (>42 weeks)
	Small for gestational age
	Large for gestational age
	Infection
	Metabolic abnormalities
	Birth trauma
	Major malformations
	Apgar score of 0–4 at 1 minute or the need for resuscitation at delivery
	Anemia

1. Maternal medications inducing neonatal depression
   a. Medications that frequently induce neonatal depression are narcotics, barbiturates, and magnesium.
   b. Neonatal effects
      (1) At birth the condition of these infants may be variable and they may or may not require resuscitation.
      (2) When an infant demonstrates general depression at birth, close observation is mandatory to determine the following:
         (a) Need for artificial ventilatory assistance
         (b) Need for parenteral fluids secondary to poor suck and swallow
         (c) Evidence of hypoglycemia
         (d) Point at which the effects of depressant drugs are diminishing
      (3) If the infant is breathing spontaneously, and after the first reactivity period has ended, the infant suffering from drug-induced depression may demonstrate the following:
         (a) Shallow breathing
         (b) Temperature instability
         (c) Poor sucking response
         (d) Decreased spontaneous activity
         (e) Delayed passage of urine and meconium
         (f) Increased tone
2. Birth by cesarean section (C/S) delivery
   a. Neonatal depression is common, and degree of depression often depends on maternal medications and indications for C/S delivery (e.g., depression more common with fetal distress).
   b. In general, the first period of reactivity is prolonged and the clinical manifestations more accentuated.
   c. Infants born by C/S delivery often have a high lung fluid volume, which may result in tachypnea, nasal flaring, grunting, mild intercostal retractions, rales, and need for supplemental oxygen during the first several hours of life (oxygen requirement beyond this period warrants further investigation).
3. Infants born to addicted mothers (see Chapter 18 for more detail): For addicted infants, the following may be seen:
   a. Moderate birth depression
   b. Evidence of withdrawal reaction (occurring with the onset of the second period of reactivity), which may include:
      (1) Accentuation of the lability characteristically seen in this period
      (2) Agitation with marked irritability, jitteriness, tremors, and inconsolable crying
4. Uteroplacental insufficiency
   a. Etiologies: Numerous causes, including insulin-dependent diabetes, hypertensive disorders, collagen vascular disorders
   b. Effects on pregnancy may include:
      (1) Decreased uterine blood flow
      (2) Decreased placental function

   c. Fetal and neonatal effects may include:
      (1) Intrauterine growth retardation
      (2) Fetal demise
      (3) Intrapartum fetal distress and perinatal asphyxia
      (4) Abnormal transition with altered cardiopulmonary adaptation
      (5) Variety of neonatal morbidities (i.e., perinatal depression, meconium aspiration, hypoglycemia, hypocalcemia, polycythemia, pulmonary hemorrhage, necrotizing enterocolitis, infection)
   5. Prematurity: Although premature infants react similarly to the challenges of adapting to extrauterine life as the term infant, they react more slowly and are at greater risk for having a complicated transition. Preterm infants, particularly those born before 34 weeks of gestation, represent the prototype of high risk infants by virtue of the immaturity of all organ systems, numerous physiologic handicaps, and significant morbidity and mortality risks.
C. **Neonatal Clinical Manifestations Signaling Abnormal Transition** (Box 5-2)
   1. Persistent tachypnea, grunting, retractions, and rales
      a. As described before, during the first period of reactivity, flaring, rapid respirations, grunting, mild retractions, and rales are accepted as normal events. Unfortunately, the same clinical manifestations with or without cyanosis are also recognized as the cardinal features of respiratory distress in the newborn.
      b. The distinction between what is considered normal transition and what represents an early onset of respiratory distress is based on severity and duration of symptoms. The respiratory score shown in Table 5-1 is useful in the evaluation of the respiratory status during the transition period. A persistent respiratory score >4 or duration of symptoms beyond the first hour of life warrants further investigation.
   2. Persistent cyanosis and prolonged oxygen requirement (Aucott, 2002)
      a. Brief cyanosis at birth lasting several minutes and transient dusky episodes during crying are considered normal during the early stages of adaptation.

● BOX 5-2
NEONATAL CLINICAL MANIFESTATIONS SIGNALING ABNORMAL TRANSITION

Persistent tachypnea, flaring, grunting, and retractions
Diffuse and persistent rales
Persistent cyanosis and prolonged oxygen requirement
Episodes of prolonged apnea and bradycardia
Marked pallor
Temperature instability
Poor capillary filling and blood pressure instability
Unusual neurologic behavior
Excessive oral secretions, drooling, and choking spells

    b. Clinical evidence of persistent central cyanosis (persistent O_2 saturation of <85%) in room air or need for supplemental oxygen after 2 hours of age in order to sustain normal oxygen saturations represents abnormal transition and requires immediate evaluation. (Note that some nurseries allow newborns 4–6 hours of supplemental oxygen need before initiating an evaluation for abnormal transition; this time limit is often determined by the experience of the nursing staff and the nurse:patient ratio).

    c. Because the causes of cyanosis may vary from trivial to life-threatening, the differential diagnosis should be approached in a systematic fashion, taking into consideration not only cardiac and pulmonary causes, but also noncardiopulmonary etiologies.

3. Apnea and bradycardia

    a. Episodes of apnea lasting longer than 20 seconds during transition, with or without associated bradycardia, should be regarded as evidence of an abnormal transition that requires further investigation.

    b. Etiologies may include maternal medications, perinatal asphyxia, infection, shock, and central nervous system (CNS) disorders.

    c. Low heart rates (as low as 80 bpm) without changes in color or respiratory pattern are often seen in transition during the period of diminished responsiveness.

    d. Persistent bradycardia needs careful evaluation.

4. Pallor

    a. Persistent pallor in the immediate postpartum period must be considered a serious sign requiring expeditious investigation (see Chapter 15 for more detail).

    b. It often reflects an underlying abnormality such as anemia or marked peripheral vasoconstriction secondary to causes such as intrapartum asphyxia and cardiovascular collapse.

    c. Differentiation of pallor due to peripheral vasoconstriction versus anemia is often difficult. However, since severe anemia may be life-threatening, prompt diagnosis and treatment are required.

5. Temperature instability (Hackman, 2001)

    a. Normal term infants kept in a neutral thermal environment are able to restore their initial drop in temperature within 2–3 hours of delivery.

    b. Persistently low body temperatures (<36.5° C) and temperature instability are evidence of compromised transition requiring evaluation.

    c. Possible etiologies include maternal medications, perinatal hypoxia, metabolic disturbances, CNS disorders, and sepsis.

6. Poor capillary filling and blood pressure instability: Marked vasoconstriction with clinical evidence of poor capillary filling (>3 seconds), generalized hypoperfusion or unstable systemic blood pressures are usually warning signs of serious underlying conditions (i.e., hypoxia, sepsis, cardiovascular instability, CNS injury).

7. Unusual neurologic behavior: While there are certain characteristic reactions and responses recognized as normal neurologic behavior during the period of transition, marked depression and lethargy, decreased activity with marked and persistent hypotonia, irritability, excessive tremors, and jitteriness are unusual neurologic behaviors and require further investigation.

8. Excessive oral secretions, drooling, and choking spells
   a. Increased salivation and oral mucus are characteristic parasympathetic reactions during the first and second periods of reactivity.
   b. Excessive amounts of oral mucus, drooling, episodes of cyanosis, choking, and coughing spells are all indicative of compromised transition needing careful evaluation (e.g., possible esophageal atresia).

D. **Specific Clinical Situations Associated with Abnormal Transition**
   1. Cardiorespiratory disorders
      a. Persistent pulmonary hypertension of the newborn (PPHN) (Walsh and Stork, 2001)
         (1) Pathophysiology
            (a) At birth, normal transition of gas exchange from the placenta to the lungs depends on a 10-fold increase in pulmonary blood flow and a sharp decline in pulmonary artery pressure secondary to a marked decrease in pulmonary vascular resistance (PVR).
            (b) In some newborn infants the transitioning pulmonary circulation reverts to the in utero pattern of circulation, resulting in PPHN (Figure 5-6). This may be due to:
               (i) A stressful insult such as hypoxia, hypotension, acidosis, or hypercarbia
               (ii) Failure for the normal development of a decrease in PVR with secondary increase in pulmonary blood flow
            (c) Resulting pathophysiologic features include:
               (i) Sustained pulmonary hypertension as a result of high PVR
               (ii) Abnormally increased pulmonary vasoreactivity
               (iii) Right-to-left shunting of blood across the patent ductus arteriosus or foramen ovale
               (iv) Severe and progressive hypoxemia
               (v) Right ventricular failure
         (2) Clinical conditions associated with PPHN include meconium aspiration syndrome, sepsis, pneumonia, respiratory distress syndrome, congenital diaphragmatic hernia, congenital heart disease, pulmonary hypoplasia, and a large group of undetermined causes (idiopathic).
         (3) Clinical manifestations may include tachypnea, respiratory distress, acidosis, cardiovascular instability, and rapidly progressing cyanosis and hypoxemia. Sometimes the clinical features are compounded by the manifestations of the precipitating disorder.
         (4) Diagnosis
            (a) Oxygenation
               (i) Diagnosis is suggested by hypoxemia and extremely labile oxygenation.

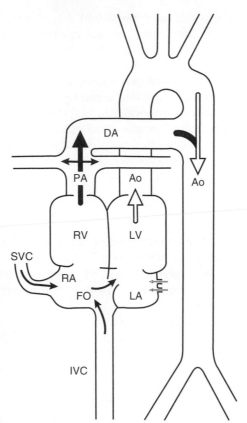

FIGURE 5-6 ● The circulation in PPHN. *IVC*, inferior vena cava; *RA*, right atrium; *LA*, left atrium; *FO*, foramen ovale; *SVC*, superior vena cava; *RV*, right ventricle; *LV*, left ventricle; *PA*, pulmonary artery; *Ao*, aorta; *DA*, ductus arteriosus. *Solid arrows* = venous blood. *Open arrows* = arterial blood.

      (ii) Preductal (i.e., right arm, right upper torso and head) and postductal (i.e., remainder of body) Pao$_2$ difference >20 mm Hg or oxygen saturation difference >10% usually supports the diagnosis of PPHN.

(b) Chest x-ray (CXR)
    (i) Diagnosis may be obscured by underlying condition.
    (ii) In idiopathic cases, the CXR often demonstrates mild-to-moderate cardiomegaly with little or no pulmonary parenchymal disease.
    (iii) Diagnosis of PPHN should be considered when hypoxemia is out of proportion to the degree of severity on CXR.

(c) Echocardiogram
    (i) Optimal method for diagnosing PPHN
    (ii) Also helps differentiate PPHN from parenchymal lung disease or cardiac lesions

b. Surfactant deficiency (Jobe, 1988)

(1) Surfactant function: Surfactant binds to the alveolar surface of the lung and markedly lessens the forces of surface tension at the air-water interphase, thereby reducing the pressure that would otherwise collapse the alveolus. By equalizing the forces of surface tension in alveolar units of varying size, surfactant is a potent anti-atelectasis factor and is essential for normal respiration.

(2) Respiratory distress syndrome (RDS): The presence of adequate amounts of lung surfactant is critical to successful pulmonary adaptation and lung stability during the period of transition. Absence or deficiency in lung surfactant disrupts this normal transition, leading to a characteristic series of clinical manifestations recognized as RDS (see below).

(3) Risk factors for surfactant deficiency: The greatest risk factor is low gestational age, with risk decreasing with advancing gestational age. RDS occurs in 60%–80% of infants born less than 28 weeks, 6%–8% of infants at 34 weeks gestation and less, and <1% at 38 weeks gestation. Other risks include maternal diabetes, maternal bleeding, pregnancy-induced hypertension, premature rupture of membranes, and perinatal birth asphyxia.

(4) Pathophysiology of RDS: Surfactant deficiency leads to the sequence of events shown in Figure 5-7.

(5) Clinical and laboratory manifestations of RDS:

(a) Infants with RDS characteristically are seen either immediately after delivery or within several hours of birth with tachypnea, nasal flaring, subcostal and intercostal retractions, cyanosis, and expiratory grunting.

(b) Although these signs are characteristic of neonatal respiratory distress, they may also result from a variety of nonpulmonary causes, such as hypothermia, hypoglycemia, anemia, or polycythemia. In addition, such nonpulmonary conditions may complicate the clinical course of RDS.

(c) The uncomplicated clinical course is characterized by a progressive worsening of symptoms, with a peak severity by days 2–3 and onset of recovery after 72 hours.

(d) Radiographic findings: Typical radiographic features include a diffuse reticulogranular pattern in both lung fields with superimposed air bronchograms.

(6) Treatment: In recent years the availability of exogenous surfactant as replacement therapy in infants with RDS has unequivocally been shown to decrease mortality and complications of RDS. The use of antenatal corticosteroids has also been found to decrease mortality in premature infants, as well as the incidence of intraventricular hemorrhage. Current studies of premature lung disease note that early use of HFOV in premature lung disease lessens parenchymal injury, improves gas exchange, and creates a more uniform lung inflation (Keszler and Durand, 2001).

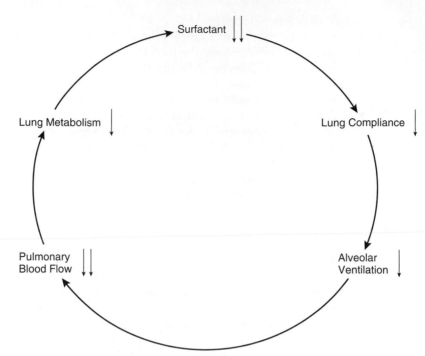

FIGURE 5-7 ● Pathophysiology of RDS.

   c. Meconium aspiration syndrome (MAS): Refers to respiratory distress
      that accompanies inhalation of meconium below the vocal cords.
      (1) Incidence: Meconium staining of the amniotic fluid occurs in
         10%–25% of all deliveries; however, MAS develops in only 1%–4%
         of all deliveries.
      (2) Pathophysiology
         (a) Passage of meconium in utero may occur secondary to fetal
            stress, particularly asphyxia. It may also occur as a physiologic
            event in infants near term.
         (b) Fetuses who undergo further stress may have gasping respira-
            tions at which time meconium is aspirated into the large air-
            ways and even into the lung itself.
         (c) Aspirated meconium may cause distress in several ways,
            including:
            (i) Mechanical obstruction of the large or small airways
            (ii) Mechanical obstruction of small airways can produce
               atelectasis if the obstruction is complete or overdistension
               of focal areas of the lung if air is inhaled but cannot be pas-
               sively exhaled past the partially-obstructing meconium
               ("ball-valve effect")
            (iii) Chemical pneumonitis can occur after a matter of hours

(iv) Overdistension of lung parenchyma secondary to meconium obstruction of the airway can result in air leak (i.e., pneumothorax or pneumomediastinum)

(v) PPHN can result from MAS-associated hypoxia

(d) Clinical findings:

(i) The infant is often post dates and with a history of in utero distress.

(ii) Symptoms include tachypnea, retractions, cyanosis, nasal flaring, and possibly grunting.

(e) Diagnosis: Usually made by suspicious history, clinical respiratory distress, and abnormal CXR (patchy hyperinflation and atelectasis, possible air leak).

(f) Treatment: Supplemental oxygen, possible mechanical ventilation, antibiotic coverage, and careful monitoring for air leak and possible PPHN.

d. Transient tachypnea of the newborn (TTN)

(1) Respiratory distress in the newborn secondary to delayed resorption of fetal lung fluid at birth

(2) Benign condition that resolves after 24–48 hours of supplemental oxygen therapy

(3) Most commonly occurs in near-term infants after cesarean delivery who do not have the benefit of passage through the vaginal canal, a process that aids in lung fluid removal

(4) Most prominent clinical findings: tachypnea and cyanosis; may also see retracting, nasal flaring

(5) Diagnosis: Respiratory distress in an infant, usually near term, in whom other treatable causes of respiratory distress have been ruled out (i.e., sepsis, pneumonia, meconium aspiration, surfactant deficiency, congenital heart disease, hyperviscosity). CXR generally shows perihilar streakiness and hyperinflation.

(6) Management: Supplemental oxygen therapy; may need IV nutrition until respiratory distress resolves

2. Perinatal asphyxia (Grow and Barks, 2002)

a. Definition: Condition following a perinatal reduction in fetal oxygen delivery that produces fetal bradycardia, impaired fetal gas exchange, and reduced tissue perfusion.

b. Fetal response to asphyxia: The mature fetus redistributes the blood flow to the heart, brain, and adrenals to ensure adequate oxygen and substrate delivery to these critical organs.

c. Impact on transition: The impact of perinatal asphyxia on the normal adaptive changes occurring at birth may be quite significant depending on the degree of asphyxia. These infants have in common a poor or unsustained response to birth stimuli, and the transitional period is prolonged, delayed, and compromised.

d. Multi-organ system injury in severe asphyxia

(1) When the severity of asphyxia exceeds the capacity of these adaptive or protective mechanisms, the shunting of blood toward initial

organs will fail, resulting in acute injury of multiple organs. After birth, these injured organs will show evidence of various degrees of functional impairment.

(2) Figure 5-8 shows the constellation of multiple organ involvement characteristic of the postasphyxic syndrome.

3. Hypoxic-ischemic encephalopathy (HIE)

a. Term used most frequently to designate the clinical and neuropathologic findings thought to occur in the full-term infant following intrapartum or postnatal asphyxia. This specific cascade of biochemical events creates an environment in which the brain becomes susceptible to excitotoxicity and free-radical injury, allowing for a propensity towards apoptotic neuronal death.

b. Table 5-2 presents the various degrees of encephalopathy and their usual clinical manifestations.

c. The diagnosis of HIE has important prognostic implications. Full-term neonates who experience an intrapartum asphyxial episode are considered at risk for developing long-term neurologic sequelae if they demonstrate neurologic dysfunction within the first week of life (especially if within the first 12 hours after birth).

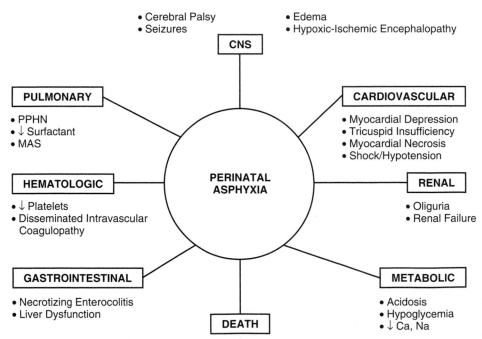

FIGURE 5-8 ● Perinatal asphyxia and its multiple effects.

● TABLE 5-2
Severity of Hypoxic-Ischemic Encephalopathy

Degree of HIE	Clinical Manifestations
Mild	Hyperalertness, uninhibited reflexes, sympathetic overactivity; duration <24 hours
Moderate	Lethargy, stupor, hypotonia, suppressed primitive reflexes, seizures
Severe	Coma, flaccid tone, suppressed brainstem function, seizures, increased intracranial pressure

From Hill A, Volpe JJ: Perinatal asphyxia: clinical aspects, *Clin Perinatol* 16[2]:436, 1989, with permission.

REFERENCES

American Academy of Pediatrics and American College of Obstetricians and Gynecologists: Perinatal care services. In Gilstrap LC, Oh W, editors: *Guidelines for perinatal care,* ed 5, Elk Grove Village, IL, 2002, American Academy of Pediatrics.

American Academy of Pediatrics, Committee on Fetus and Newborn: Routine evaluation of blood pressure, hematocrit, and glucose in the newborn, *Pediatrics* 92: 474-476, 1993.

Aucott, S: Physical examination. In Fanaroff AA, Martin RM, editor: *Neonatal-perinatal medicine: diseases of the fetus and infant,* ed 7, St Louis, 2002, Mosby.

Behring A, Vezeau TM, Fink R: Timing of the newborn first bath: a replication, *Neonatal Network* 22(1):39-43. 2003.

Clark DA: Times of first void and first stool in 500 newborns, *Pediatrics* 60:457-459, 1977.

Cornblath M, Hawdon JM, Williams AF, et al: Controversies regarding definition of neonatal hypoglycemia: suggested operational thresholds, *Pediatrics* 105: 1141-1145, 2000.

Desmond MM, Rudolph AJ, Philaksphraiwan P: The transitional care nursery—mechanism for preventive medicine in the newborn, *Pediatr Clin North Am* 13:651-668, 1966.

Gritton JR: The transition to extrauterine life and disorders of transition, *Clin Perinatol* 25:271-294, 1998.

Grow J, Barks JDE: Pathogenesis of hypoxic-ischemic cerebral injury in the term infant: current concepts, *Clin Perinatol* 29:585-602, 2002.

Hackman RS: Recognizing and understanding the cold-stressed term infant, *Neonatal Network* 20:35-41, 2001.

Jobe A: The role of surfactant in neonatal adaptation, *Semin Perinatol* 12:113-123, 1988.

Keszler M, Durand DJ: Neonatal high-frequency ventilation: past, present and future, *Clin Perinatol* 28:579-607, 2001.

Padbury JR, editor: Neonatal adaptation: the transition to postnatal life, *Semin Perinatol* 12, 1988.

Siassi B: Normal and abnormal transitional circulation in the IUGR infant, *Semin Perinatol* 12:80-83, 1988.

Walsh MC, Stork, EK: Persistent pulmonary hypertension of the newborn: rational therapy based on pathophysiology, *Clin Perinatol* 28:609-627, 2001.

6 Birth Injuries

Meica M. Efird, MD ▪ *Jacinto A. Hernandez,* MD, MHA

A birth injury refers to any injury resulting from the natural processes of labor and delivery or from any iatrogenic processes used to aid in delivery. Birth injuries are subdivided into those due to hypoxia and those due to mechanical factors or birth traumas. Predisposing factors for birth injury include precipitous labor, fetal macrosomia, prematurity, cephalopelvic disproportion, abnormal presentation, forceps and vacuum extractions, and shoulder dystocia.

EPIDEMIOLOGY

The true incidence of birth injuries is uncertain, but estimates range from 1 to 7.2 per 1000 live births. The overall incidence has decreased over the past two decades, and obvious trauma resulting from labor and delivery is rare. However, birth injuries continue to occur and represent an important problem for the clinician (Perlow, Wigton, and Hart, 1996).

SIGNIFICANCE

Many birth injuries are self-limited and require no special treatment. However, some have the potential for permanent sequelae (mortality and morbidity) in the neonate. The clinician should be able to recognize the most frequent types of birth injuries and be able to provide necessary treatment and support.

PRESENTATION

Birth injuries are frequently noted during the newborn's initial physical examination (Taeusch and Sniderman, 1998). An injury may be recognized as a skin lesion (abrasion, laceration, or ecchymosis) or may be noted by lack of movement of the extremities or face. An injured newborn may experience obvious pain upon palpation of a fractured bone. Other signs and symptoms suggestive of a birth trauma may include unexplained pallor, anemia, shock, or generalized hypotonia.

COMMON BIRTH INJURIES

    A. Head and Facial Traumas (King and Boothroyd, 1998; Medlock and Hanigan, 1997).

        1. Cephalhematoma (Figure 6-1)

            a. Cephalhematoma is the most frequent type of cranial injury in neonates. It occurs in up to 2.5% of all live births and is associated with forceps delivery and vacuum extraction.

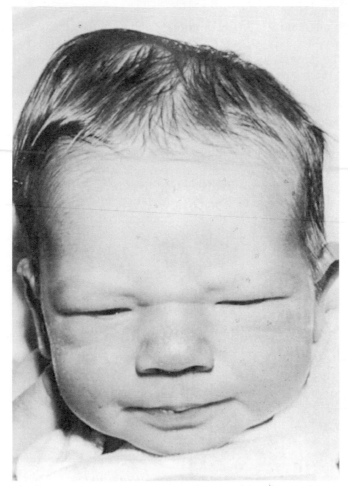

FIGURE 6-1 ● Cephalhematoma: also milia on the nose. (From Beischer NA, Mackey EV, Colditz PB: *Obstetrics and the newborn,* ed 3, Philadelphia, 1997, WB Saunders, p 602.)

b. Disruption of the superficial communicating veins under the periosteum leads to hemorrhage and subsequent swelling. Suture lines confine the cephalhematoma and therefore limit the extent of the bleeding.

c. Clinically, the infant presents with swelling over the site within the first few hours to the first few days of life. The site may feel soft and fluctuant initially, becoming tense as the cephalhematoma resolves.

d. An underlying linear skull fracture may be present in 10%–25% of cephalhematomas.

e. Prognosis is good, with most of the lesions reabsorbing between 2 weeks to 3 months.

2. Skull fracture

   a. Skull fracture is an uncommon birth injury. The fracture usually presents as either a depressed fracture or a linear fracture (Figures 6-2 and 6-3). The parietal and frontal bones are most often involved. Skull fracture is often a result of forceps use during delivery.

   b. A depressed fracture is the most common type of skull fracture. This fracture is associated with intracranial bleeding; therefore, a head CT is indicated to evaluate the extension of the fracture. If the head CT is otherwise negative and the infant is asymptomatic, only expectant management is recommended. A depressed fracture usually improves spontaneously over several weeks. However, if an infant has any neurologic symptoms in the setting of a depressed skull fracture, a neurosurgeon should be consulted (Loeser, 1976).

   c. Linear fracture is usually asymptomatic with a good prognosis. However, a leptomeningeal cyst may develop within the fracture and become a focus of seizure activity.

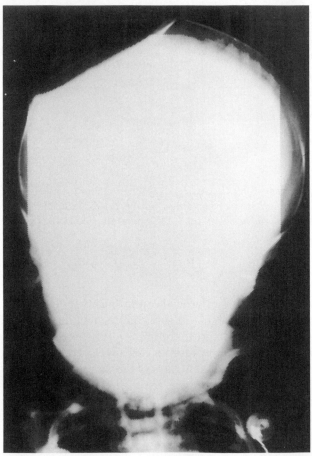

FIGURE 6-2 ● Depressed skull fracture. (Courtesy Jacinto Hernandez.)

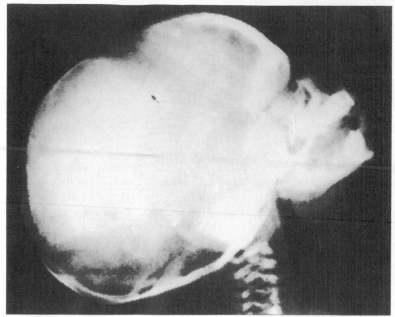

FIGURE 6-3 ● Linear skull fracture. (Courtesy Jacinto Hernandez.)

3. Nasal trauma (Jablon and Hoffman, 1997; Jeppesen, 1972).
   a. A fracture of the nose may lead to early respiratory distress and feeding difficulties in the newborn. It requires immediate attention by an otolaryngologist or plastic surgeon.
   b. Transient flattening of the nose has been described in 30%–60% of all newborn infants.
   c. Some form of nasal septal deformities are seen in 0.9%–4% of neonates. The most significant factor causing septal dislocation is intrauterine pressure stress and strain.
   d. By manipulating the tip of the nose, the clinician is able to differentiate between a septal dislocation and transient nasal flattening (Figure 6-4). If the septum can be returned to midline, the diagnosis is most likely nasal flattening.
   e. If a true septal dislocation exists, the septum needs to be corrected by the third day of life by an otolaryngologist to prevent permanent disfiguration.

B. **Fractures**
   1. Clavicle fracture
      a. Fracture of the clavicle is the most frequent type of birth injury (Color Plate 20). The incidence is 4.5 per 1000 live births. Most clavicle fractures are greenstick-type fractures.
      b. The injury is due to compression of the shoulder or manipulation of the ipsilateral arm during delivery.

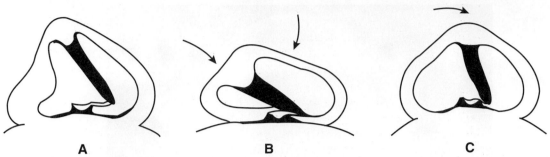

A   **B**   **C**

FIGURE 6-4 ● Diagram of basal view of nose. **A,** Dislocation of triangular cartilage of the nasal septum. **B,** Compression test showing further evidence of dislocation of triangular cartilage. **C,** Return of nasal septum to midline and failure of cartilage to relocate. (From Silverman, Leibow, Sheldon: Dislocation of the triangular cartilage of the nasal septum, *J Pediatr* Sept:458, 1975.)

      c. During physical examination, the clinician may feel crepitus upon palpation of the clavicle. Affected newborns may be asymptomatic, or they may cry with manipulation of the arm. On examination the affected infant may exhibit an asymmetric Moro reflex and have limited use of the arm.

      d. For comfort, the arm and shoulder may be immobilized by pinning the infant's T-shirt in a natural position across the chest for approximately 2 weeks.

      e. Clavicular fracture is not related to permanent sequelae; it heals without treatment. Parents should be told to expect a small bump over the fracture as a callus forms at approximately 7 to 10 days of life.

      f. Clavicular fracture must be distinguished from a condition known as congenital pseudoarthrosis. If there is no history of a difficult delivery and the lesion occurs on the right side, congenital pseudoarthrosis is the likely diagnosis. Congenital pseudoarthrosis of the clavicle is usually painless. Surgical correction of these lesions may be an option for affected infants.

    2. Fracture of the humerus

      a. The humerus is the second most common bone fractured during birth. The fracture is most often a greenstick type of fracture, although complete fractures can occur.

      b. Clinically, the infant has immobility of the affected arm, along with tenderness and crepitus on palpation. The Moro reflex is absent on the affected side.

      c. Prognosis is good. Treatment consists of immobilization, with the arm in adduction for approximately 2 to 4 weeks.

C. Nerve Injuries

    1. Etiology

      a. Most nerve injuries occur as a result of shoulder dystocia. Shoulder dystocia occurs in 0.15%–3.0% of all deliveries when the fetal shoulders become impacted at the pelvic inlet and the descent of the fetus is halted. Subsequent nerve injury is caused by the downward lateral traction of the head and neck away from the shoulder (Gherman, 2002).

   b. Risk factors for shoulder dystocia include maternal obesity, maternal diabetes, post-term pregnancy, prolonged second stage of labor, and fetal macrosomia. Most cases occur in infants greater than 3500 g.

2. Brachial plexus injuries (Bennet, 1976; Wilson and Kenyon, 2002).

   a. Paralysis occurs as a result of nerve compression from either hemorrhage or edema. Permanent paralysis can occur from tearing of the nerve or avulsion of the nerve root from the spinal cord.

   b. Clinical types (Jennett, Tarby, and Krauss, 2002; Sandmire and DeMott, 2002).

   (1) Duchenne-Erb upper brachial palsy, also referred to as Duchenne palsy or Erb palsy (C5–C6), is the most common type of brachial plexus injury, accounting for 70%–80% of plexus injuries. Clinically, the infant has no motion of the ipsilateral shoulder. The involved arm is adducted, prone, and internally rotated (Color Plate 43). Additional involvement of the seventh cervical root (C7) leads to weakness of the wrist extensors and contraction of the flexors, giving the characteristic "waiter's tip" position of the hand. Hand muscles are intact and there is no sensory deficit.

   (2) Klumpke palsy (C8–T1) is rare, accounting for <5% of brachial plexus injuries. These infants present with weakness of the wrist flexors, lack of wrist movement, and paralysis of the hand muscles. In addition, Horner syndrome (eyelid ptosis, miosis, and enophtalmos) may be present if the lesion involves the sympathetic nervous system.

   (3) Entire arm paralysis (C5–T1) occurs in 20%–25% of plexus injuries.

   c. Treatment for brachial plexus injuries is supportive and consists of exercises and splinting of the arm. Pinning the T-shirt sleeve across the chest is a good method for splinting the arm in the appropriate position.

   d. Prognosis is related to the severity of the injury and is better for upper arm paralysis. The faster the recovery of the injury, the more complete the functional return. Of affected infants, 80% recover by 4 months and 93% recover by 18–24 months. Permanent lesions are associated with muscle atrophy, contractures, and poor limb growth.

   e. Follow-up with a rehabilitation specialist or a neurologist should occur within 6 weeks if symptoms persist. If the infant continues to have paralysis at 3 months of age, nerve conduction studies should be performed.

3. Phrenic nerve palsy

   a. Phrenic nerve paralysis occurs as a result of the overstretching of nerve roots C3–C5 by lateral hyperextension of the neck during a breech birth or other difficult delivery.

   b. Most cases are associated with an ipsilateral Erb palsy. Only 25% of phrenic nerve palsies are isolated cases.

      c. Clinically, the infant presents with respiratory distress within the first month of life. The chest radiograph typically reveals an elevated diaphragm. Fluoroscopy of the diaphragm shows paradoxical movement.

      d. If the infant is asymptomatic, it is recommended that he or she be followed for 4 to 6 months to see whether there is recovery before any surgical procedure is performed. If the infant is symptomatic (e.g., pneumonia, atelectasis), surgical plication of the involved diaphragm is recommended within 2 to 3 weeks.

   4. Facial palsy

      a. Facial palsy is caused either by direct pressure over the seventh cranial nerve by the sacral promontory during the delivery or by forceps application.

      b. The incidence of facial palsy is approximately 0.6 per 1000 live births.

      c. The infant presents with loss of movement of the facial muscles on the affected side (Color Plate 19).

      d. The palsy is usually self-limited but may be associated with lifelong disabilities.

      e. Liquid tears are recommended to prevent drying of the eyes.

D. Ocular Trauma

   1. Multiple types of eye trauma may be associated with delivery, especially with forceps-assisted deliveries. Trauma to the eye may include eyelid edema, retinal hemorrhages, intraorbital hemorrhages (traumatic hyphema), corneal opacifications (a break in Descemet membrane), and fractures at the base of the orbit. Among these, a break in Descemet membrane is the most severe. Injuries to this membrane require immediate consultation by an ophthalmologist, because they can result in permanent visual loss.

E. Subgaleal Hemorrhage (Cavlovich, 1995).

   1. The subgaleal (subaponeurotic) space is located between the periosteum and the galea aponeurotica. This space extends from the orbital ridges to the nape of the neck and laterally to the ears. A subgaleal hemorrhage is rare; however, it is a potentially fatal complication in the newborn (Figure 6-5).

   2. The incidence is 4 in 10,000 deliveries, but it may be higher in centers where vacuum extraction is used. Mortality associated with subgaleal hemorrhage is approximately 20%–25%.

   3. The bleeding associated with subgaleal hemorrhages can be extensive. Bleeding is caused by damage to the large emissary veins located in the subaponeurotic layer.

   4. The subgaleal space is very large and can accommodate up to approximately 260 mL of blood (more than a newborn's total blood volume).

   5. Most subgaleal hemorrhages are diagnosed during the first 24 hours, with many diagnosed within the first 4 hours of life.

   6. Clinically, the infant may present with pallor and hypotonicity, followed by tachycardia, tachypnea, and hypotension. The scalp appears tight and boggy. Many of the infants progress to hypovolemic shock.

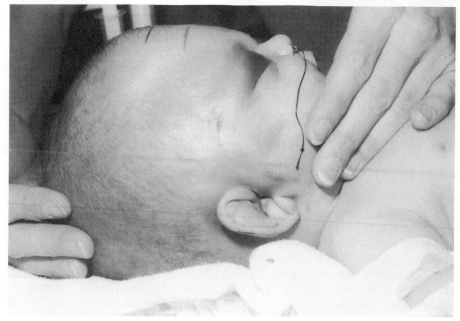

FIGURE 6-5 ● Subgaleal hemorrhage. (Courtesy Jacinto Hernandez.)

7. Frequent measurements of head circumference, hematocrit level, blood pressure, and platelet count should follow. A head CT scan can help to determine the extent of the injury.

8. Treatment consists of following lab values and transfusing blood products as needed.

F. **Soft Tissue Injuries**

1. Subcutaneous fat necrosis (Burden and Krafchik, 1999).

   a. Subcutaneous fat necrosis can present as demarcated, subcutaneous nodules on the extremities, face, trunk, or buttocks within the first few weeks of life.

   b. Etiologies may include a defect in subcutaneous fat, birth hypoxia, local trauma, hypothermia, maternal gestational diabetes, preeclampsia, or maternal ingestion of calcium antagonists.

   c. The nodules or lesions may persist for several weeks to months.

   d. No treatment is necessary; however, some cases have been associated with hypercalcemia.

2. Lacerations

   a. Forceps may cause small lacerations on the face. If the lacerations are of full thickness, they should be approximated with either adhesive strips or 6-0 nylon sutures.

REFERENCES

Altemus LA, Ferguson AD: The incidence of birth injury, *J National Med Assoc* 58:333, 1966.

Bennet GC: Prognosis and early management of birth injuries to the brachial plexus, *Brit Med J* 1:1520-1521, 1976.

Bhalla M: Birth injuries in the newborn, *Indian J Pediatr* 43:297-305, 1976.

Burden AD, Krafchik BR: Subcutaneous fat necrosis of the newborn: a review of 11 cases, *Pediatr Dermatol* 16:384-387, 1999.

Carlan SJ, Angel JL, Knuppel RA: Shoulder dystocia, *AFP* 43:1307-1311, 1991.

Cavlovich FE: Subgaleal hemorrhage in the neonate, *JOGNN* 24:397-404, 1995.

Gei AF, Belfort MA: Forceps-assisted vaginal delivery, *Obstetr Gynecol Clin North Am* 26:345-370, 1999.

Gherman RB: Shoulder dystocia: an evidence-based evaluation of the obstetric nightmare, *Clin Obstetr Gynecol* 45:345-362, 2002.

Jablon MJH, Hoffman JF: Birth trauma causing nasal vestibular stenosis, *Arch Otolaryngol Head Neck Surg* 123:1004-1006, 1997.

Jennett RJ, Tarby TJ, Krauss RL: Erb's palsy contrasted with Klumpke's and total palsy: different mechanisms are involved, *Am J Obstet Gynecol* 186:1216-1220, 2002.

Jeppesen F: Dislocation of the nasal septal cartilage in the newborn, *Arch Obstet Gynecol Scand* 51:5, 1972.

King SJ, Boothroyd AE: Cranial trauma following birth in term infants, *Brit J Radiol* 71:233-238, 1998.

Loeser JD: Management of depressed skull fracture in the newborn, *J Neurosurg* 44:62-66, 1976.

Medlock MD, Hanigan WC: Neurologic birth trauma: intracranial, spinal cord, and brachial plexus injury, *Clin Perinatol* 24:845-857, 1997.

Nakahara T, Sakoda K, Uozumi T, et al: Intrauterine depressed skull fracture, *Pediatr Neurosci* 15:121-124, 1989.

Perlow JH, Wigton T, Hart, et al: Birth trauma: a five-year review of incidence and associated perinatal factors, *J Reproduct Med* 41:754-760, 1996.

Sandmire HF, DeMott RK: Erb's palsy causation: a historical perspective, *Birth* 29:52-54, 2002.

Schullinger JN: Birth trauma, *Pediatr Surg* 40:1351-1358, 1993.

Taeusch HW, Sniderman S: Initial evaluation, history, and physical examination of the newborn. In Taeusch HW, Ballard RA, editors: *Avery's diseases of the newborn,* ed 7, Philadelphia, 1998, WB Saunders, p 342.

Wilson P, Kenyon P: Congenital brachial plexus lesions, *Newsletter Child Hosp Physical Med Rehab* 6, 2002.

7 Physical Assessment of the Newborn

Jacinto A. Hernandez, MD, MHA ■ *Sharon M. Glass*, RNC, MS, NNP

Early recognition of existing or potential problems is important to initiate appropriate treatment as soon as possible. A comprehensive physical assessment must be performed on every newborn infant. Information collected can be reassuring to the newborn's family or can identify problems that must be treated. This chapter discusses a systematic approach to conducting a physical examination and reviews the clinical estimation of gestational age.

PHYSICAL EXAMINATION OF THE NEWBORN

The initial physical examination of the newborn should be done in the delivery room to detect significant anomalies, birth injuries, and cardiorespiratory disorders that may compromise a successful adaptation to extrauterine life. A more detailed examination should then take place in the nursery before the infant's status is discussed with the parents. This examination should take place within 12 to 18 hours after birth. Ideally, a final physical should be performed within 24 hours of discharge, preferably in the presence of the parents. However, in this era of early hospital discharge after delivery, many infants undergo only one complete physical examination before leaving the hospital (Phibbs, 1991; Rosenberg, 1997).

 The newborn examination must be carried out in a comfortable environment (i.e., thermoneutral temperature, good light, minimal noise). General inspection and observation of activity and skin color should be made first, without disturbing the sleeping or quiet infant. Next, listen to the heart and lungs while the infant is still peaceful; then finally move to a more thorough and "careful" examination of the body parts and organs.

   A. **Skin**
    1. General appearance: The skin should be soft, smooth, and opaque. Vernix caseosa is a whitish, greasy material that covers the body after 35 weeks gestation, decreasing in quantity as it is shed into amniotic fluid with increasing gestational age (Color Plate 1). Discolored vernix occurs with hemolytic disease and meconium staining as a result of in utero fetal distress. The skin of a post-term infant may be dry and peeling. The skin should be warm to touch after the infant has been warmed postpartum. Petechiae seen over the head and neck or above the nipple line may be secondary to pressure from a nuchal cord or from the delivery process.

2. Color

    a. Plethora (deep rosy red color; Color Plate 2): Plethora is more common in infants with polycythemia but may also be seen in overoxygenated or overheated infants. It is best to obtain a venous hematocrit for plethoric infants (see Chapter 15).

    b. Jaundice (yellow color): With obvious jaundice, bilirubin levels in the blood are usually higher than 5 mg/dL. This is abnormal in infants under 24 hours of age and may signify blood group incompatibility or infection (see Chapter 14).

    c. Pallor (washed-out, pale white appearance): May be secondary to anemia, birth asphyxia, or shock (see Chapter 15).

    d. Cyanosis (blue or dusky appearance of the skin):

        (1) Usually perceived clinically when O_2 saturation is reduced to less than 85%.

        (2) Often, the most difficult task in dealing with cyanotic neonates is recognizing that cyanosis exists.

        (3) Infants suspected of being cyanotic are best observed when they are quiet or sleeping in a thermoneutral environment under a white light (preferably daylight).

        (4) The clinical presentation of cyanosis is best detected during examination of the tongue, oral and buccal mucosa, and peripheral skin.

           (a) Peripheral cyanosis, a blue discoloration or duskiness confined to the skin of the extremities, is usually ascribed to "vasomotor instability" (acrocyanosis). It is frequently seen in normal infants but may be due to cold environment, a high hematocrit, or local obstruction. It may persist for days or weeks.

           (b) Central cyanosis, a blue discoloration of the mucous membranes and periphery due to the presence of 3 g/dL or more of reduced hemoglobin in arterial blood. It may indicate a pathologic condition; persistent central cyanosis always requires immediate evaluation.

        (5) Since the causes of cyanosis may vary from trivial to life-threatening, the differential diagnosis should be approached in a systematic fashion.

    e. Extensive bruising is usually associated with traumatic delivery and may result in early jaundice.

3. Transient cutaneous lesions

    a. Milia (Figure 7-1; also see Figure 6-1): Approximately 40% of full-term infants have multiple yellow or pearly white 1-mm papules (pinhead-sized). They are usually scattered on the chin, nose, forehead, and cheeks. They are benign, represent tiny epidermal cysts in connection with a sebaceous follicle, and disappear within a few weeks.

    b. Sebaceous gland hyperplasia: Tiny white or yellow lesions visible at the opening of each pilosebaceous follicle. They are more prominent on the nose, upper lip, and over the malar regions. They likely represent

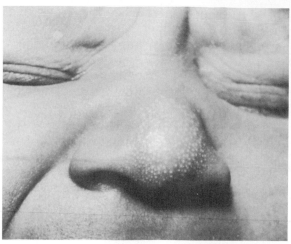

FIGURE 7-1 ● Milia (vernix-filled sebaceous glands). (From Beischer NA, Mackey EV, Colditz PB: *Obstetrics and the newborn,* ed 3, Philadelphia, 1997, WB Saunders, p 599.)

hyperplastic sebaceous glands. They spontaneously diminish in size after birth and are no longer visible after the first weeks of life.

c. Erythema toxicum (Color Plate 3, *A* and *B*): Numerous small areas of red skin with a yellowish white papule in the center. They are most noticeable at 48 hours but can appear as late as 7 to 10 days. Wright staining of the papule reveals eosinophils. The rash resolves spontaneously within 4 to 5 days after appearance. It may be confused with *Candida* dermatitis (Color Plate 3, *C*), miliaria rubra, and pustular melanosis.

d. Mongolian spot (Color Plate 4): Dark blue or purple macular spots resembling bruises, usually located over the lumbosacral area. Present in 90% of African-American, Native American, and Asian infants; 85% of Hispanics; and 5%–10% of Caucasians. They usually fade during late infancy or at least by 4 years of age but may persist to adulthood.

e. Macular hemangioma (also referred to as telangiectatic nevus, nevus flammeus, "salmon patch," or "stork bite"; Color Plate 5): A true vascular nevus normally seen on the occipital area, eyelids, and glabella (forehead area over the eyebrows). The lesions disappear spontaneously within the first year of life except those on the nape of the neck, many of which persist. The most common type of birthmark, macular hemangioma occurs in 60%–70% of all infants.

f. Harlequin phenomenon (Color Plate 6): A clear line of demarcation with an area of redness and an area of paleness. The cause of harlequin coloration is usually unknown; it is most likely due to vasomotor instability. The condition may be benign and transient or may indicate that shunting of blood is occurring, as in sepsis or persistent pulmonary hypertension of the newborn. There may be varying degrees of redness and perfusion. The line of demarcation may run from the head to the abdomen, dividing the body into left and right halves.

g. Cutis marmorata (lacy red pattern): May be seen in a normal infant or one with cold stress, hypovolemia, or sepsis. Persistent mottling is seen in infants with a variety of chromosomal abnormalities.

h. Miliaria

    (1) Transient lesions that commonly occur in a warm environment as the result of obstruction of the sweat gland ducts. Can be confused with candida dermatitis and erythema toxicum. There are two principal types:

        (a) Miliaria crystallinia: Clear, superficial tiny vesicles without inflammation (Color Plate 8).

        (b) Miliaria rubra: Small, erythematous, grouped papules on a red base.

    (2) Sites of predilection are the intertriginous areas, face, and scalp. Rapid resolution occurs following removal to a cooler environment.

i. Petechiae (Color Plate 9): Small pinpoint hemorrhagic skin lesions frequently seen on the presenting part and on the face if there is a history of a nuchal cord. Petechiae occurring on the torso are more likely to be associated with thrombocytopenia or congenital infection.

j. Pustular melanosis (Color Plate 10, *B*): Transient condition of unknown cause; characterized by pustules, vesicles, and hyperpigmented macules, presenting individually or in combination, singly or in clusters, at birth. New lesions do not occur, but the existing pustules or vesicles may form a brownish crust or rupture, producing a fine white scale around the lesion. Vesicles and pustules usually resolve in several days, whereas pigmented macules may take weeks to months to disappear. There is no associated erythema, which distinguishes it from erythema toxicum. Pustular melanosis rarely affects the hands and feet.

4. Birthmarks: Very common, occurring in >99% of neonates. Most are classified as hamartomas, which are collections of cells of one or more elements of normal skin. For example, salmon patches and port wine stains are vascular birthmarks. Salmon patches and Mongolian spots (see descriptions under "Transient cutaneous lesions" above) are 100 times more common than all other birthmarks.

a. Port wine stain (nevus flammeus): Deep red or purple in color, port wine stains are usually present at birth, blanch only minimally with pressure, and do not disappear with time. If the lesion appears over the forehead and upper eyelid (distribution of the first branch of the trigeminal nerve), Sturge-Weber syndrome (associated with glaucoma, seizures, and mental retardation) must be ruled out. Other syndromes can be associated with port wine stains. Can be treated with laser therapy.

b. Hemangioma: Many hemangiomas are not visible at birth, but 90% are present by 1 month of age. Proliferation occurs for 6 to 8 months, but involution may take years (50% at 5 years, 90% by 9 years).

Periocular lesions require ophthalmologic consultation and aggressive treatment. Lumbosacral lesions may indicate underlying tethered cord. Large facial lesions may be associated with Dandy-Walker syndrome. 80% of lesions involve spontaneously. When therapy is required, systemic steroid and laser treatment are the most common.

(1) Cavernous hemangioma: Usually appears as a large, red, firm, ill-defined mass resembling a cyst, located anywhere on the body.

(2) Strawberry hemangioma (Figure 7-2): Usually appears within a few days of birth as a raised pink or red macule that is sharply demarcated and most commonly found on the face. They enlarge during the first 5 to 6 months, blanching incompletely with pressure, and usually regressing spontaneously (70% by 7 years of age).

B. Cardiorespiratory System

1. Heart

   a. Check heart rate. Normal rate is 100–180 beats/minute (usually 120–160 when awake).

   b. Note PMI (point of maximum cardiac impulse).

   c. Listen for murmurs.

   (1) Ventricular septal defect: The most common heart defect, accounting for 25% of cases of congenital heart disease. Typically, a loud, harsh,

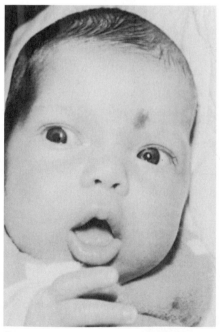
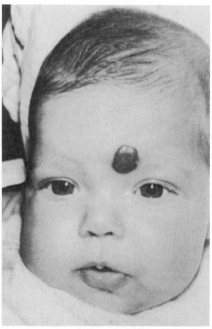

A   B

FIGURE 7-2 ● Strawberry nevus. **A,** Appearance 4 days after birth. **B,** Appearance 6 weeks later. (From Beischer NA, Mackey EV, Colditz PB: *Obstetrics and the newborn,* ed 3, Philadelphia, 1997, WB Saunders, p 599.)

blowing pansystolic murmur, best heard over the lower left sternal border, usually on the second or third day of life.

(2) Patent ductus arteriosus: A harsh, continuous, machinery-type or "rolling thunder" murmur that is localized to the second left intercostal space. It may radiate to the left clavicle or down the left sternal border. It usually presents on the second or third day of life. A hyperactive precordium, bounding pulses, and wide pulse pressure may be found.

(3) Coarctation of the aorta: A systolic ejection murmur that radiates down the sternum to the apex and also to the interscapular area. It is often heard loudest in the back. May also detect diminished to absent femoral pulses.

(4) Peripheral pulmonic stenosis: A systolic murmur is heard bilaterally in both axillae and across the back. It is secondary to turbulence caused by blood flow from the main pulmonary arteries to the peripheral pulmonary arteries, which are smaller than usual. This murmur is benign, although it may persist until 3 months of age.

(5) Hypoplastic left heart syndrome: A short midsystolic murmur can be heard beginning on day 1 or 2. A gallop is usually heard.

d. Palpate the pulses (femoral, pedal, radial, and brachial) and assess capillary refill.

(1) Femoral pulses should be felt for, but they are often only fair in the first day or two of life. If still questionable by discharge, check the blood pressure in the legs.

(2) Bounding pulses can be seen with patent ductus arteriosus.

(3) Absent or delayed femoral pulses are associated with coarctation of the aorta.

(4) Check the capillary refill time by pressing one finger against the sole of the infant's foot or the palm of the hand for 1 second. Return of pink color normally takes 2 seconds. Refill of 2 or 3 seconds is considered delayed refill; longer than 3 seconds should be investigated.

e. Check for signs of congestive heart failure, which may include hepatomegaly, gallop, tachypnea, wheezes and rales, tachycardia, abnormal pulses, and diaphoresis with feeding.

2. Chest and lungs

a. Check respiratory rate. Normal rate in the newborn is 30–60/min.

b. The chest should be round and symmetric and wider than its anterior-posterior dimension. The chest circumference is normally 1 to 2 cm smaller than the infant's occipital-frontal circumference (OFC).

c. It is normal for infants' abdomens to rise and fall as they breathe, because they use their diaphragm more than their intercostal muscles.

d. Breathing pattern

(1) Most newborn infants breathe irregularly and at varying depths. Respirations are periodic (i.e., episodes of 5–10 seconds without breathing) rather than regular, particularly if the infant is premature.

(2) *Apnea* refers to a cessation of breathing >20 seconds in duration, during which an infant's color changes from normal to cyanotic. This is abnormal and requires investigation and treatment.

e. Asymmetry of the chest may signify a tension pneumothorax, skeletal disorders, diaphragmatic hernia, overdistended lobes of the lung, intrathoracic masses, or simply compression by the infant's own arm in utero.

f. Respiratory distress may be evidenced by tachypnea, intercostal retractions, grunting on expiration, cyanosis, and flaring nostrils.

g. Pectus excavatum is a congenital structural depression of the sternum and is usually of no clinical concern.

h. Breasts in both male and female newborns may be enlarged secondary to the effects of maternal estrogen (Color Plate 11). The breast may also secrete a milk-like substance (also known as "witch's milk"); although unusual, this is a normal finding (Figure 7-3), lasts only 1 to 2 weeks, and is of no clinical concern.

i. Widespread nipples occur if the distance between the nipples is greater than 25% of the chest circumference. This finding may be associated with congenital disorders such as Turner syndrome.

j. Supernumerary nipples: Raised, pigmented areas found vertical and medial to the true nipple; these require no treatment and often gradually become imperceptible. Several studies have demonstrated a weak correlation with renal anomalies in Caucasian populations.

C. **Head**: Assess the size, shape, symmetry, and general appearance relative to the rest of the body and face; include distribution and character of the hair and

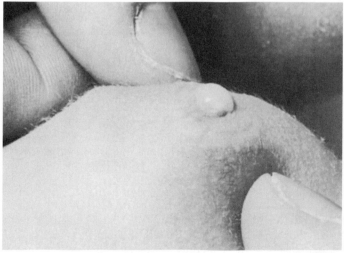

FIGURE 7-3 ● Witch's milk. (From Beischer NA, Mackey EV, Colditz PB: *Obstetrics and the newborn*, ed 3, Philadelphia, 1997, WB Saunders, p 599.)

the underlying scalp. For most term infants, the occipital-frontal circumference (OFC) is 32–36 cm and is usually 2 cm larger than the newborn's chest. Any departure more than 2 standard deviations above or below these normal values should be investigated (microcephaly, anencephaly, hydrocephalus, etc).

1. Sutures (Figure 7-4): Strong, flexible fibrous tissue connecting the five major bones of the skull. These include the coronal, lamboidal, sagittal, and frontal (or metopic) sutures.
2. Fontanelles (see Figure 7-4).
   a. Anterior: Located at the junction of the sagittal and coronal sutures, diamond-shaped, and measuring from 4 to 6 cm at the largest diameter. The size of the fontanelles varies widely. Large fontanelles may be seen with hypothyroidism, hydrocephaly, in utero malnutrition, rickets, and some genetic disorders. A bulging or tense anterior fontanelle may be associated with hydrocephalus, birth injury, intracranial bleeding, infection, or a late sign of increased intracranial pressure.
   b. Posterior: Located at the junction of the lambdoid and sagittal sutures; usually triangular-shaped and barely admits a fingertip.
   c. A third fontanelle may be located between the anterior and posterior fontanelles; varies in size and may be associated with congenital anomalies.
   d. A depressed fontanelle is a late sign of dehydration.

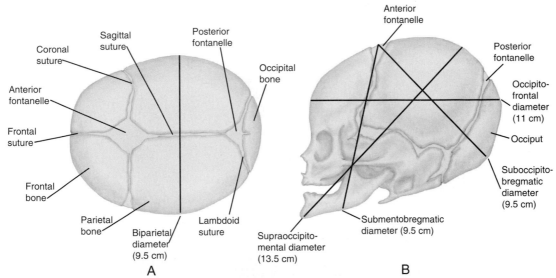

FIGURE 7-4 ● **A,** Bones, sutures, and fontanelles of the fetal head. Note that the anterior fontanelle has a diamond shape, whereas the posterior fontanelle is triangular. **B,** Lateral view of the fetal head, demonstrating how anterior-posterior diameters vary with the amount of flexion or extension. (From Gorrie T, McKinney E, Murray S: *Foundations of maternal newborn nursing,* ed 2, Philadelphia, 1998, WB Saunders, p 276.)

3. Molding (Color Plate 12): A temporary asymmetry of the skull resulting from the birth process; most often seen with prolonged labor. It is more common with vaginal delivery, although it may occur in C-section delivery if labor is prolonged. The head of a newborn delivered in the breech position may be flat on top with an increased anterior-posterior measurement (Color Plate 13).

4. Caput succedaneum (Figure 7-5): A diffuse edematous swelling of the soft tissues of the scalp, which may extend across suture lines. It is secondary to pressure of the uterus or vaginal wall on areas of the fetal head bordering the caput, and usually resolves within several days.

5. Cephalhematoma (see Figures 7-5 and 6-1). A subperiosteal hemorrhage that never extends across a suture line; usually resulting from a traumatic or forceps delivery. Skull films should be obtained if an underlying skull fracture is suspected (approximately 5%–10% of cephalhematomas). In large hematomas, the hematocrit and bilirubin levels should be followed in these infants. Most cephalhematomas resolve within 6 weeks to several months.

6. Craniosynostosis: A premature closure of one or more sutures of the skull; it should be considered in an infant with an asymmetric skull where the mobility of the sutures seems restricted. On palpation of the skull, a bony

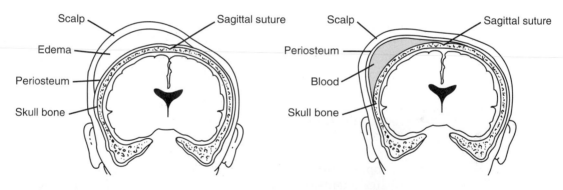

UNDERSTANDING THE DIFFERENCES

CAPUT SUCCEDANEUM
- Condition marked by localized soft tissue edema with poorly defined outline
- Caused by pressure of the fetal head against the cervix during labor, which decreases blood flow to the area and results in edema
- Present at birth; does not increase in size
- Swelling crosses suture lines
- Disappears after birth within a few hours to several days
- Complications are rare

CEPHALHEMATOMA
- Condition marked by soft, fluctuant, localized swelling with well-defined outline
- Caused by subperiosteal hemorrhage
- Appears after birth; increases in size for 2–3 days
- Swelling does not cross suture lines
- Disappears from several weeks to even months after birth
- Complications include defective blood clotting, underlying skull fracture or intracranial bleeding, jaundice

FIGURE 7-5 ● Characteristics of caput succedaneum and cephalhematoma. (From Nichols FM, Zwelling E: *Maternal-newborn nursing: theory and practice*, Philadelphia, 1997, WB Saunders, p 1105.)

ridge may be felt over the suture line, and it may not be possible to move the cranial bones freely. Mobility of the sutures is checked by putting each thumb on opposite sides of a suture and pushing in alternately while feeling for motion.

7. Craniotabes: An occasional finding; a soft "ping-pong ball" effect of the skull bones (usually the parietal bones). It is most commonly found in dysmature infants. If physiologic, it will disappear within a few weeks. Pathologic craniotabes occur with syphilis and rickets.

8. Subgaleal hematoma: A bleeding that may feel crepitant, with less pitting than the edema of caput succedaneum. Because there is little anatomic restriction to subgaleal fluid accumulation, large volumes may redistribute and deplete total body volume. Monitor blood pressure and hematocrit for signs of bleeding or shock. May require emergency transfusion. Observe for hyperbilirubinemia.

   a. Auscultate: Listen for bruits over the temporal arteries and anterior fontanelle if there is reason to suspect conditions involving high-output cardiac failure or neuropathology.

9. Scalp

   a. Observe for abrasions or lacerations, which may have occurred during delivery or from an internal monitor probe.

   b. Observe for cutis aplasia, which is a localized congenital absence of skin. Lesions may be solitary or multiple and are located just lateral to the midline.

   c. Inspect hair for color, texture, distribution, and directional patterns.

      (1) Hair color may change, but there should be racial concordance; reddish or blond hair in a dark-skinned race baby may indicate albinism. Hair color should be fairly uniform; random patches of white hair are familial, but white forelocks with other pigment defects and anomalies are sometimes associated with deafness and retardation (i.e., Waardenburg syndrome).

      (2) The hairline may vary at the frontal margin. Normal but hirsute infants may have hair well down the forehead (Figure 7-6). Synophrys (fusion of the eyebrows in the midline) is common in hirsute infants but may also be associated with Cornelia de Lange syndrome. The posterior hairline has a more consistent limitation, and hair roots below the neck creases (beyond lower pole of ear lobes), particularly at the lateral margins, suggest syndromes associated with short or webbed necks.

      (3) Growth direction of hair is normally consistent with a single parietal hair whorl just off center, usually 1–2 cm anterior to the posterior fontanelle and most commonly on the left (56%). If there is more than one whorl, if it is midline, or if it is posterior to the posterior fontanelle, there may be abnormal development of the underlying brain (Smith and Gong, 1973).

      (4) If there is extremely unruly hair, particularly if associated with unusual facies, microcephaly, or SGA status, there may be poor

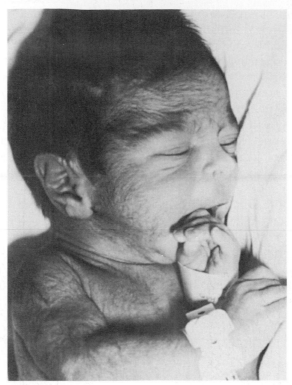

FIGURE 7-6 ● Hirsute infant. (From Beischer NA, Mackey EV, Colditz PB: *Obstetrics and the newborn*, ed 3, Philadelphia, 1997, WB Saunders, p 600.)

brain growth of early fetal onset. This is typical of a number of genetic disorders, including Cornelia de Lange syndrome and Down syndrome.

D. **Face:** Look for obvious abnormalities, noting symmetry, size, shape, and location of eyes, ears, nose, mouth, and chin, as well as how the infant holds or uses them. The face can be divided into thirds, with one third encompassing the forehead, one third the eyes and nose, and one third the mouth and chin. An unusual appearance requires an analysis of the individual components of the facies to determine whether the constellation represents malformation (structural abnormality), deformation (abnormality caused by mechanical forces such as pressure in a structure in utero), a syndrome (recognized pattern of malformations with a single and specific etiology), or merely a familial likeness.

   1. Eyes

      a. Examination technique: The eyes may be edematous for several days following delivery, making the initial examination difficult. In subdued light, while sucking on a pacifier or being held vertically, most infants will open their eyes, making them easier to examine for general appearance.

b. Sclera: Normally white, although the thinner sclera of a premature infant may appear bluish. If the sclera is deep blue, osteogenesis imperfecta should be ruled out.

c. Subconjunctival hemorrhage (Color Plate 14): Rupture of small conjunctival capillaries, which can occur normally (5% of newborns) but is more common following traumatic delivery. The hemorrhages usually clear within a few days.

d. Mongoloid slanting (upward slant of the outer edge of the eye) and antimongoloid slanting (downward slant of the outer edge of the eye): Mongoloid slant may be indicative of trisomy 21 (Box 7-1 provides details about Down syndrome). Both types of slant may be seen in a number of syndromes.

e. Epicanthal fold (skin fold over the medial aspect of the eye): May be familial but occurs in <1% of the population. Seen in Down syndrome and other syndromes.

f. Hypertelorism (widely separated eyes) and hypotelorism (narrowly separated eyes): This diagnosis should be based on the measurement of the inner canthal distance (Figure 7-7). The inner canthal angles are

---

● BOX 7-1
DOWN SYNDROME

Diagnosis

Usually diagnosed prenatally by triad screening (low maternal serum alpha-fetoprotein and estriol levels, high human chorionic gonadotropin levels) with targeted ultrasound or postnatally by identification of physical stigmata (Color Plate 15):

- Flat facial profile (90%)
- Poor Moro reflex (85%)
- Excess skin on back of neck (80%)
- Generalized muscular hypotonia (80%)
- Characteristic facies with eyes that show epicanthal folds and upward- and outward-slanting palpebral fissures (80%)
- Joint laxity (80%)
- Small, low-set ears; anomalous auricles (60%)
- Short hands with simian creases (45%; see Color Plate 40) and clinodactyly of fifth finger (50%)
- Brushfield spots on the iris (speckling of the iris)
- Small, upturned nose with saddle bridge
- Small mouth with protruding tongue

Major Anomalies

- Mental deficiency (40%)
- Congenital heart disease (40%)
- Gastrointestinal abnormalities (37%)
- Hearing loss (conductive, mixed, or sensorineural; 66%)

(Continued)

● BOX 7-1
DOWN SYNDROME—cont'd

Incidence
- Most common pattern of human malformation: 1 in 660 live births worldwide; 1 in 1100 in United States.
- Male predominance: 3:2 male-to-female ratio.
- Incidence increases with increasing maternal age; however, fewer infants overall are born to women >35 years, so most infants with Down syndrome are born to younger women.

Life Span
- High incidence of neonatal deaths.
- 40% die in <5 years from congenital heart disease/infection.
- Survivors at 5 years have a mean survival of 45 years.

Expected Developmental and Physical Problems
- Poor physical growth
- Delayed development (milestones, speech, secondary sex characteristics, intelligence)
- Frequent infections (respiratory, otitis)
- Transient leukemoid reactions and polycythemia in neonatal period; lifelong increased risk for leukemia
- Thyroid disorders
- Premature senility and aging
- Ophthalmologic abnormalities (strabismus, cataracts, glaucoma, refraction abnormalities)
- Atlantoaxial instability

Ethical Issues
- Withholding critical care on the basis of Down syndrome can no longer be supported ethically or legally (U.S. Commission on Civil Rights, 1989).
- Institutional placement, common before the mid-1980s, is no longer an option for the newborn.
- Early care/correction for disabilities (cardiac, gastrointestinal, hearing, vision, thyroid) leads to improved quality of life.
- Improved care and family living lead to increased life expectancy, broadened life skills, and accomplishments (education, employment, community life opportunities).

Referral
- See "Parental Care When the Child Has a Chromosomal Abnormality" in Chapter 10.
- Genetic consult; chromosome analysis of infant and parents to rule out translocation (recurrence risk increases to 5%–10%).
- If diagnosed prenatally, consult with staff already involved with family. Notify primary care provider for immediate follow-up and support to the family.
- Provide family with written information on local and national support groups (many will not be ready for referral during the first few days of life).

From American Academy of Pediatrics: Clinical practice guideline: early detection of developmental dysplasia of the hip, *Pediatrics* 105:896-905, 2000; Cronk C, Crocker AC, Pueschel SM, et al:. Growth charts for children with Down syndrome: 1 month to 18 years of age, *Pediatrics* 81:102-110, 1988.

Facial measurements

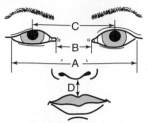

A = Outer canthal distance
B = Inner canthal distance
C = Interpupillary distance

Percentile (%)	Distance (cm)		
	A	B	C
3	5.5	1.5	3
25	6.0	1.8	3.5
50	6.5	2.0	4.0
75	7.0	2.3	4.25
97	7.5	2.5	4.5

FIGURE 7-7 ● Facial measurements used to determine hyper- and hypotelorism. (From Feingold M, Bossert WH: *Birth defects* 10[suppl 13]:57, 1974. John Wiley & Sons, New York and the March of Dimes Foundation, White Plains, New York.)

normally 2 cm apart (1.5 cm is the lower normal limit; 2.5 cm, the upper normal limit). In the case of epicanthal folds, the outer angles or the interpupillary distance should be used as reference for this diagnosis. Hyper- and hypotelorism may be isolated findings but sometimes are present in association with other anomalies.

g. The iris often appears dark blue until 3–6 months of age when eye color may change.

h. Observe for pupil response to light and symmetry of eye movements. Pupils should be rounded and regular and react to light. Pupil reaction occurs consistently only after 32 weeks of gestation, but may develop as early as 28 weeks. Bright lights or a flashlight beam will usually cause a blink, indicating at least grossly intact vision.

i. Brushfield spots: A "salt and pepper" speckling of the iris often seen in Down syndrome.

j. Tearing is not normal until 2 months of age. Chemical blepharo-conjunctivitis caused by silver nitrate may produce copious secretions and edema, but it is self-limited. Tearing or persistent eye crusting after the first 2 days requires evaluation for glaucoma, infection, corneal abrasion, mass lesions with obstructions of the nasolacrimal duct, or absence of the puncta. Signs of congenital glaucoma observable during a neonatal examination include photophobia, excessive tearing, cloudy cornea, or eyes that appear large.

k. Integrity of the iris and the presence of a red reflex may be more easily evaluated the day of discharge rather than immediately after birth.

The red reflex is normally present and represents an intact lens. Its absence may indicate congenital cataracts or other abnormalities. Cataracts may be the result of intrauterine viral infection or can be inherited as a dominant trait from an affected parent (Color Plate 16).

2. Ears (Figure 7-8 illustrates landmarks).

   a. Ear position at term should be similar on both sides; normal location is determined by drawing an imaginary horizontal line from the inner canthi of the eyes perpendicular to the vertical axis of the head. If the helix (topmost curve) of the ears lies below this line, the ears are low-set; this can be associated with other ear abnormalities or anomalies on other parts of the body (Color Plate 17).

   b. Preauricular skin tags (Color Plate 18) and dimples are common and usually benign, although they may be associated with renal problems or hearing loss (Box 7-2).

   c. Hairy ears are seen in infants of diabetic mothers.

   d. Observe for patency of the ear canals, although visualization of tympanic membranes is not necessary unless indicated by history or other findings.

   e. Hearing: An infant who becomes alert and stops moving or fretting in the presence of conversation or noise from a rattle or a bell can probably hear. However, a more definitive hearing assessment can be done by a newborn/infant screening program.

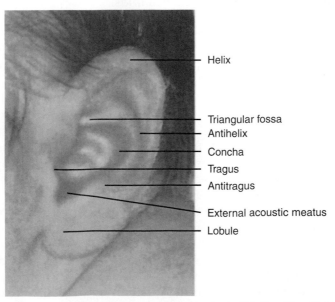

FIGURE 7-8 ● Landmarks of the external ear. (From Nichols FM, Zwelling E: *Maternal-newborn nursing: theory and practice*, Philadelphia, 1997, WB Saunders, p 1094.)

● BOX 7-2
● **EAR ANOMALIES**

- Can include external ear abnormalities, nonpatent canals, preauricular skin tags (see Color Plate 18), branchial sinuses/fistulas, pits.
- Approximately 1 in 200 infants with preauricular abnormalities also have hearing loss and should receive an initial hearing screening before discharge.
- Majority of abnormalities (approximately 80%) are isolated defects, but the infant should be examined for the possibility of syndrome association, which might also include vertebral, cardiac, and renal abnormalities.
- Tags can be removed before discharge by simple ligation at the parents' request.
- Branchial sinuses/fistulas may present as preauricular or lateral neck lesions, which usually are remnants of the second branchial cleft. Tracts extend from an external opening and may end in a blind pouch or continue to an internal opening at the tonsillar fossa.
- Otorhinolaryngologic/surgical consult may be indicated for mucus-draining fistulas.

From American Academy of Pediatrics: Hearing assessment in infants and children: recommendations beyond neonatal screening, *Pediatrics* 111:436-440, 2003.

3. Nose
    a. The nose is assessed for shape, size, position on the face, patency, presence of swelling over the nasolacrimal duct, the size of the philtrum, and definition of the nasolabial folds.
    b. Nasal positional deformities may be a result of the birth process, and most will resolve without treatment; however, they should be examined to be sure that dislocation of the triangular cartilage has not produced a true septal deviation (Silverman and Leibow, 1975). With depression of the tip of the nose, a dislocated septum appears more angled within the nares, but a normal septum merely compresses. After release, a dislocated septum does not return to normal. A dislocated septum requires surgical relocation within the first week of life.
    c. Abnormal shape of the nose may include hypoplastic nares, an extremely thin nose, or a depressed, wide or prominent nasal bridge; these may be associated with congenital syndromes.
    d. Nasal patency should be verified since infants are obligate nose breathers. Most often this can be done by observing comfortable and quiet respirations. An appropriate-sized catheter may be passed through the nares to be sure there is no choanal atresia/stenosis (membranous or bony blockage, which may be unilateral or bilateral); however, many nurseries no longer pass catheters to assess patency if an infant appears to be breathing comfortably because of the nasal trauma that may be induced. A cold, flat metal object may also be held under the nose to observe for fogging, or a thread may be held in front of the nostrils to watch for fluttering of the thread with breaths.

      e. Flaring of nostrils may be indicative of respiratory distress. Cyanosis, apnea, or noisy breathing may be evident with choanal atresia.

      f. Dacryocystocele is a dilation of the lacrimal drainage system due to obstruction at its proximal and distal ends, resulting in filling of the enclosed space. Dacryocystoceles present at birth as tense, blue-gray cystic swellings about 1 cm in diameter located just below the medial canthal tendon.

   4. Mouth and chin

      a. External observations

        (1) The shape and size of the mouth are best determined by looking at the mandible and how well it fits the maxilla. It should open at equal angles bilaterally.

        (2) For the mouth to develop properly, there must be muscle activity of the tongue against an intact hard palate. If not, the mandible recedes and micrognathia results. Microgranthia is also seen in some genetic conditions such as Pierre-Robin syndrome.

        (3) The shape of the mouth is a marker of uterine position and neuromuscular activity. If the uterine position tilts the head laterally, there may be asynclitism, in which the jaw opens at an angle. This deformation resolves spontaneously, although it may cause temporary feeding problems.

        (4) Asymmetry with crying occurs with facial nerve paresis (Color Plate 19), in which the nasolabial folds are asymmetric, or with the absence of the depressor anguli oris muscle, in which the folds are symmetric. This muscle absence is also palpable as a thin lower lip.

      b. Internal examination of the mouth

        (1) Should be examined using a small tongue blade to visualize the tongue, buccal surface, palate, uvula, and back of the mouth. The gums and hard palate are best assessed with a gloved finger to feel for masses or submucous defects and to allow evaluation of the sucking and gag reflexes.

        (2) Check hard and soft palates, gums, and lips for clefts, which can vary from a niche in the lip to a complete separation extending up into the nostril (Box 7-3 provides more details about cleft lip and palate; Table 7-1 covers feeding infants with cleft lip/palate; Color Plate 20).

        (3) Epstein pearls: Small white inclusion cysts clustered about the midline at the juncture of the hard and soft palates; a normal finding that resolves spontaneously with sucking.

        (4) Mucocele: Small lesion on the oral mucosa that occurs secondary to trauma of the salivary gland ducts; usually benign and subsides spontaneously.

        (5) Alveolar cysts with or without natal teeth: Natal teeth (usually lower central incisors) present in approximately 1 in 3500 live births; may require radiographs to determine whether they are supernumerary teeth or prematurely erupted decidual teeth.

● BOX 7-3
CLEFT LIP/PALATE

Initial Diagnosis and Referral
- Birth of a child with an orofacial cleft can be a particularly devastating experience for a family. Judgments concerning character, personality, and in particular, intellect are often made based on facial appearance. Understandably, the parents' concern for the well-being of their child and the level of the family's stress are high during the newborn period.
- Ongoing care of the infant and family must begin in the hospital, if possible, under the direction of specialists who will be able to assist the primary care provider with all aspects of the infant's long-term care (audiology, genetics, nursing, oral/maxillofacial surgery, orthodontia, otolaryngology, dentistry, pediatrics, plastic/reconstructive surgery, psychology, social services, speech/language pathology).
- Prenatal ultrasound diagnosis may allow early referral and initial preparation and counseling of the family.

Presentation
- Cleft lip and palate are separate fusion abnormalities that often occur simultaneously as a result of developmental progression.
- Midline fusion of the developing upper lip occurs at 6–8 weeks gestation. Failure of migration of supporting tissue can result in the development of cleft lip.
- Palatal fusion, also in progress at this time, may be disrupted if a cleft lip is present, allowing the tongue to protrude higher in the oral cavity and obstruct palatal closure.

Incidence
- Ranges from 0.8 to 2.7 in 1000 live births. Isolated cleft palate affects approximately 1 in 2000 live births.
- Native Americans infants have the highest incidence, followed by Japanese, Maoris, and Chinese. Caucasians have an intermediate incidence, and African-Americans have the lowest incidence of clefts.
- In addition to race, other risk factors include advanced maternal age, chromosomal abnormalities, syndromic development, and environmental teratogens (alcohol, thalidomide).
- Although several autosomal dominant conditions lead to clefting, overall this is believed to be a multifactorial defect, requiring genetic predisposition in combination with environmental factors.
- Recurrence risk is approximately 2% if parents and siblings have no clefts; approximately 2%–7% if either parent or a sibling has a cleft; and approximately 14%–17% if either parent and a sibling has a cleft.

Immediate Care Needs
- Resuscitation at birth is usually not an issue unless the cleft is associated with Pierre Robin syndrome, which involves micrognathia and airway obstruction.
- Parents should be assured in the delivery room that the cleft will not threaten the infant's survival and that it is surgically correctable. If the infant's condition is stable, allow the parents to begin the normal attachment process in the delivery room and explain that a thorough examination will be done when the infant is admitted to the nursery.
- Physical examination includes assessment of all systems to detect or exclude other abnormalities that would indicate the cleft is associated with a chromosome abnormality or syndrome, which might limit prognosis.

● BOX 7-3
CLEFT LIP/PALATE—cont'd

Feeding Difficulty
This is the most common problem encountered in the nursery. Although infants suck abnormally because of the anatomic defect, swallowing is normal and many infants can breast-feed successfully. Long-term weight gain is a significant problem and often lags behind established norms.

Breast-feeding
- Isolated cleft lip: The breast conforms to the defect and sucking usually generates adequate negative pressure.
- Isolated cleft palate: Usually successful with soft palate cleft or narrow hard palate cleft.
- Cleft lip and palate: Most likely to have difficulty; breast milk may be pumped and fed through a supplemental nursing system that drips milk through a thin tubing inserted into the mouth along the side of the mother's nipple. This supplemental system stimulates sucking reflex (which promotes continued muscular development) and milk production while ensuring adequate milk delivery to the infant.

Formula Feeding
- When the infant has an isolated cleft lip, a soft, wide-based nipple might conform to the defect to allow adequate sucking.
- When the infant has an isolated cleft palate or cleft lip and palate combination, the wide-based nipple will also require enlargement of the holes for easy milk delivery because the infant will have an inefficient suck. Infants fed by a combination of nipple hole enlargement, suck stimulation, and rest following suck, known as the ESSR method (see Table 7-1), showed greater mean weight gain when compared with a group of infants fed by nipple enlargement alone.
- Successful feeding by parents must occur before hospital discharge in order to assure parents of their ability to care for their infant. Close follow-up with the craniofacial team is essential for long-term success.

From American Cleft Palate–Craniofacial Association: Parameters for the evaluation and treatment of patients with cleft lip/palate or other craniofacial anomalies, *Cleft Palate Craniofac J* 30:S1-S16, 1993.

Dental consultation and extraction should be undertaken prior to discharge if the teeth are supernumerary or are loose, suggesting poor root formation (approximately 30%), since this poses an aspiration risk.

(6) Ranulae: Uncommon sublingual cysts that are benign but may rupture with vigorous sucking.

(7) Bifid uvula: Associated with submucous cleft palate.

(8) Macroglossia: Enlarged tongue, which may be congenital or acquired. Localized macroglossia is usually secondary to congenital hemangioma. Macroglossia can be seen in association with several disorders including Beckwith syndrome, Pompe disease, hypothyroidism, and Down syndrome.

● TABLE 7-1
The ESSR Feeding Method*

Action	Effect
E Enlarge precut nipple hole by placing tip of sharp manicure scissors into hole and cutting in four directions.	Allows infant to receive formula to the back of the throat for swallowing without relying on ineffective suction.
S Stimulate the suck reflex by gently rubbing the nipple against the lower lip; insert and then invert bottle	Prepares infant for feeding. Because of enlarged nipple, inverting after inserting prevents spillage and waste.
S Swallow fluid normally.	Receives an adequate amount of formula without using excess energy and will meet nutritional requirements for proper weight gain.
R Rest after signal; infant will exhibit a facial expression indicating that a short break in feeding is necessary	Allows infant to finish swallowing formula already in back of throat and avoid uncomfortable gagging or nasal regurgitation.

*Repeat process until infant has eaten normal amount of formula in normal amount of time.
From Richard ME: Feeding the newborn with cleft lip and/or palate: the enlargement, stimulate, swallow, rest (ESSR) method, *J Pediatr Nurs* 6(5):319, 1991.

    (9) Ankyloglossia: Commonly known as "tongue-tie," the frenulum on the underside of the tongue prevents complete tongue protrusion; it may extend to papillated surface of the tongue or cause a fissure in the tip of the tongue. Rarely, this requires surgical intervention in the neonatal period (if feeding is severely impaired) or later in life (if speech is affected).

  E. Neck: Elicit the rooting reflex by lightly stroking the cheek lateral to the edge of the mouth, causing the infant to open its mouth and turn its head to the stroked side in anticipation of sucking; this will allow easier examination of the neck. The infant's head should be able to turn as far as the shoulder in both directions and slightly farther if premature.

    1. Palpate the neck to rule out sternocleidomastoid hematoma, thyroid enlargement, or thyroglossal duct cysts. If the head is persistently drawn to one side, suspect torticollis.

    2. Webbing should alert the examiner to possible Turner syndrome or other syndromes.

    3. A pouch of redundant skin may be found at the base of the neck posteriorly; this is seen in syndromes such as trisomy 21.

    4. Inspect the clavicles for fractures, which may have occurred during delivery (Color Plate 21). A palpable mass, crepitus, or tenderness may be evident at the site (Box 7-4 provides more information on clavicle fracture).

    5. The most common neck mass is a cystic hygroma, which is a multiloculated cyst arising from lymphatic channels usually posterior to the

● BOX 7-4
CLAVICLE FRACTURE (see Color Plate 21)

- Most frequent birth injury. Crepitus is felt during palpation of the clavicles, making radiographic confirmation unnecessary in most cases. Most are greenstick fractures and will heal without treatment.
- Newborns may be asymptomatic, or they may show limited use of the arm, an asymmetric Moro reflex, and/or cry with manipulation of the arm.
- If the infant displays discomfort, the arm can be immobilized by pinning the T-shirt sleeve in a natural position across the chest.
- Care should be taken to support the back and arm when lifting the infant.
- Parents should be told to expect a small bump over the fracture site that will disappear as healing occurs.

sternocleidomastoid muscle and extending into the scapula and axillary and thoracic compartments. Most hygromas occur in the neck (65%) and may invade and distort local anatomy including the airway, making respiratory distress evident at birth.

F. **Abdomen:** Examination of the abdomen is best accomplished during the first 24 hours of life and at a time when the infant is quiet or is feeding. The newborn abdomen is mildly protuberant compared with the chest and should be softly rounded, with a diameter slightly greater above the umbilicus than below. The abdominothoracic relation is reversed in diaphragmatic defects with herniation of abdominal contents into the thorax, leaving a scaphoid abdomen.

1. General inspection
   a. Supraumbilical fullness is increased in the presence of duodenal atresia, gastric distention, or hepatomegaly. Infraumbilical fullness is increased with distention of the urinary bladder.
   b. Asymmetry, unless it is due to a large stomach bubble (often just after eating or crying), may be a clue to an abnormal abdominal mass.
   c. The veins in the skin over the upper abdomen often appear dilated.
   d. A flabby abdomen may be associated with the depressant effects of residual maternal medication, immaturity, or the absence of muscles in the abdominal wall. "Prune belly syndrome" is sometimes used to describe the condition in which there are no muscles in the abdominal wall; this is associated with other anomalies of the gastrointestinal (GI) and genitourinary (GU) tracts.
   e. Diastasis recti is the nonunion of the two rectus muscles from the umbilicus to the xiphoid; it often causes a mild herniation in the midline.
   f. Abdominal distention may be due to obstruction, infection, masses, or enlargement of an abdominal organ (Color Plate 22).
2. Umbilicus
   a. Normally positioned midway between the xiphoid and the pubis.

    b. The cord should contain two arteries and one vein. A single artery may be associated with an increased incidence of congenital abnormalities, usually of the GI and GU system.

    c. The diameter of the cord varies in relation to the quality of Wharton jelly and is an indicator of the in utero nutritional status. In the neonatal stage, the umbilicus is normally relatively protuberant with redundant skin; this is no indication of the adult appearance.

    d. If the cord itself is broad or remains fluctuant after pulsations have stopped and the umbilicus is centrally located, it may indicate the presence of an omphalocele, in which the abdominal contents are herniated into the cord to one degree or another. The herniation may be small and present with just an enlarged cord, or it may be an obvious omphalocele.

    e. Umbilical hernia: intestinal muscles fail to close around the umbilicus. Intestines protrude into the weaker area. More common in term African-American (30%) infants than in Caucasian (4%) infants. Rarely associated with trisomies. Requires no intermediate intervention; closure is not enhanced by taping or using belly bands. Usually will close spontaneously by 2 to 3 years of age; larger hernias may require surgical intervention (Color Plate 23).

    f. Discharge, redness, foul odor, or edema around the base of the cord may indicate a patent urachus (Color Plate 24) or omphalitis (Color Plate 25).

    g. A persistently moist cord base may indicate a granuloma of the umbilical cord (Color Plate 26) or a patent urachus. A granuloma can be treated with topic silver nitrate therapy; if this fails to treat the granuloma, rule out a patent urachus. Patent urachus is a persistence of the urachus, a fetal connection between the umbilicus and the bladder, with physical findings that ranges from a persistently moist cord to obvious urinary drainage. This requires surgical intervention to prevent urinary tract infection.

3. Auscultate the abdomen for the presence of bowel sounds. Auscultation may reveal the existence of a bruit over the liver (indicating an arteriovenous malformation) or over the kidneys (indicating renal artery stenosis).

4. Palpation

    a. Liver

        (1) Begin in the right lower quadrant and progress upward with the thumb pad so that an enlarged liver edge will not be missed. Hepatomegaly may be associated with congenital heart disease, infection, or hemolytic disease.

        (2) The lower liver edge is normally palpable 1.0–3.5 cm below the costal margin in the midclavicular line and across the midline, where the left lobe is distinguishable from the lobulated spleen, which may be felt more laterally. A left lobe larger than the right may reflect situs inversus.

        (3) At term the normal liver span is 5.9 ± 0.8 cm in the midclavicular line by percussing the upper and lower margins. An estimation of hepatomegaly based on the lower border alone is inaccurate.

      (4) It is possible to outline the liver (or any solid mass) by scratching lightly across the skin surface, while auscultating for change in pitch with the diaphragm of the stethoscope held directly over the mass.

      (5) The normal edge of the liver is sharp and soft, and the hepatic surface is smooth. A full or firm edge may represent a marked increase in total blood volume, increased extramedullary hematopoiesis, chronic infection, an infiltrative process, and sometimes congestive heart failure.

   b. Spleen: The normal spleen is rarely palpable; a palpable spleen tip more than 1 cm below the left costal margin is abnormal and may indicate infection or extramedullary hematopoiesis.

   c. Kidneys

      (1) Only routinely palpable during the first 1–2 days of life with any ease or reliability. The kidneys are moderately firm and lobulated with a normal measurement at full-term of 4.5–5.0 cm pole to pole. On palpation, the infant will normally demonstrate pain by a grimace, cry, or drawing up of the legs.

      (2) Placing the third finger of one hand posteriorly in the lowest costovertebral angle, the left kidney can almost always be palpated by trapping it against that finger with the index and third finger of the other hand. The lower pole of the right kidney may not be palpable, but if it is enlarged it will be noted.

      (3) Enlarged kidneys or absence of palpable kidneys requires further evaluation.

   d. Genitourinary system

      (1) The bladder may be palpated 1–4 cm above the symphysis, and gentle pressure over the bladder may initiate a urinary stream.

      (2) An enlarged ureter simulates a large loop of bowel, although it is less mobile.

      (3) Abnormal abdominal masses are most frequently of GU tract origin.

G. Genitalia and Anus

  1. Genitalia: Genital abnormalities are relatively uncommon but cause significant parental stress. It is important to identify the variations of normal, which occur more frequently than pathologic malformations.

   a. Female

      (1) Genitalia should be inspected for size and location of the labia, clitoris, meatus, and vaginal opening, as well as the relation of the posterior fourchette to the anus.

      (2) The labia majora in the term female infant are enlarged and usually cover the labia minora, clitoris, urethral meatus, and external vaginal vault. In the preterm female infant the labia majora may not cover the labia minora, and the clitoris will be prominent. Palpate the labia majora for masses that may be hernias or ectopic gonads.

      (3) Ecchymosis and edema of the labia are common in breech deliveries.

      (4) The vaginal orifice should be pink and glistening and should be assessed for patency. It is likely to have a creamy white or slightly

blood-tinged discharge (Color Plate 27). Virtually all female newborns have redundant hymenal tissue. The hymen is usually annular (80%) with a smooth or fimbriated edge and a central or ventrally displaced opening. An enlarged Bartholin gland often mimics an imperforate hymen. Vaginal mucosal skin tags are a common finding and may extend beyond the rim of the hymen; they will disappear within the first few weeks of life.

(5) The clitoris should be examined for size and palpated for diameter. An unusually large clitoris may indicate pseudohermaphroditism.

(6) Assessment of virilization of the female is difficult: both labia should be spread to ensure no labioscrotal fusion is present. Clitoral size is fully developed by 27 weeks gestation but with little deposition of fat in the labia. Masculization causes posterior fusion of the labioscrotal folds independent of clitoral hypertrophy.

(7) Occasionally, 0.5- to 1.0-cm vesicles (similar to milia) with no erythematous base are seen. They are usually clustered around the genitalia, and their surface is frequently broken.

(8) Measurement should be made between the posterior fourchette and the anus. This result should be divided by the distance from the coccyx to the fourchette with the hips flexed and the infant relaxed so that the perineum does not bulge. In the term infant, normal findings thus determined should be 0.44 ± 0.05 cm, with <0.34 cm being an anteriorally placed anus (Color Plate 28).

b. Male

(1) The glans should be completely covered by the foreskin at birth, and the newborn male usually has marked phimosis. The foreskin is unable to be retracted until 3–10 years of age.

(2) The penis should be examined to identify the meatal opening, although completely retracting the foreskin is unnecessary.

(a) Hypospadias exists if the urethral opening is located on the ventral surface (underside) of the penis (Color Plate 29; Box 7-5 provides more detail regarding GU abnormalities in the male infant).

(b) Epispadias exists if the urethral opening is located on the dorsal surface (top side) of the penis.

(3) The penis should be stretched and measured for an expected term length of 2.5–3.5 cm, with <2.5 cm being abnormally short. In obese infants, the shaft may be retracted and covered by suprapubic fat, appearing abnormally small unless stretched.

(4) The scrotum and testes

(a) The scrotum should be inspected for size, rugae (present after 37 weeks gestation), and presence of testes. If the testis is not located within the scrotal sac or the inguinal canal, use a lubricated finger to sweep from the anterior iliac crest along the canal while palpating the scrotum. Failure to palpate a testicle should prompt evaluation for an undescended testicle (or cryptorchidism) (Figure 7-9; see Box 7-5).

● BOX 7-5
GENITOURINARY ABNORMALITIES OF THE MALE INFANT

Early Treatment

Earlier surgical repair for genital anomalies is now standard between 6 and 12 months of age without increased risk to the child if performed by those with pediatric training. Earlier repair is advantageous for the following reasons:

- Limits the perception of the child's "defective status," which can ultimately alter interactions between the child and caregiver
- Diminishes distortions of body image
- Diminishes postoperative emotional difficulties seen in older children

Major Anomalies

Cryptorchidism

- Also called undescended testicles (UDT; see Figure 7-9).
- Incidence related to birth weight: approximately 3% in term male >2500 g; approximately 20% in infants <2500 g. 70% of testes will descend by 3 months of age, leaving the overall incidence of cryptorchidism at 1 year of age at 1%. Approximately 4% will eventually be found to have anorchidism; 10% are affected bilaterally.
- Testicular descent occurs between the seventh and ninth months of gestation and therefore should be complete at term.
- 40% of UDTs show structural abnormalities. Men with a history of unilateral UDT have lower sperm counts, and 40% experience infertility; men with a history of bilateral UDT have a 70% incidence of infertility; 10% have an increased incidence of testicular cancer.
- True cryptorchidism must be differentiated from retractile testes (testes can be manipulated into the scrotum and will remain momentarily); retractile testes are more common and do not require surgical intervention. Abdominal testes have an increased propensity for malignant degeneration and should be brought down to the scrotal sac or removed.
- Earlier age of surgical intervention (< 1 year) may positively impact fertility. Notify primary care provider for follow-up examination.

Hypospadias/chordee

- Hypospadias (incomplete formation of the anterior urethra, resulting in placement of the urethral meatus anywhere between the tip of the glans and the perineum) occurs in approximately 1 in 300 male infants (see Color Plate 29).
- The penis should be examined for meatal opening at the tip of the glans. Hypospadias should be suspected anytime an infant is noted to have a shawl prepuce, sometimes referred to as a "natural circumcision."
- Abnormalities are classified as anterior (65%), in which the urethral meatus is malpositioned at the glanular, coronal, or distal third of the shaft; midshaft (15%); and posterior (20%), occurring on the posterior third of the shaft.
- Preputial skin is preferred for reconstruction; it is therefore essential that the infant with hypospadias *not* be circumcised.
- Chordee (the presence of fibrotic tissue that causes a ventral curvature of the erect penis) may be associated with hypospadias or can occur alone. Because plastic repair may be required, circumcision also should not be performed on infants with chordee.
- Urologic consult should be discussed with the parents and primary care provider. Surgical repair is usually undertaken between 6 and 18 months.

From American Academy of Pediatrics: Timing of elective surgery on the genitalia of male children with particular reference to the risks, benefits, and psychological effects of surgery and anesthesia, *Pediatrics* 97:590-594, 1996.

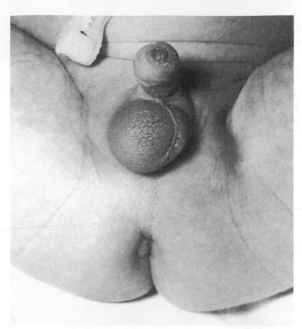

FIGURE 7-9 ● Left undescended testis. (From Beischer NA, Mackey EV, Colditz PB: *Obstetrics and the newborn*, ed 3, Philadelphia, 1997, WB Saunders, p 678.)

      (b) The volume of the testes should be estimated (1–2 mL is normal).

      (c) If the scrotum or a testis is distended, transillumination may reveal a hydrocele, which may be unilateral or bilateral and is usually transient. A mass which does not transilluminate may be a tumor or a torsion of the testes, the latter being a surgical emergency.

      (d) Discoloration suggests a hematoma or torsion. This requires immediate surgical evaluation unless it represents only superficial ecchymosis following a breech presentation.

      (e) The scrotum of African-American, Native American, or Hispanic male infants will appear darker than the rest of their skin.

      (f) Bifid scrotum (Figure 7-10): May be a normal variant but is also seen with a variety of genetic syndromes and may represent ambiguous genitalia.

      (g) Nonpalpable testes in a phenotypic term male should raise a question of virilizing adrenal hyperplasia in a female.

  (5) Hydrocele of the cord may be a forerunner of inguinal hernia (Color Plate 30) (Box 7-6 and Figure 7-11 provide more information on inguinal hernias).

  (6) Assessment of the distance from the anus to the scrotum divided by the distance from the coccyx to the scrotum should result in a measurement of 0.58 ± 0.06 cm, with a distance <0.46 cm being abnormal.

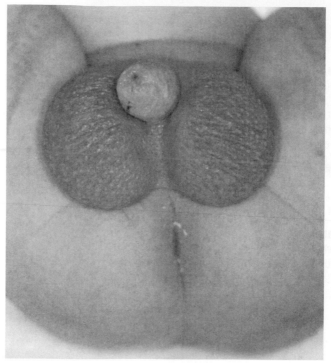

FIGURE 7-10 ● Bifid scrotum.

c. Gender assignment: **Never assign gender without palpating for testes**. In a presumed female infant, palpate the labia for testes. In a presumed male infant, if no testes are palpated in the scrotum or inguinal canal, do not assign gender until further work-up is completed. Various examples of ambiguous genitalia are shown in Color Plates 31–33.

2. Anus and rectum
   a. The anus and rectum should be checked carefully for patency, position, and size (normal diameter is 10 mm; Color Plate 34).
   b. Occasionally, large fistulae are mistaken for a normal anus, but fistulae are usually anterior or posterior to the normal location of the anus.

H. **Musculoskeletal System**
   1. General inspection
      a. Place the resting infant in a prone position for inspection. Examination of the spine involves observation for abnormal curvature, gross defects, and cutaneous manifestations of underlying deformities such as sacral agenesis or spina bifida.
      b. A pilonidal sinus is suspected if the bottom of a sacral pit is not visible or if there is moisture around an otherwise dry dimple, perhaps belying a small meningomyelocele or other anomaly (Color Plate 35).

● BOX 7-6
● **INGUINAL HERNIA (see Color Plate 30)**

Incidence/Etiology
- Accounts for approximately 80% of all hernias in newborns; occurs more frequently in males (90%)
- Caused by persistence of the processus vaginalis (tube of peritoneum that precedes the testicle through the inguinal canal into the scrotum); following testicular descent, the upper portion atrophies, leaving the distal portion (tunica vaginalis) to envelop the testicle (see Figure 10-1).
- Failure of obliteration of the upper portion of the processus vaginalis allows abdominal fluid or intestinal protrusion into the inguinal canal or scrotum, creating a palpable mass.

Assessment
- Should be reducible by gentle compression

Incarceration
- Incarcerated inguinal hernia is a surgical emergency.
- Symptoms include intestinal obstruction, irritability, and tenderness.
- Vascular occlusion can lead to gangrene and gonad destruction.
- Parents should be taught signs and significance of incarceration. Timing of surgical consult should be discussed with the parents and primary care provider.

From Hockenberry M et al.: *Wong's nursing care of infants and children*, ed 7, St Louis, 2003, Mosby.

    c. Abnormal pigmentation, overlying hemangioma, pigmented nevus, or dark hairy patches over the lower spine suggest an underlying vertebral anomaly.

    d. A palpable mass usually indicates a lipoma if it is covered with normal skin and moves with the skin.

    e. A sacrococcygeal teratoma tends to be just lateral to midline, whereas spinal dysraphism presents as a midline mass.

2. Extremities: Place the infant in a supine position. Examine the hands, arms, and legs with close attention to the digits and palmar creases. Length, contour, symmetry, size, and range of active and passive motion of extremities should be evaluated for obvious deformity, as well as to rule out unexpected fractures resulting from difficult delivery.

    a. Hands and feet

      (1) The length of the upper extremities should allow the hand to reach the upper thighs on extension.

      (2) Oligodactyly: Missing digits. May be seen as a result of amniotic bands (Color Plate 36) or syndromes. Complete absence or hypoplasia of the thumb is often associated with autosomal recessive syndromes, which may also include radial, renal, cardiac, and hematologic defects. Rehabilitation consult should be considered if prosthetic devices will enhance normal development and function.

      (3) Syndactyly: Abnormal fusion of the digits (fingers or toes) (Color Plate 37).

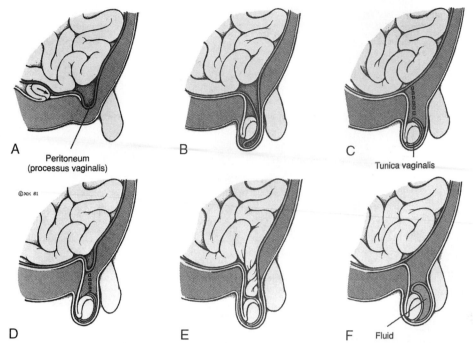

FIGURE 7-11 ● Development of inguinal hernias. **A** and **B,** Prenatal migration of processus vaginalis. **C,** Normal. **D,** Partially obliterated processus vaginalis. **E,** Hernia. **F,** Hydrocele. (From Wong DL: *Whaley & Wong's nursing care of infants and children,* St Louis, 1995, Mosby, p 494.)

(4) Polydactyly: Extra digits (finger or toes) (Figure 7-12) (Color Plate 38). An x-ray will reveal any bony structures in the digit. If bony structures are not present, a suture can be tied tightly around the digit until it falls off. If bony structures are present, surgical removal will be necessary, if desired or indicated.

(5) The digits should be scrutinized for any abnormalities of the nails, clubbing, edema, unusual creases, or curvature.

    (a) The creases of the fifth digit should be parallel. If there is shortening of the midphalanx, the nonparallel creases indicate a radial deviation (also known as clinodactyly) (Color Plate 39).

    (b) Any curve <8 degrees is normal.

(6) The hand maintains a fairly constant proportion throughout life; the distance from the tip of the index finger to the base of the thumb should be roughly one half the distance of the index finger to the carpal crease, and the thumb should reach just beyond the base of the index finger.

(7) Simian crease (Color Plate 40): A single transverse palmar crease seen bilaterally is highly associated with chromosomal and congenital abnormalities. Unilaterally, it is seen in 5%–10% of the normal population.

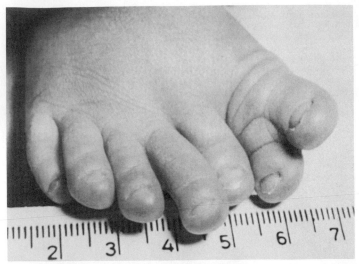

FIGURE 7-12 ● Extra digits. (From Beischer NA, Mackey EV, Colditz PB: *Obstetrics and the newborn*, ed 3, Philadelphia, 1997, WB Saunders, p 611.)

(8) Talipes equinovarus (club foot; Color Plate 41): The foot is turned downward and inward, and the sole is directed medially. If the angle can be corrected with gentle force, the condition will resolve spontaneously over time. If not, orthopedic treatment is necessary and should be arranged within the first 1–2 weeks of life. Can occur as an isolated defect or in association with congenital hip dysplasia or other more serious defects. More common in males.

(9) Metatarsus adductus: Adduction of the forefoot; if correctable with passive range of motion, it will probably correct itself in time; if not able to passively return to normal position, an orthopedic consult should be obtained. Most common congenital foot deformity; usually a result of abnormal intrauterine positioning.

(10) Calcaneovalgus: Foot is dorsiflexed at a sharp angle with the top of the foot in contact with the anterior surface of the tibia. Occurs secondary to abnormal in utero positioning, and requires orthopedic consultation if postnatal positioning appears fixed.

(11) "Rocker-bottom" foot (Color Plate 42): May be associated with genetic syndromes, particularly trisomies.

b. Upper extremities: Any deficit in motor activity of the upper extremities should be investigated for the possibility of brachial nerve injury (Box 7-7 provides details on brachial plexus injuries).

c. Lower extremities and hips (Box 7-8 provides more information on developmental dysplasia [DDH] of the hip): Examine the infant in supine position.

(1) Check the lower leg for tibial bowing or torsion.

(2) Hips: The anatomy of normal and dislocated hips is shown in Figure 7-13. Compare symmetry of creases over the back of the

● BOX 7-7
BRACHIAL PLEXUS INJURIES

Incidence/Etiology

- 80% of infants with brachial plexus injuries suffer damage to the fifth or sixth cervical roots.
- Improved obstetric practices have decreased the incidence of injuries. Risk factors include large-birth-weight infant, prolonged and difficult labor, and heavy maternal sedation. Nerve injury most often results from shoulder traction during breech delivery or from turning the head away from the shoulder in difficult cephalic presentation.
- Transient paralysis occurs as a result of nerve compression from hemorrhage or edema; permanent paralysis may result from nerve tearing or avulsion of the roots from the spinal cord.

Erb-Duchenne Palsy

- Clinically, the arm is in a position of tight adduction and internal rotation at the shoulder, with extension and pronation at the elbow (Color Plate 43).
- Additional involvement of the seventh cervical root causes weakness of the wrist extensors, leading to persistent contraction of the flexors that gives the characteristic "waiter's tip" position of the hand.
- The infant will show absent or diminished Moro reflex on the affected side but intact palmar grasp.

Klumpke Paralysis

Presentation

- Rare injury to the lower brachial plexus (<2.5% of plexus injuries) involves paralysis of the muscles of the hand and weakness of the wrist and finger flexors.
- Grasp reflex is absent, and often a unilateral Horner syndrome (eyelid ptosis) is present.

Treatment

- Immobilization of the arm by pinning the T-shirt sleeve to the chest in a natural position provides comfort and allows brachial plexus injuries to heal.

Prognosis

- Prognosis is uncertain initially.
- Transient lesions show return of motor function beginning by 1–2 weeks of age, with full recovery expected over a period of weeks to months; permanent lesions are associated with eventual muscle atrophy, contractures, and poor limb growth.

Follow-up

- Notify primary care provider for follow-up exam and further referral for permanent disability.

---

thigh; asymmetry suggests dislocation of the hip. With the infant in a supine position, the knees flexed and the feet resting on the flat surface, compare leg length; if the legs appear to be of unequal length, suspect dislocation of the shorter leg (Galeazzi sign). Two commonly used maneuvers should be performed sequentially to assess for dislocation:

(a) Barlow maneuver (Figure 7-14): With the newborn in a supine position and the knees flexed, the thigh is grasped and adducted

● BOX 7-8
DEVELOPMENTAL DYSPLASIA OF THE HIP (DDH)

Prognosis
- Early detection and treatment significantly alter the outcome and cost of congenital hip dislocation by diminishing the need for surgical correction and helping to ensure normal development. Late presentation or detection (>6 months) is associated with prolonged, complicated treatment and poor outcome.

Etiology
- DDH occurs when the upper rim of the acetabulum fails to develop and the femoral head is malpositioned (see Figure 7-13).

Presentation
- Dislocation ("clunk"): Femoral head lies above and lateral to the acetabulum; adductor muscles shorten; knee and inguinal creases are higher.
- Subluxation or ligament laxity ("click"): Femoral head lies within the acetabulum but can be moved to the edge of the acetabulum with manipulation (approximately 60% of unstable hips become clinically normal by 1–4 weeks of age).

Incidence
- Ranges from 1.5 to 2.7 per 1000 live births.
- Female-to-male ratio of approximately 4:1; 20%–30% genetic transmission. Increased incidence in Caucasians, Eskimos, and Native Americans; decreased incidence in African-Americans and Chinese. In utero position (particularly breech presentation; Color Plate 44), birthing, swaddling, and infant-carrying positions may all affect the incidence rate.
- Left hip involvement, 65%; right hip involvement, 9%; bilateral involvement, 26%.
- Risk factors include breech delivery, positive family history, foot deformities, and race.

Examination Techniques
- Ortolani maneuver: Gentle abduction test can detect dislocated hips (head of femur is outside the acetabulum and can be reduced with abduction and lifting of the greater trochanter).
- Barlow maneuver: Gentle manipulation test can detect dislocatable hips (head of femur is in the acetabulum and can be subluxated or dislocated by pushing posteriorly on the femur in adduction).
- Radiographs: Identify bony landmarks of the pelvis, acetabulum, and femoral shaft. Femoral head is not ossified in the newborn and therefore cannot be visualized; position must be inferred from relationship of bony parts. Delaying radiograph examination until 2 weeks of age prevents unnecessary examination in transiently unstable hips that resolve spontaneously.
- Ultrasound: Allows visualization of the cartilaginous femoral head and contour of the acetabulum. Allows dynamic evaluation of the hip if performed in real time during Ortolani/Barlow maneuvers. Delaying ultrasound examination until 2 weeks of age prevents unnecessary examination in transiently unstable hips that resolve spontaneously.
- Vibration arthrometry (currently under investigation): Detects vibrations produced when joints are manipulated; can differentiate pathologic vibrations.

Treatment and Follow-Up Recommendations
- Any abnormal finding at birth or presence of risk factors should be communicated to the parents and primary care provider for follow-up examination at no later than 2 weeks of age.

● BOX 7-8
DEVELOPMENTAL DYSPLASIA OF THE HIP (DDH)—cont'd

- Goal: Concentric relocation of the femoral head in the acetabulum is necessary to allow normal growth and development (concave shape of acetabulum develops in response to the presence of the femoral head).
- Pavlik harness
  1. Harness with stirrups; holds hip and knee joints in flexion; hip extension is prevented, but all other motions of the hip are possible (Color Plate 45).
  2. Most widely used therapy; success depends on type of hip abnormality. Small risk for damage to the growth of the upper end of the femur (avascular necrosis).
  3. Hip stability usually apparent after 2–3 weeks of treatment, and harness can be removed after 6 weeks.
  4. If not improved after 3 weeks, other methods (traction, open or closed reduction, spica casts) are usually necessary.

From American Academy of Pediatrics: Clinical practice guideline: early detection of developmental dysplasia of the hip, *Pediatrics* 105:896-905, 2000.

while applying downward pressure. Dislocation of the femoral head from the acetabulum is considered a positive Barlow maneuver.

(b) Ortolani maneuver (Figure 7-15): Intended to reduce the dislocation. With the hip and knee flexed, the thigh is grasped with the third finger over the greater trochanter, the thumb near the lesser trochanter, and the other hand stabilizing the pelvis. The thigh is abducted while pressure is applied to the greater trochanter to reduce the dislocated femoral head into the acetabulum with a clunking sensation. Benign hip "clicks," possibly caused by movement of the ligamentum teres in the acetabulum, are much more common than the "clunk" that is observed when the femoral head dislocates.

I. **Neonatal Neurologic Examination** (Table 7-2): Neurologic evaluation begins with the initial observations of the infant and continues as the infant is positioned and stimulated throughout the remainder of the physical examination. Always observe the newborn for neurologic deficits while simultaneously studying the organs and physiologic systems. Symmetry of movement and posturing, body tone, and response to being handled and disturbed can all be observed during the sequence of physical assessment. An abnormal examination should be repeated to validate findings and document changes over time. The approach to examination of neurologic status includes the motor system, reflexes, sensory system, and cranial nerves.

  1. External evaluation
     a. Examine for signs of birth trauma (cephalhematoma, forceps marks, lacerations, abrasions, bruising, localized swelling); dysmorphic features

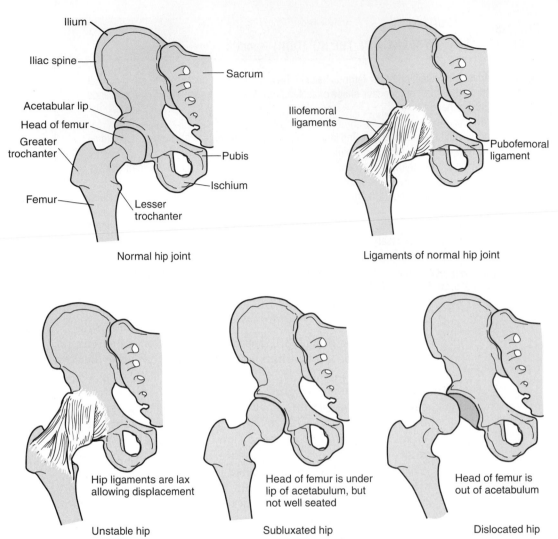

FIGURE 7-13 ● The normal hip, the moderately stretched "dislocatable" hip, and the overly stretched dislocated hip. (From Clarren S, Smith DW: Congenital deformities, *Pediatr Clin North Am* 24:665, 1977.)

(more than six café-au-lait spots may indicate the presence of neurofibromatosis; a nevus flammeus involving skin innervated by the trigeminal nerve may indicate the presence of Sturge-Weber syndrome with underlying arteriovenous malformations); skin lesions; posture; and activity.

b. Assess quality of the cry, symmetry of facial movement, and facial expression. A loud, lusty cry is normal in the term newborn. A weak cry may indicate a depressed, ill, or premature infant. A high-pitched cry

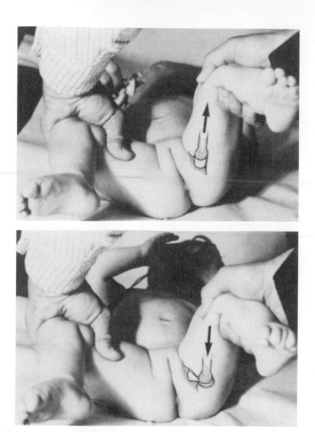

FIGURE 7-14 ● Technique of the Barlow maneuver, which assists in detecting the unstable dislocatable hip in the acetabulum. The leg is forcibly pulled up during the upper maneuver. Passage over the rim (lower maneuver) usually yields a noticeable "clunk." (Courtesy Dr. Lynn Staheli, University of Washington.) (From Smith DW: *Recognizable patterns of human deformations*, Philadelphia, 1981, WB Saunders, p 23.)

may be present in infants with neurologic or metabolic abnormalities or those experiencing drug withdrawal.

2. Resting posture: Influenced by gestational age. The term newborn lies with knees flexed and hips abducted and partially flexed. The arms are adducted and flexed at the elbow. The fists are loosely clenched with the thumb resting in the palm or lying adjacent to the fingers. Abnormal posture includes persistent extension of the neck (opisthotonus), obligate flexion of the thumb (cortical thumb), and frog-leg positioning in infants >36 weeks gestation.

3. Spontaneous movements: Movements should be smooth. All limbs should move in an alternating fashion. Mass movements occur in response to environmental stimuli and discomfort. Coarse tremors or brief trembling of the chin may occur normally. Jitteriness is characterized by rhythmic tremors of equal amplitude around a fixed axis, as in an extremity or in the jaw.

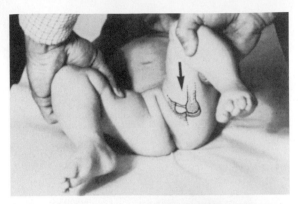

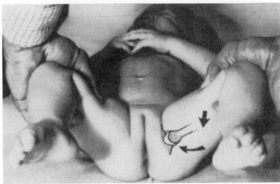

FIGURE 7-15 ● Technique of the Ortolani maneuver. This maneuver assists in detecting the dislocated hip, which can be repositioned into the acetabulum. **Top,** Downward pressure further dislocates the hip. **Bottom,** Inward rotation of the hip will force the femoral head over the acetabular rim, leading to a noticeable "clunk." (From Smith DW: *Recognizable patterns of human deformations*, Philadelphia, 1981, WB Saunders, p 24.)

This occurs more often when the infant is awake and after a startle or crying; jitteriness may be distinguished from tonic-clonic seizure activity because it can usually be stopped by the infant sucking on the extremity or by the examiner holding the extremity.

4. State of alertness: Perform the examination when the infant is in the quiet alert state (optimally 30–60 minutes before a feeding). Note state of alertness before, during, and after the examination. State is affected by gestational age, feeding schedule, prior handling, and stimulation. The infant may pass through several state changes during the examination (deep and light sleep, drowsy, quiet alert, active alert, crying). Persistent irritability or lethargy is not normal.

5. Muscle tone

    a. Phasic tone is tested by evaluating the resistance of the upper and lower extremities to movement (scarf sign; arm and leg recoil). Tendon reflexes are tested by sharp percussion with examiner's finger over the

● TABLE 7-2
Neonatal Neurologic Evaluation

Test	Technique	Normal for Term	Deviant for Term
Resting posture	Observe unswaddled infant without contact in quiet awake, quiet active, or light sleep states	Moderate flexion of four limbs, held off bed Equal side-to-side and upper-to-lower if head is in midline Extension of neck in face presentation or legs in breech presentation	Constant tight flexion Full extension, flaccid or forced Knees abducted to bed (i.e., frog-leg) Elbows flexed with dorsum of hands on bed Tight, persistent fisting ATNR persistent ≥30 sec
State	Deep sleep Light sleep Awake, light peripheral movements Awake, large movements, not crying Awake, crying	Moves from one to the other with appropriate stimuli Self-calms Modulated cry with expression	Strong lateral preference; difficult to move from one state to the other Stays too alert or cries without physical reason Does not come to fully awake state Weak or monotonous cry
Motor activity	Observe throughout physical examination	Appropriate for state of alertness Symmetric, fairly smooth Expressive face with yawn or cry	Bicycling, swatting without stimulus Asymmetric, weak Jittery while sucking Flat facial expression
Phasic (i.e., passive) tone: resistance to movement	Measure resistance to extension (limb recoil) Scarf, heel to ear	Response appropriate for gestational age	Resists too much or too little Asymmetry
Tendon reflexes	Test patellar reflex with head midline	Patellar reflex is only reflex reliably present at birth	Sustained clonus
Postural (i.e., active) tone: resistance to gravity			
Traction response	Pull to sitting while grasping infant's hands	Infant pulls back with flexion at elbows, knees, and ankles Head comes with body with minimal lag and falls forward when sitting is obtained	Asymmetry in pulling back No resistance Full head lag Pull to stand instead Head does not fall forward as infant goes past upright

ATNR, asymmetrical tonic neck reflex.

(Continued)

● TABLE 7-2
Neonatal Neurologic Evaluation—cont'd

Test	Technique	Normal for Term	Deviant for Term
Vertical suspension	Suspend infant facing examiner with both hands in axillae	Infant supports self then yields slowly Holds head erect, flexes hips, knees, ankles Eyes open	Infant falls through immediately Legs extend Eyes fail to open Infant fails to relax and fall through after 1 min
Horizontal suspension	Hold infant under chest and suspend in prone position Galant: stroke adjacent to spine Landau: stroke caudalcephalad along spine	Flexes arms, extends neck, holds back straight Curves toward side of stimulus Extends back, lifts head and pelvis, micturates	Hangs limply or excessively rigidly Asymmetric incurving Weak or absent response
Positive support	Hold infant to support trunk with feet touching firm, flat surface	Infant extends hips to bear own weight and relaxes after 1 min	Infant fails to bear weight or extends too much or too long
Integrated reflexes			
Moro reflex	Hold infant in supine position; support head and neck with hand; allow head to drop while still supporting it	Spreading: arms abduct, extend; hands open Hugging: arms abduct and flex; hands close	Absence of spread Asymmetry Exaggeration with disorganization in state
Tonic neck reflex	Infant in supine, neutral position; turn head to one side; repeat opposite side	Mental extension, occipital flexion primarily of arms; does not remain in position for >30 sec	Exaggerated response and stays in position >30 sec
Withdrawal reflex	Painful stimulus to one foot	Withdrawal of stimulated foot; variable extension of opposite leg	Absence of flexion in stimulated leg

From Avery G, editor: *Neonatology—pathophysiology and management of the newborn*, ed 4, Philadelphia, 1994, JB Lippincott, pp 284-285.

tendon. The biceps reflex and the patellar (knee jerk) reflex can be tested in the newborn. Weak or absent reflexes may be seen with birth asphyxia, sepsis, or dysfunction of the motor unit. Sustained clonus (>8–10 beats) is abnormal and may be seen in drug withdrawal or cerebral irritation.

b. Postural tone is tested by evaluating the resistance to gravity. It is best tested by the traction response (pull-to-sit maneuver; Figure 7-16).

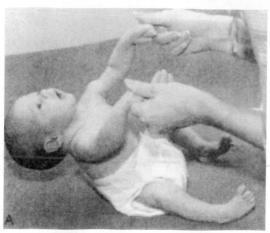

FIGURE 7-16 ● Pull-to-sit maneuver with grasp reflex and normal infant head lag. (From Schulte EB, Price DL, James SR, editors: *Thompson's pediatric nursing: an introductory text*, ed 7, Philadelphia, 1997, WB Saunders, p 59.)

By grasping the neonate's hands and pulling slowly from the supine position, the infant will pull back with flexion at elbows, knees, and ankles. The head comes with the body with minimal lag and falls forward when sitting is obtained. In the term newborn, more than minimal head lag is abnormal and may indicate hypotonia.

    c. Abnormalities of tone may indicate hypo- or hypertonia. Hypotonia is the most frequent abnormality observed during the neurologic examination. Further work-up is necessary if abnormalities of tone persist.

6. Muscle strength: Directly correlates with muscle tone. Upper extremity strength is tested using the grasp reflex and the pull-to-sit maneuver. Lower extremity strength is assessed by observing the stepping reflex; when newborn is held upright with the soles of the feet touching a flat surface, alternating stepping movements can be observed (Figure 7-17).

7. Assessment of development reflexes
    a. Sucking reflex (Figure 7-18): Present at birth. After touching or stroking the lips, the mouth opens and sucking movements begin. A gloved finger gently inserted into the mouth can evaluate strength and coordination of the suck reflex.
    b. Rooting reflex (Figure 7-19): After the cheek or corner of the mouth is stroked, the infant's head should turn toward the stimulus and the mouth should open.
    c. Palmar grasp (Figure 7-20): Stroking the palm of the infant's hand with a finger should cause the infant to grasp the finger. The grasp will tighten with attempts to withdraw the finger. Palmar grasp can be tested bilaterally and the infant can be lifted off the bed for several seconds.
    d. Plantar grasp (Figure 7-21): Elicited by stimulating the ball of the foot by firm pressure.

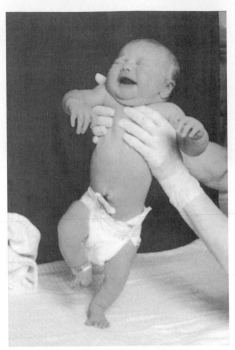

FIGURE 7-17 ● Stepping reflex. (From Nichols FM, Zwelling E: *Maternal-newborn nursing: theory and practice*, Philadelphia, 1997, WB Saunders, p 1117.)

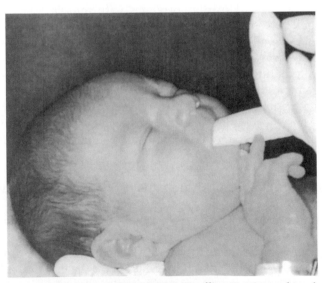

FIGURE 7-18 ● Sucking reflex. (From Nichols FM, Zwelling E: *Maternal-newborn nursing: theory and practice*, Philadelphia, 1997, WB Saunders, p 1115.)

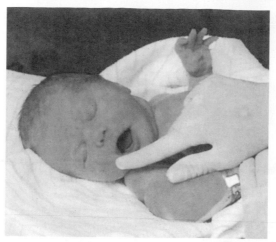

FIGURE 7-19 ● Rooting reflex. (From Nichols FM, Zwelling E: *Maternal-newborn nursing: theory and practice*, Philadelphia, 1997, WB Saunders, p 1115.)

  e. Tonic neck reflex (also known as fencing position; Figure 7-22): With the infant in a supine, neutral position, turn head to one side. The upper extremity on the side the head is turned toward is extended and the upper extremity on the opposite side should flex. An exaggerated response or inability to elicit the reflex can indicate an abnormality.
  f. Moro reflex (also known as the startle reflex; Figure 7-23): Hold infant in a supine and neutral position several centimeters off the bed.

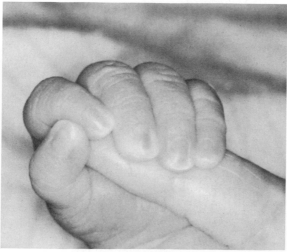

FIGURE 7-20 ● Palmar grasp. (From Nichols FM, Zwelling E: *Maternal-newborn nursing: theory and practice*, Philadelphia, 1997, WB Saunders, p 1116.)

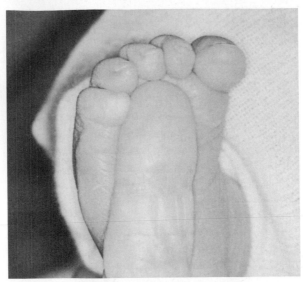

FIGURE 7-21 ● Plantar grasp. (From Nichols FM, Zwelling E: *Maternal-newborn nursing: theory and practice*, Philadelphia, 1997, WB Saunders, p 1116.)

Support the head and neck with hand. Allow head to drop into examiner's hand while still supporting it. In the first response, the arms extend and abduct and hands open. That response is followed by an inward movement with flexion of the arms and closing of the hands. A cry may follow. Complete absence of the reflex is abnormal. Asymmetric movements may indicate a localized neurologic defect.

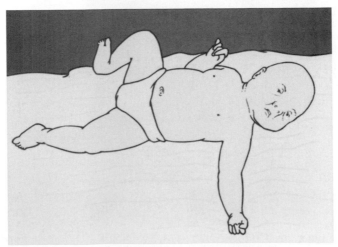

FIGURE 7-22 ● Tonic neck reflex. (From Nichols FM, Zwelling E: *Maternal-newborn nursing: theory and practice*, Philadelphia, 1997, WB Saunders, p 1118.)

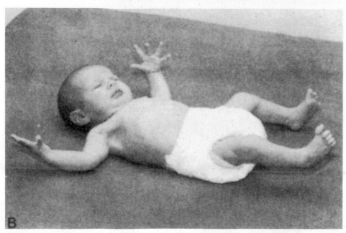

FIGURE 7-23 ● Moro reflex. (From Schulte EB, Price DL, James SR, editors: *Thompson's pediatric nursing: an introductory text*, ed 7, Philadelphia, 1997, WB Saunders, p 59.)

    g. Stepping reflex (see Figure 7-17): When the infant is held upright with the soles of the feet touching a flat surface, alternating stepping movements can be observed.

    h. Truncal incurvation (also known as Galant reflex; Figure 7-24): Hold infant under the chest and suspend in prone position. Stroke adjacent to the spine with cotton swab or thumb. Flexion of the pelvis toward the side of the stimulus is a positive response.

    i. Babinski reflex (Figure 7-25): Plantar flexion occurs after stimulation of the sole of the foot. A positive response occurs if extension or flexion of the

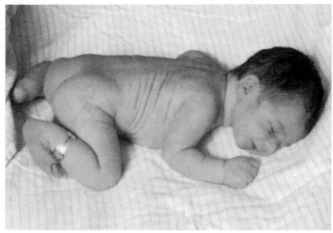

FIGURE 7-24 ● Truncal incurvation (Galant reflex). (From Nichols FM, Zwelling E: *Maternal-newborn nursing: theory and practice*, Philadelphia, 1997, WB Saunders, p 1117.)

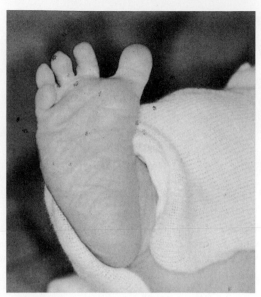

FIGURE 7-25 ● Babinski reflex. (From Nichols FM, Zwelling E: *Maternal-newborn nursing: theory and practice*, Philadelphia, 1997, WB Saunders, p 1118.)

toes occurs. Consistent absence of the reflex is abnormal and may indicate central nervous system depression or a spinal nerve innervation problem.

  j. Placing reflex: The infant is held upright and suspended by the examiner with hands under both axillae. The infant is slowly raised until the dorsum of the foot touches a protruding edge, usually the bassinet edge. Infant replaces the ipsilateral foot back on the edge after hip and knee flexion.

8. Sensory function

  a. Touch: A painful stimulus to a foot elicits a withdrawal reflex. Touch the sole of the foot with a pin to provoke flexion of the limb and extension of the contralateral limb. Absence of flexion in the stimulated leg is abnormal.

  b. Response to light: A penlight shone in infant's eye results in eyelid closure.

  c. Response to sound: A bell is rung sharply within a few inches of the infant's ear while infant is lying supine. Response is based on observable attentiveness to the sound. A formal brainstem auditory-evoked response may be needed if there are concerns about hearing or a family history of hearing loss.

9. Evaluation of the cranial nerves

  a. Olfactory (I): Test by placing a strong-smelling substance (oil of cloves, peppermint, or anise) under the nose and evaluating for startle, grimace, or sniffing.

b. Optic (II): Test by checking pupils for size and constriction in response to light. Also evaluate the ability of the neonate's eyes to fix on an object and follow it over an arc of 60 degrees.

c. Oculomotor (III), trochlear (IV), and abducens (VI): These nerves supply the pupil and the extraocular muscles. Test by observing pupillary response to light. Evaluate spontaneous movements of the eye, its size, and symmetry. Movement of the eyes as the head is turning is evaluated. The "doll's eye" test consists of rotating the head from side to side and evaluating for movement of the eyes away from the direction of rotation. A normal response is the eyes deviating to the left when the head turns to the right. If eyes remain in a fixed position, or move in the same direction as the head, brainstem or oculomotor nerve dysfunction may be present.

d. Trigeminal (V): Supplies the jaw muscles and sensory innervation of the face. Test by touching the cheek. The infant should turn the cheek toward the stimulus. Also evaluate the biting portion of the suck by placing a gloved finger in the neonate's mouth.

e. Facial (VII): Controls facial expression. Note asymmetric facial movements. Severe injury can result in obvious facial weakness or an inability to wrinkle the brow or close the eyes with crying.

f. Auditory (VIII): Tested grossly as described in "Sensory function" above.

g. Glossopharyngeal (IX): Evaluate by inspecting tongue movement and eliciting a gag reflex.

h. Vagus (X): Supplies soft palate, pharynx, and larynx. Evaluate by listening to the cry and assessing presence of hoarseness, stridor, or aphonia. Assess ability to swallow.

i. Accessory (XI): Supplies sternocleidomastoid and trapezius muscles. Test by turning supine infant's head to one side; infant should attempt to bring head to midline.

j. Hypoglossal (XII): Supplies muscles of the tongue. Evaluate sucking, swallowing, and gagging.

ASSESSMENT OF GESTATIONAL AGE

A gestational age examination should be performed on each infant. Knowing the gestational age assists in determination of appropriateness of physical findings, helps identify potential morbidities that are more common with various gestational ages, and determines neonatal mortality risk (Amiel-Tison, 1968; Dubowitz et al., 1970).

A. **Prenatal Determination of Gestational Age**

1. Date of last menstrual period is the most commonly used method.

2. Date of first reported fetal activity: "Quickening" usually occurs at 16–18 weeks.

3. First reported heart sounds: 10–12 weeks by Doppler ultrasound.

4. Ultrasound examination: Very reliable if obtained before 20 weeks.

B. **Classification by Gestational Age and Size**
1. Classification by gestational age
   a. Term: >37 to <42 weeks
   b. Preterm: <37 weeks
   c. Post-term: ≥42 weeks
2. Classification by size (fetal growth)
   a. Small for gestational age (SGA): Weight <10th percentile for gestational age
   b. Appropriate for gestational age (AGA): Weight between 10th and 90th percentile for gestational age
   c. Large for gestational age (LGA): Weight >90th percentile for gestational age
C. **Postnatal Assessment of Gestational Age by Physical and Neurologic Criteria**: The New Ballard Score (Figure 7-26): Based on six physical and six neurologic criteria; for infants >20 weeks gestation, this scoring system is accurate within 2 weeks of gestational age whether the infant is sick or well (Ballard et al., 1991).
   1. Timing of examination
      a. Most accurate when performed <12 hours after delivery for infants 20–26 weeks gestation.
      b. Valid for the first 96 hours of life for infants >26 weeks gestation.
   2. Examination technique
      a. The examination is administered twice by two separate examiners to ensure objectivity. This New Ballard Score form is available in most nurseries.
      b. The 12 scores (physical + neuromuscular maturity) are totaled, and maturity rating is expressed in weeks of gestation using the chart provided on the form.
   3. Physical maturity scoring
      a. Skin: The skin becomes less transparent, thicker, and tougher with increasing gestational age. Extremely premature infants have sticky, transparent skin and are given a score of –1.
      b. Lanugo (Figure 7-27): Examined on the infant's back, between and over the scapulae. A fine downy hair covers the body of the fetus from 20 to 28 weeks with only few patches over the shoulder present at term.
      c. Plantar surface of the foot: Measure foot length from the tip of the great toe to the back of the heel (Color Plate 46).
      d. Breast tissue: Observe for nipple size and development and for amount of breast tissue.
      e. Eye and ear: Loosely fused eyelids are those that open with gentle traction; tightly fused eyelids are defined as inseparable by gentle traction. The pinna in the term ear is well formed and quickly returns to position. In the preterm infant the pinna shows little curving and recoils slowly (Figure 7-28).
      f. Genitalia (Figures 7-29 and 7-30): Use the New Ballard Score chart (see Figure 7-26).

Neuromuscular Maturity

	-1	0	1	2	3	4	5
Posture							
Square Window (wrist)	>90°	90°	60°	45°	30°	0°	
Arm Recoil		180°	140°-180°	110°-140°	90°-110°	<90°	
Popliteal Angle	180°	160°	140°	120°	100°	90°	<90°
Scarf Sign							
Heel to Ear							

Physical Maturity

Skin	sticky friable transparent	gelatinous red, translucent	smooth pink, visible veins	superficial peeling &/or rash. few veins	cracking pale areas rare veins	parchment deep cracking no vessels	leathery cracked wrinkled
Lanugo	none	sparse	abundant	thinning	bald areas	mostly bald	
Plantar Surface	heel-toe 40-50mm:-1 <40mm:-2	>50mm no crease	faint red marks	anterior transverse crease only	creases ant. 2/3	creases over entire sole	
Breast	imperceptible	barely perceptible	flat areola no bud	stippled areola 1-2mm bud	raised areola 3-4mm bud	full areola 5-10mm bud	
Eye/Ear	lids fused loosely:-1 tightly:-2	lids open pinna flat stays folded	sl. curved pinna; soft; slow recoil	well-curved pinna; soft but ready recoil	formed &firm instant recoil	thick cartilage ear stiff	
Genitals male	scrotum flat, smooth	scrotum empty faint rugae	testes in upper canal rare rugae	testes descending few rugae	testes down good rugae	testes pendulous deep rugae	
Genitals female	clitoris prominent labia flat	prominent clitoris small labia minora	prominent clitoris enlarging minora	majora & minora equally prominent	majora large minora small	majora cover clitoris & minora	

Maturity Rating

score	weeks
-10	20
-5	22
0	24
5	26
10	28
15	30
20	32
25	34
30	36
35	38
40	40
45	42
50	44

FIGURE 7-26 ● Maturational assessment of gestational age (New Ballard Score). (From Ballard JL, Khoury JC, Wedig K, et al: New Ballard Score, expanded to include extremely premature infants, *J Pediatr* 119:417-423, 1991.)

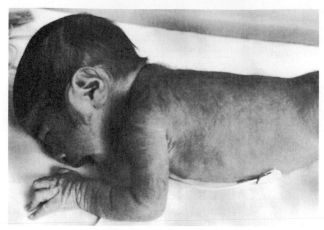

FIGURE 7-27 ● Lanugo. (From Gorrie T, McKinney E, Murray S: *Foundations of maternal newborn nursing*, Philadelphia, 1994, WB Saunders, p 541.)

4. Neuromuscular maturity: Neuromuscular criteria are based on the understanding that passive tone is more useful than active tone in determining gestational age.
   a. Posture (Figure 7-31): Score while the infant is quiet and relaxed.
   b. Square window (Figure 7-32): Flex the hand on the forearm between the thumb and index finger of the examiner. Apply sufficient pressure to

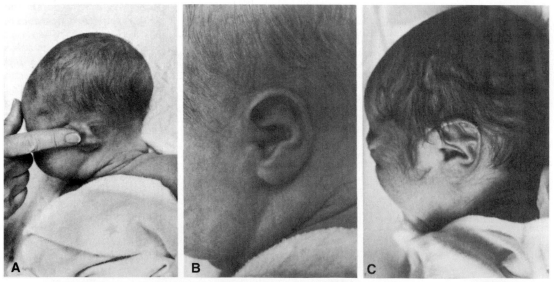

FIGURE 7-28 ● Ear maturation. **A** and **B,** Full-term infant. **C,** Preterm infant. (From Gorrie T, McKinney E, Murray S: *Foundations of maternal newborn nursing*, Philadelphia, 1994, WB Saunders, p 542.)

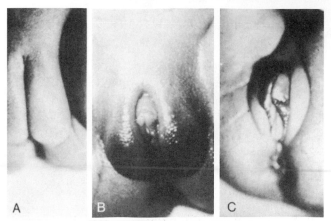

FIGURE 7-29 ● Female genitalia. **A,** Full-term infant. **B,** Near-term infant. **C,** Preterm infant. (From Gorrie T, McKinney E, Murray S: *Foundations of maternal newborn nursing,* Philadelphia, 1994, WB Saunders, p 542.)

get as much flexion as possible and visually measure the angle between the hypothenar eminence and the ventral aspect of the forearm.

   c. Arm recoil (Figure 7-33): Flex the forearms for 5 seconds. Then grasp the hand and fully extend the arm and release. Score based on arm position after release.

   d. Popliteal angle (Figure 7-34): Hold the thigh in the knee-chest position with the left index finger and the thumb supporting the knee.

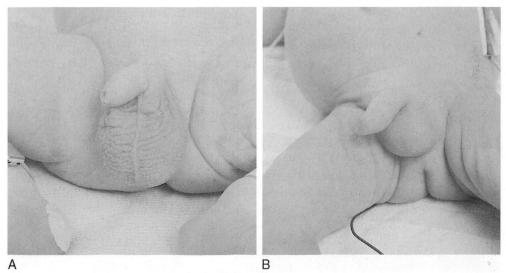

FIGURE 7-30 ● Male genitalia. **A,** Full-term infant. **B,** Preterm infant. (From Gorrie T, McKinney E, Murray S: *Foundations of maternal newborn nursing,* Philadelphia, 1994, WB Saunders, p 543.)

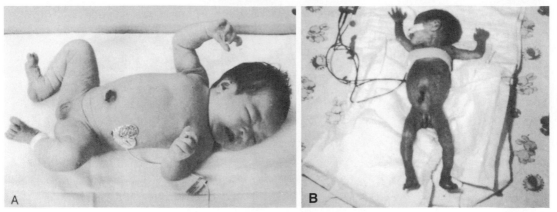

FIGURE 7-31 ● **A,** Term posture (flexed). **B,** Preterm posture (extended). (From Gorrie T, McKinney E, Murray S: *Foundations of maternal newborn nursing,* Philadelphia, 1994, WB Saunders, p 537.)

Then extend the leg by applying gentle pressure from the right index behind the ankle. Measure the angle at the popliteal space and score accordingly.

   e. Scarf sign (Figure 7-35): Take the infant's hand and try to put it around the neck posteriorly as far as possible over the opposite shoulder while keeping the infant's back flat on the examination surface.

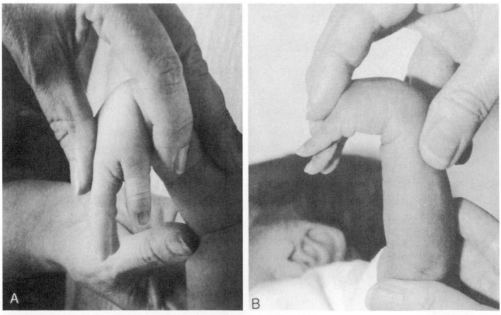

FIGURE 7-32 ● Square window sign. **A,** Term infant. **B,** Preterm infant. (From Gorrie T, McKinney E, Murray S: *Foundations of maternal newborn nursing,* Philadelphia, 1994, WB Saunders, p 538.)

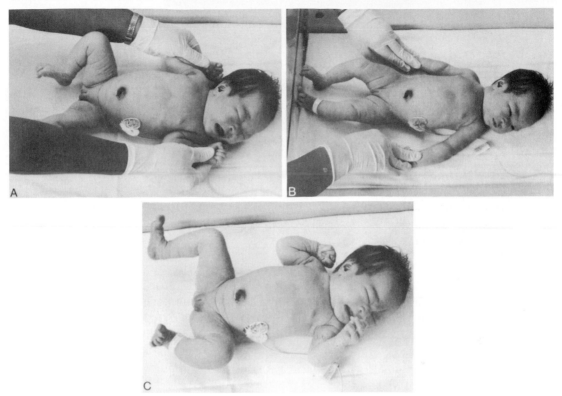

FIGURE 7-33 ● Arm recoil. **A,** Arms flexed. **B,** Arms extended. **C,** Recoil in full-term infant. (From Gorrie T, McKinney E, Murray S: *Foundations of maternal newborn nursing,* Philadelphia, 1994, WB Saunders, p 541.)

      f. Heel to ear (Figure 7-36): Keeping the pelvis flat on the table, take the infant's foot and try to put it as close to the head as possible without forcing it.

D. Postnatal Assessment of Gestational Age by Examination of the Anterior Vascular Capsule of the Lens (Hittner et al., 1977)

    1. Technique

      a. Uses direct ophthalmoscopy of the lens.

      b. For best results, the pupil should be dilated under the supervision of an ophthalmologist.

      c. The assessment must be performed within 24–48 hours of birth before the vessels atrophy.

    2. Examination scoring (Figure 7-37)

      a. Grade 4 (27–28 weeks): Vessels cover the entire anterior surface of the lens, or the vessels meet in the center of the lens.

      b. Grade 3 (29–30 weeks) Vessels do not meet in the center but are close. Central portion of the lens is not covered by vessels.

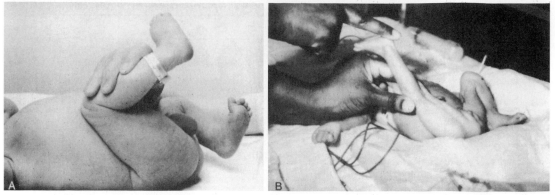

FIGURE 7-34 ● Popliteal angle. **A,** Full-term infant. **B,** Preterm infant. (From Gorrie T, McKinney E, Murray S: *Foundations of maternal newborn nursing,* Philadelphia, 1994, WB Saunders, p 539.)

    c. Grade 2 (31–32 weeks): Vessels reach only to the middle-outer part of the lens. The central clear portion of the lens is larger.

    d. Grade 1 (33–34 weeks): Vessels are seen only at the periphery of the lens.

  3. Accuracy

    a. Good correlation between the vessel changes and gestational age between 27 and 34 weeks.

    b. Before 27 weeks, the cornea is too opaque to allow visualization; after 34 weeks, atrophy of the vessels of the lens occur.

    c. The correlation between examination and gestational age does not appear to be affected by size at birth (i.e., same accuracy in SGA, AGA, and LGA infants).

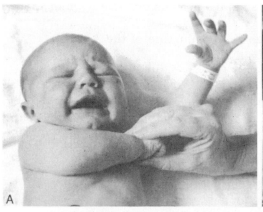
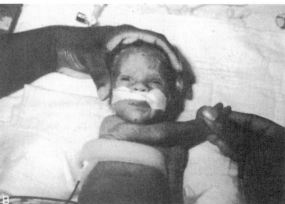

FIGURE 7-35 ● Scarf sign. **A,** Full-term infant. **B,** Preterm infant. (From Gorrie T, McKinney E, Murray S: *Foundations of maternal newborn nursing,* Philadelphia, 1994, WB Saunders, p 539.)

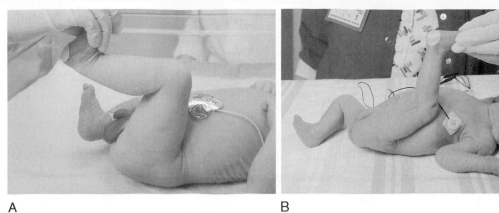

A   B

FIGURE 7-36 ● Heel-to-ear. **A,** Full-term infant. **B,** Preterm infant. (From Gorrie T, McKinney E, Murray S: *Foundations of maternal newborn nursing,* Philadelphia, 1994, WB Saunders, p 540.)

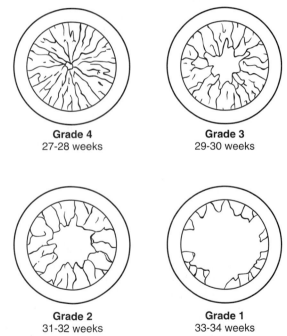

Grade 4
27-28 weeks

Grade 3
29-30 weeks

Grade 2
31-32 weeks

Grade 1
33-34 weeks

FIGURE 7-37 ● Grading system for assessment of gestational age by examination of the anterior vascular capsule of the lens. (From Hittner HM, Hirsch NJ, Rudolph AJ: Assessment of gestational age by examination of the anterior vascular capsule of the lens, *J Pediatr* 91:455, 1977.)

REFERENCES

American Academy of Pediatrics: Timing of elective surgery on the genitalia of male children with particular reference to the risks, benefits, and psychological effects of surgery and anesthesia, *Pediatrics* 97:590-594, 1996.

American Academy of Pediatrics: Clinical practice guideline: early detection of developmental dysplasia of the hip, *Pediatrics* 105:896-905, 2000.

American Academy of Pediatrics: Health supervision for children with Down syndrome, *Pediatrics* 107:442-449, 2001.

American Academy of Pediatrics: Hearing assessment in infants and children: recommendations beyond neonatal screening, *Pediatrics* 111:436-440, 2003.

American Cleft Palate–Craniofacial Association: Parameters for the evaluation and treatment of patients with cleft lip/palate or other craniofacial anomalies, *Cleft Palate Craniofac J* 30:S1-S16, 1993.

Amiel-Tison C: Neurological evaluation of the maturity of newborn infants, *Arch Dis Child* 43:89-93, 1968.

Avery G, editor: *Neonatology-pathophysiology and management of the newborn,* ed 4, Philadelphia, 1994, JB Lippincott.

Ballard JL, Khoury JC, Wedig K, et al: New Ballard Score, expanded to include extremely premature infants, *J Pediatr* 119:417-423, 1991.

Cloherty JP, Stark AR, editors: *Manual of neonatal care,* ed 3, Boston, 1991, Little, Brown.

Cronk C, Crocker AC, Pueschel SM, et al: Growth charts for children with Down syndrome: 1 month to 18 years of age, *Pediatrics* 81:102-110, 1988.

Driscoll JM: Physical examination and care of the newborn. In Fanaroff M, editors: *Neonatal perinatal medicine,* ed 5, St Louis, 1992, Mosby Year Book, pp 325-345.

Dubowitz LMS, Dubowitz V, Goldberg C: Clinical assessment of gestational age in the newborn infant, *J Pediatr* 1970; 77:1-10.

Duc G, Largo RH: Anterior fontanel: size and closure in term and preterm infants, *Pediatrics* 1986, 78:904-908.

Gornella TL, editor: *Neonatology,* ed 2, Norwalk, CT, 1994, Appleton and Lange.

Hittner HM, Hirsch NJ, Rudolph AJ: Assessment of gestational age by examination of the anterior vascular capsule of the lens, *J Pediatr* 91:455-458, 1977.

Hockenberry MJ: *Wong's nursing care of infants and children,* ed 7, St Louis, 2003, Mosby.

Klaus MH, Fanaroff AA, editors: *Care of the high-risk neonate,* ed 4, Philadelphia, 1993, WB Saunders Co.

Merenstein GB, Gardner SL, editors: *Handbook of neonatal intensive care,* ed 3, St Louis, 1993, CV Mosby.

Ogawa GSH, Gonnering RS: Congenital nasolacrimal duct obstruction, *J Pediatr* 119:12-17, 1991.

Phibbs, RH: The newborn infant. In Rudolph AM, editor: *Rudolph's pediatrics,* ed 19, Norwalk, CT, 1991, Appleton and Lange, pp 165-210.

Rosenberg AA, Thilo EH: The newborn infant. In Hay WW Jr, editor: *Current pediatric diagnosis and treatment,* ed 12, Norwalk, CT, 1995, Appleton and Lange.

Scanlon JW, editor: *A system of newborn physical examination,* Baltimore, 1979, University Park Press.

Silverman SH, Leibow SG: Dislocation of the triangular cartilage of the nasal septum, *J Pediatr* 87:456-458, 1975.

Smith DW, Gong BT: Scalp hair patterning as a clue to early fetal brain development, *J Pediatr* 83:374-380, 1973.

Wahrman JE, Honig PJ: Hemangiomas, *Pediatr Rev* 15:266-271, 1994.

Post-Transition Care

With the trend toward early discharge for the family with an uncomplicated post-partum and newborn course, the time for consideration of post-transition care may be as short as hours. The goals of this critical time period include continued intensive observation for indicators of illness, assessment of unique needs of the individual newborn, establishment of a basis for successful feeding and care of the newborn, and identification and initiation of necessary follow-up care.

8 Feeding the Newborn

Sharon M. Glass, RNC, MS, NNP

BREAST-FEEDING

The American Academy of Pediatrics (AAP) recommends human milk as the ideal source of nutrition for all infants, stating that "all substitute feeding options differ markedly from it" (AAP, 1997). National health initiatives have set goals to increase both the initiation and duration of breast-feeding. A recent survey of breast-feeding prevalence in the United States shows initiation of breast-feeding near the national goal of 75%; however, continuation of breast-feeding to 6 and 12 months falls far short of the desired goals (Li et al., 2003).

A. **Benefits**
   1. Natural, convenient, easily digested, optimal for infant growth and development, species-specific.
   2. Enhances mother-infant interaction and attachment.
   3. Strong evidence for conferring protection against illness: diarrhea, otitis media, lower respiratory tract infections, bacteremia, bacterial meningitis, botulism, urinary tract infections, necrotizing enterocolitis.
   4. Possible protective effect: sudden infant death syndrome, insulin-dependent diabetes, chronic digestive diseases, lymphoma, some allergic diseases.
   5. Related to enhanced cognitive development.
   6. Possible maternal health benefits: release of oxytocin, aiding uterine involution and decreasing postpartum bleeding; earlier pregnancy weight loss; increased child spacing due to ovulation delay; improved bone remineralization; decreased risk for ovarian and breast cancer.
   7. Societal/economic benefits from improved health status.

B. **Contraindications**
   1. Maternal HIV infection: risk for transmission to infant (may not be a consideration in countries where the highest mortality risks are due to infectious diseases and nutritional deficiencies).
   2. Active herpes infection of the breast.
   3. Maternal active tuberculosis infection (if untreated).
   4. Debilitating maternal disease in which lactation would worsen maternal condition.
   5. Infant galactosemia disorder.
   6. Certain maternal medication or illicit drug ingestion (AAP, 2001).
      a. Prescription medications rarely preclude breast-feeding.
         (1) See Appendix B for drugs that are contraindicated during breast-feeding.

    (2) Nuclear radiopharmaceuticals for diagnostic studies require temporary cessation of breast-feeding until radioactivity clears breast milk.

    (3) Cytotoxic drugs may cause immune suppression.

    (4) Effect of psychotropic drugs on nursing infants is unknown but may be of concern with long-term maternal use.

b. Some over-the-counter medications, environmental agents, or foods may also have adverse effects on the nursing infant and should be avoided or used with caution (see Appendix B).

c. Mothers should be counseled against breast-feeding if they use illicit drugs or regularly consume alcoholic beverages.

d. When maternal drug therapy is necessary, the physician should ensure that: (1) the safest drug is used; (2) if there is an associated risk to the infant, measuring infant blood concentrations is considered; (3) infant exposure is minimized by instructing mother to take medications just after breast-feeding; and (4) adverse effects encountered in infants are communicated to the AAP Committee on Drugs and the Food and Drug Administration.

e. Maternal smoking results in milk concentrations of nicotine 1.5–3 times the maternal plasma concentration. Although there is no evidence documenting infant health risk, smoking cessation should be urged for maternal health reasons.

f. Silicone breast implants do not contraindicate breast-feeding. Cow milk and formula have higher silicone concentrations than that found in the milk of mothers with implants. Simethicone, used for infant colic without reports of toxicity, is similar to the silicone in implants.

TECHNIQUES FOR SUCCESSFUL BREAST-FEEDING

A. Positioning During Breast-Feeding

  1. Side-lying (Figure 8-1): Infant and mother face each other lying on their sides. Infant is brought to the lower breast or mother leans over infant to present the upper breast. Mother uses her opposite hand to support the breast with her fingers underneath and thumb on top of the breast in a "C" configuration (Figure 8-2).

  2. Football hold (Figure 8-3): Position infant on pillows at mother's side. Mother cradles the infant's head in her hand and brings infant to her breast on that side.

  3. Cradle hold (Figure 8-4): Mother cradles infant across her abdomen with the infant's head in the antecubital fossa and arm behind mother.

  4. Cross-cradle hold (Figure 8-5): Infant lies across mother's abdomen facing the breast. She cradles the infant's head with the hand opposite the side of the breast and holds her breast with the other hand. The other arm supports the infant's body and allows mother to guide the infant to the breast.

B. Latching-On (Figure 8-6): Process by which infants learn to establish appropriate suckling by taking the entire nipple/areola area into their mouths.

  1. Mother-infant pair should assume a comfortable position.

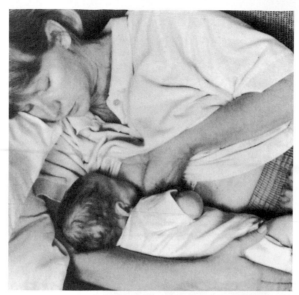

FIGURE 8-1 ● Side-lying position. (From Gorrie TM, McKinney ES, Murray SS: *Foundations of maternal newborn nursing,* Philadelphia, 1994, WB Saunders, p 571.)

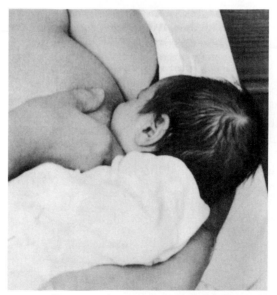

FIGURE 8-2 ● "C" position of hand on breast. (From Gorrie TM, McKinney ES, Murray SS: *Foundations of maternal newborn nursing,* Philadelphia, 1994, WB Saunders, p 571.)

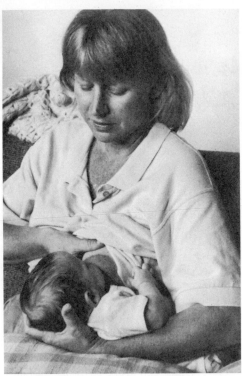

FIGURE 8-3 ● Football hold. (From Gorrie TM, McKinney ES, Murray SS: *Foundations of maternal newborn nursing*, Philadelphia, 1994, WB Saunders, p 570.)

2. Mother supports breast with fingers below and thumb on top, well behind the nipple/areola.
3. Gently stroke the infant's lower lip and cheek with nipple.
4. Wait until infant's mouth is wide open and then insert nipple and areola as far as possible in the center of the infant's mouth.
5. Pull the infant close so that the tip of the nose touches but is not occluded by the breast.
6. Mother should be cautioned against allowing infant to chew on the nipple.
7. As the infant suckles, let-down will be triggered, followed by long sucks and repeated swallowing.

C. **Feeding Frequency and Duration**
1. Breast-feeding should begin immediately after birth if mother and infant are well. Ideally, the infant should not be separated from the mother to accommodate routine transitional procedures such as observation, weight, measurements, medications, or bathing. Delay in breast-feeding or decrease in frequency during the first postpartum day can initiate a cycle that leads to maternal engorgement, breast-feeding failure, and infant hyper-bilirubinemia, thus leading to further separation (AAP, 1997; Slusser and Frantz, 2001).

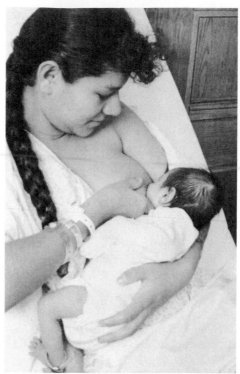

FIGURE 8-4 ● Cradle hold. (From Gorrie TM, McKinney ES, Murray SS: *Foundations of maternal newborn nursing,* Philadelphia, 1994, WB Saunders, p 569.)

2. Encourage 8–12 feedings per 24 hours for the first few weeks.
   a. Frequent feedings establish maternal milk supply and minimize breast-feeding jaundice.
   b. Human milk protein is easily digested, which leads to rapid stomach emptying time and necessitates frequent feedings.
   c. Milk should "come in" by 2–4 days after delivery (breasts will feel full and tight before the infant nurses).
3. Both breasts should be offered at each feeding.
   a. Babies get more milk from nursing at both breasts even though they usually do not nurse as vigorously or as long on the second breast.
   b. Alternate starting breast to ensure that both breasts get adequate stimulation and emptying.
4. Feeding interval should be approximately 1.5–3 hours, with one 4- to 5-hour interval at night (initially some infants may need to be awakened if they do not demand).
5. Feedings are most successful when the infant indicates hunger (awake, rooting, sucking on fists). Crying is a late indication.
6. In the absence of maternal discomfort, duration of feeding should not be limited; infant should be allowed to nurse until satisfied. By 3–5 days of

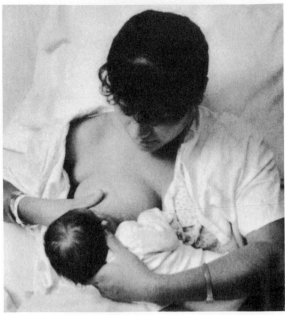

FIGURE 8-5 ● Cross-cradle hold. (From Gorrie TM, McKinney ES, Murray SS: *Foundations of maternal newborn nursing*, Philadelphia, 1994, WB Saunders, p 570.)

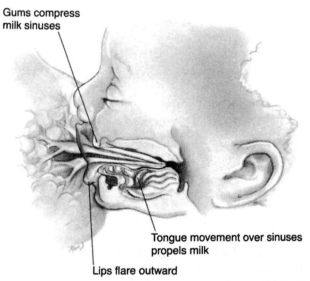

FIGURE 8-6 ● Infant's mouth position while sucking. (From Gorrie TM, McKinney ES, Murray SS: *Foundations of maternal newborn nursing*, Philadelphia, 1994, WB Saunders, p 572.)

age, the infant should be suckling approximately 10 minutes per breast per feeding.

7. Need for supplementary feedings
   a. Unless medically indicated, no supplementary water or formula should be given until breast-feeding is successfully established.
   b. For jaundice or excessive weight loss, increase frequency of breast-feeding. Supplement with formula only if deemed medically necessary or if mother's preference.
   c. For mild hypoglycemia, increase frequency of breast-feeding and supplement with formula.

8. Determining adequate milk supply: Assure parents that after the milk comes in, they can determine whether infant is getting enough milk by the following:
   a. Infant's urine will be colorless to pale yellow, with six to eight wet diapers per day.
   b. Stools are usually frequent (four or more per day) and look like "cottage cheese and mustard" by 4–5 days of age.
   c. Infant should appear satisfied after nursing and frequently will fall asleep at the second breast.
   d. Breasts should feel full before feedings and softer after nursing.
   e. By 2–3 weeks the let-down reflex will be recognized (breasts will feel "tight" or "tingle" as milk begins to flow, infants may gulp or drip milk from the mouth while sucking, milk may drip from other breast).
   f. Consistent weekly weight gain will be noted after the first 7–10 days of life (expected initial weight loss is <7% of birth weight; expected gain is approximately 1 oz/day in the first month after milk is in).

D. **Preventing Common Problems**
   1. Provide mother with written information regarding breast-feeding expectations for home reference (Table 8-1) and a list of local resources to call for breast-feeding information, support, and equipment.
   2. The breast-feeding couple should be seen by a health care practitioner when the infant is 2–4 days of age and evaluated for successful breast-feeding (feeding behaviors, hydration, jaundice, urination, and stooling).
   3. Provide lactation consultation as available and as needed.
   4. Sore nipples
      a. This is the most common problem and a frequent cause of cessation.
      b. Mild discomfort at the beginning of feedings during the first week is expected and requires no treatment.
      c. Persistent or severe pain is abnormal and requires evaluation. Also abnormal are red, cracked, or blistered nipples. Limiting breast-feeding does not improve nipple soreness. Commonly, the cause is poor positioning and incorrect latching-on. Observe the mother-infant pair and assist with the following:
         (1) Latch-on and position properly as outlined above.
         (2) Begin feeding on the least sore side; this will allow the infant to satiate slightly, and nursing will be less vigorous on the sore side. Return to alternating the beginning breast as soon as possible.

● TABLE 8-1
Example of Breast-Feeding Support Information Given to Mother Before Discharge

	First 8 Hours	8–24 Hours	Day 2	Day 3	Day 4	Day 5	Day 6 Onward
Milk supply	You may be able to express a few drops of milk.			Milk *should* come in between days 2 and 4.		Milk should be in. Breasts may be firm and/or leak milk. You should be able to hear your baby swallow your milk.	Breasts should feel softer after nursing. Baby should appear satisfied after feedings.
Baby's activity	Baby is usually wide awake in first hour of life. Put baby to breast within a half-hour of birth.	Wake up your baby. Babies may not wake up on their own to feed.	Baby should be more cooperative and less sleepy.	Look for early feeding cues such as rooting, lip smacking, hands to face.			
Feeding routine	Baby may go into a deep sleep 2–4 hr after birth.	Feed your baby every 1 1/2 to 3 hr, as often as wanted, a minimum of 8–10 times each day.	Use chart to write down time of each feeding.			May go *one* longer interval (up to 5 hr) between feeds in a 24-hr period.	
Breast-feeding	Baby will wake up and be alert and responsive for several more hours after initial deep sleep.	If you are comfortable, nurse at both breasts as long as baby is actively suckling.	Try to nurse both sides each feeding, aiming for 10 min on each side. Expect some nipple tenderness.	If the breast is too firm for the baby to latch on, consider hand expressing or pumping a few drops of milk to soften the nipple.	Nurse a minimum of 10–15 min on each side every 2–3 hr for the first few months of life.		Nipple tenderness should be gone or at least improving.
Baby's urine output		Baby must have a minimum of 1 wet diaper in first 24 hr.	Baby must have a minimum of 1 wet diaper every 8–12 hr.	You should see an increase in wet diapers to 4–6 times in 24 hr.	Baby's urine should be light yellow.	Baby should have 6–8 wet diapers each day with colorless or light yellow urine.	
Baby's stools		Baby should have a black-green stool (meconium stool).	Baby may have a second very dark (meconium) stool.	Baby's stools should be changing color from black-green to yellow.		Baby should have 3–4 yellow, soft stools a day.	Number of stools may decrease gradually after 4–6 weeks of life.

Prepared by Lisbeth Gabrielski, RN, BSN, CLE. Copyright 1994. All rights reserved. May be purchased from Lactation Support Services, The Children's Hospital, 1056 East 19th Avenue, B535, Denver Colorado, 80218. Telephone: (303) 861-6548.

Record number of minutes you breast feed on each side and the number of wet and dirty diapers your baby has each day.

BREAST FEEDING CHART
Date _____

	Minutes/side (Left/Right)	# urines/ stools
MNight	/	/
1:00 a.m.	/	/
2:00	/	/
3:00	/	/
4:00	/	/
5:00	/	/
6:00	/	/
7:00	/	/
8:00	/	/
9:00	/	/
10:00	/	/
11:00	/	/
Noon	/	/
1:00 p.m.	/	/
2:00	/	/
3:00	/	/
4:00	/	/
5:00	/	/
6:00	/	/
7:00	/	/
8:00	/	/
9:00	/	/
10:00	/	/
11:00	/	/

BREAST FEEDING CHART
Date _____

	Minutes/side (Left/Right)	# urines/ stools
MNight	/	/
1:00 a.m.	/	/
2:00	/	/
3:00	/	/
4:00	/	/
5:00	/	/
6:00	/	/
7:00	/	/
8:00	/	/
9:00	/	/
10:00	/	/
11:00	/	/
Noon	/	/
1:00 p.m.	/	/
2:00	/	/
3:00	/	/
4:00	/	/
5:00	/	/
6:00	/	/
7:00	/	/
8:00	/	/
9:00	/	/
10:00	/	/
11:00	/	/

BREAST FEEDING CHART
Date _____

	Minutes/side (Left/Right)	# urines/ stools
MNight	/	/
1:00 a.m.	/	/
2:00	/	/
3:00	/	/
4:00	/	/
5:00	/	/
6:00	/	/
7:00	/	/
8:00	/	/
9:00	/	/
10:00	/	/
11:00	/	/
Noon	/	/
1:00 p.m.	/	/
2:00	/	/
3:00	/	/
4:00	/	/
5:00	/	/
6:00	/	/
7:00	/	/
8:00	/	/
9:00	/	/
10:00	/	/
11:00	/	/

BREAST FEEDING CHART
Date _____

	Minutes/side (Left/Right)	# urines/ stools
MNight	/	/
1:00 a.m.	/	/
2:00	/	/
3:00	/	/
4:00	/	/
5:00	/	/
6:00	/	/
7:00	/	/
8:00	/	/
9:00	/	/
10:00	/	/
11:00	/	/
Noon	/	/
1:00 p.m.	/	/
2:00	/	/
3:00	/	/
4:00	/	/
5:00	/	/
6:00	/	/
7:00	/	/
8:00	/	/
9:00	/	/
10:00	/	/
11:00	/	/

(3) Frequent, shorter feedings might lessen discomfort.

(4) Avoid excessive nipple drying.

(5) Lanolin or hind milk (secreted late in the feeding with a very high fat content) can be used to lubricate and soften nipples.

(6) Evaluate for infection; *Staphylococcus aureus* has been associated with nipple fissures.

5. Engorgement (Walker, 2000)

a. Temporary condition in which breasts become swollen, hard, and tender. Often secondary to hormonal changes and increased vascularity/lymphatic congestion associated with milk production. Usually subsides by the end of the second week when supply and demand become more balanced.

b. May be due to vascular stasis and subsequent inflammatory process. Overdistension causes storage cells to flatten, stretch, and even rupture. Circulation slows with the increased pressure, and congested vessels leak into the interstitium, worsening the edema. Lymphatic drainage is obstructed, predisposing the breasts to mastitis. Milk production can be diminished or abolished through progressive glandular degeneration.

c. Lack of engorgement in the first week can be associated with insufficient milk production. Women with hypoplastic breasts (intramammary space >1 inch) may have <50% of the appropriate milk production in the first week.

d. Risk factors:

(1) Infrequent or inadequate breast drainage: The higher the number of minutes breast-feeding, the lower the incidence of painful engorgement.

(2) Small breast size: Does not limit production but decreases storage capacity. More frequent feedings may be necessary.

(3) Previous breast-feeding: Earlier engorgement, faster resolution.

(4) Hyperlactation: Volume exceeds removal.

(5) Decreased mother/baby contact: Decreased emptying.

e. Current research is examining association with antepartum medications (epidurals/magnesium sulfate).

f. Heat application to breasts 5–10 minutes before nursing can either provide comfort or increase discomfort.

g. Application of cold gel packs or cold cabbage leaves for 20 minutes between feeding may give more relief than heat because of vasoconstriction, decreased edema, and subsequent improved lymphatic drainage. The Cochrane review (Snowden et al., 2001) showed no benefit of cabbage leaves or cabbage cream over gel packs.

h. Gentle massage improves lymphatic drainage, thus reducing edema and improving cellular function.

i. Frequent nursing (1 1/2- to 3-hour intervals) without supplements helps minimize engorgement.

j. Manual expression before feeding may be needed to soften breasts and enhance latching-on.

6. Mastitis (Berens, 2001)
   a. Breast infection resulting in pain and redness in the affected area of the breast, usually accompanied by flu-like symptoms (fever, chills, headache).
   b. Predisposing factors
      (1) Most commonly caused by incomplete breast emptying resulting from an abrupt change in feeding frequency, missed feedings, a clogged duct that prevents draining, or an obstruction of the milk flow by a tight-fitting bra.
      (2) Other factors include infection entering through cracked nipples, breast trauma (teething, incorrect latching-on, improper breast pumping), and maternal exhaustion.
      (3) Usually unilateral with breast erythema.
   c. Treatment
      (1) Antibiotic therapy that includes staphylococcal coverage (usually 10–14 days). Incomplete treatment can result in recurrent mastitis.
      (2) Analgesics may be required for several days to enable continuation of breast-feeding, which will help to prevent abscess formation, a complication that requires surgical drainage.
      (3) Breast-feeding more frequently to ensure emptying of affected breast.
      (4) Apply moist heat before nursing.
      (5) Assistance from an electric breast pump may be needed to empty the breast if breast-feeding is too uncomfortable.
7. Bloody nipple discharge
   a. Postpartum bloody discharge; usually caused by nipple trauma.
   b. Not harmful if feedings continue to be tolerated.
   c. Blood is a cathartic, which can increase intestinal peristalsis, causing liquid bloody stools in the infant.
   d. If no further complications, should resolve within 1 week.
8. Inverted nipples usually are not a problem once breast-feeding is established.
   a. Initially, breast shields worn 30 minutes before the feeding may aid nipple protrusion.
   b. If shields are used long-term, reduction in milk supply and infant weight loss can occur because of diminished transfer of milk.
9. Ensuring adequate milk supply
   a. Factors affecting milk supply
      (1) Effective sucking stimulates milk glands to produce milk.
      (2) Regular and complete emptying of breasts stimulates milk production.
      (3) Supply and demand are interrelated: the more milk removed from the breast, the more milk will be produced.
   b. Frequent causes of insufficient supply
      (1) Maternal factors
         (a) Separation from infant during the first week of life.
         (b) Regular use of formula supplement.

   (c) Maternal stress or illness, postpartum complications, sore nipples.

   (d) Previous breast surgery that severed ducts and nerves; supplemental nursing apparatus may be needed to augment supply.

   (e) Small percentage of women are unable to produce an adequate supply of milk despite proper techniques and a vigorous infant; this is most likely a result of hypoplastic glandular development.

   (f) Use of inhibitory substances (nicotine, estrogen-containing birth control).

  (2) Infant factors

   (a) Intrapartum analgesics may cause infant sedation.

   (b) Inadequate suckling; incomplete emptying of breasts.

   (c) Neuromuscular or CNS dysfunction.

   (d) Prematurity; usually, infants <35 weeks who do not require neonatal intensive care will need close monitoring for effective feeding behaviors and weight gain. Also, preterm infants may need to be awakened for more frequent feedings because of fatigue and incomplete emptying. These infants are at risk for excessive weight loss, hypoglycemia, hyperbilirubinemia.

 c. Methods to increase milk supply

  (1) Sleeping in a skin-to-skin position, rooming-in, feeding frequently.

  (2) Switch breasts every 5 minutes to awaken and arouse infant with each breast change.

  (3) Avoid supplements.

  (4) Use breast pump after or between feedings to assist emptying if infant is unable to nurse frequently.

 10. Breast-feeding and breast milk jaundice (see Chapter 16)

E. Maternal Diet to Encourage Breast-Feeding: Quality of breast milk is usually constant, but the quantity produced can be affected by maternal diet.

 1. Diet should be varied; include fresh fruits/vegetables, whole grain breads/cereals, dairy products, and protein-rich meats/fish/legumes.

 2. Mothers should intake extra liquids each day to supply additional water required for milk production.

 3. Continue prenatal vitamins or multivitamin supplement while breast-feeding; strict vegetarians may also need vitamin B_{12} supplementation.

 4. Limit caffeine (may cause infant irritability) and any other foods that seem to upset the infant when they are included in the maternal diet. If a food group intolerance (i.e., dairy) is suspected in the infant, consult a dietitian regarding appropriate substitutes to ensure adequate intake of essential nutrients.

F. Infant Supplements

 1. Vitamin D content of human milk is low (22 IU/L); supplementation of 200 IU/day is recommended for all infants beginning in the first 2 months of life to prevent rickets and vitamin D deficiency associated with decreased sunlight exposure. Regular use of sunscreens (recommended for skin cancer protection) significantly decreases vitamin D production in the skin (AAP, 2003).

2. There is no evidence that vitamin A or E supplementation is necessary for healthy, breastfed term infants.
3. Iron content of human milk is low (0.3 mg/L) but deficiency rarely occurs in the exclusively breastfed newborn because of enhanced absorption of ferritin. By 6 months additional iron sources are required. Addition of iron-fortified cereal or elemental iron supplementation, 2-3 mg/kg per day, is recommended (AAP and ACOG, 2002).
4. Fluoride supplementation is controversial. Dental fluorosis (tooth staining that can range from white specks to pitting and brownish-gray staining) can be caused by excess fluoride ingestion during tooth formation. The AAP (1997) favors initiating supplementation after 6 months of age if the local water supply contains <0.3 ppm of fluoride.
5. Multivitamin supplements should be given to breast-fed infants whose mothers are malnourished; appropriate counseling regarding diet and access to available nutritional resources is also essential.

G. **Milk Collection and Storage** (Slusser and Frantz, 2001)
   1. If infant is hospitalized or unable to nurse regularly and/or vigorously, milk collection (breast pumping) and storage may be required.
   2. If collection for an extended period of time is anticipated or if low milk supply is a problem, a pump that mimics the infant's sucking pattern (1 suck/second) and includes positive and negative pressure to mimic the peristaltic pattern of the suck will be the most efficient. An electric pump that pumps both breasts at the same time stimulates the highest prolactin levels and provides the most efficient, most effective, and least time-consuming method for breast milk collection. A prescription from the medical provider stating the need and reason for the electric pump might enhance attainment and coverage by Medicaid/private insurance.
   3. To encourage or maintain an adequate supply, the pumping schedule should mimic the feeding schedule of every 2–3 hours with one longer interval of 5–6 hours at night. A frequency of 8 or more times in 24 hours for a 10-minute period of pumping is the most efficient for maintaining adequate milk production.
   4. Let-down may be compromised in the absence of infant suckling. Possible enhancing techniques include relaxation exercises, music, visualization of the infant, gentle massage of the chest wall progressing toward the nipple, nipple stimulation, warm shower, or warm breast compresses.
   5. After the first week of pumping, obtaining approximately 20–24 oz of milk per day signifies adequate milk production for a full-term infant.
   6. Storage and handling of human milk (Box 8-1).

BOTTLE FEEDING

A. **Feedings and Frequency**
   1. Most newborns will take 0.5–1 oz of formula per feeding every 2–4 hours in the first 24–48 hours of life (approximately 60–100 mL/kg/day); thereafter, volume of feedings in the first month will increase to 12–24 oz/day.

● BOX 8-1
STORAGE AND HANDLING OF BREAST MILK FOR WELL NEWBORN INFANTS

It is preferable for you to be available to your infant for each nursing. However, circumstances may arise that take you away from your baby for occasional or regular, brief or extended periods of time. During these times, it is desirable for your baby to be fed your expressed breast milk when he or she cannot be breast-fed. Following are guidelines for expressing and safely storing your breast milk for later use.

Preparation and Hygiene
1. Always wash your hands thoroughly before pumping your breasts.
2. A daily shower or bath is adequate to maintain breast cleanliness. Avoid using soap on your nipples.
3. Wash all pump parts that come into contact with your milk in hot soapy water and rinse well after each use.
4. Notify your own and your baby's doctor if you become ill or need to take any medication.

Collection of Milk
1. Pour the milk expressed during one pumping session into a sterile container (glass or plastic bottle or disposable bottle bag), taking care to avoid touching the inside of the container. It is best to double-line bottle bags to prevent milk loss through tears or holes.
2. If milk will be frozen, allow room for expansion at the top of the container.
3. Tightly cap bottles (do not store with nipples attached). Bottle bags are best sealed with a clean rubber band after the top edges are folded over a few turns.
4. Label each container with the date and time the milk was expressed. If your infant is hospitalized, also mark your infant's full name on the container.
5. Place multiple bottle bags in a larger Zip-lock bag to prevent them from sticking to the freezer shelf.

Milk May Be Stored
1. In the refrigerator for up to 48 hours after expressing or thawing (1-5° C or 34°–40° F).
2. In an "inside refrigerator" freezer for up to 3 weeks (–4° C or 20°–28° F).
3. In a "separate-door" freezer for up to 3 months (–12° C or 5°–15° F).
4. In a deep freezer for up to 6 months (–20° C or 0° F or below).

Milk May Be Thawed
1. Slowly in the refrigerator. Volumes of 3 oz or more may take several hours to thaw.
2. Relatively quickly under running warm water in a clean bowl or cup. Be sure the top of the bag or container remains above the water level at all times.
3. Once thawed, milk can be refrigerated for up to 24 hours.

Milk May Be Heated
1. Under running warm water.
2. In a pan of warm water (not over direct heat).
3. In a commercial bottle warmer.
4. Authorities generally recommend **against** using a microwave to either thaw or warm expressed milk. Inadvertent overheating of milk occurs easily in a microwave, and infants have been burned accidentally. In addition, many of the immune properties of human milk are heat-sensitive and can be destroyed by overheating.

● BOX 8-1
STORAGE AND HANDLING OF BREAST MILK FOR WELL NEWBORN INFANTS—cont'd

Additional Recommendations
1. Do **not** thaw milk at room temperature by letting it sit out for hours.
2. Do **not** overheat milk (it will curdle, and some of the immune components will be destroyed).
3. Do **not** leave milk at room temperature for more than 1 hour.
4. Do **not** refreeze thawed milk.
5. Do **not** store milk in the door of your freezer, where the temperature is less stable.
6. **Always** transport milk on ice in an insulated cooler.
7. Milk may be reheated and used for the next feeding if it has not been left at room temperature for more than 1 hour. Any milk remaining after the second feeding should be discarded.
8. For healthy babies who are not in the hospital, it is safe to "layer" milk collected on the same day by adding milk from more than one pumping session to the same bottle. Chill freshly expressed milk in the refrigerator before adding it to previously frozen milk.

Adapted from Neifert M: *The storage and handling of breast milk for nonhospitalized infants,* Information sheet developed for the Lactation Program at Presbyterian–St. Luke's Medical Center, Denver, Colorado, December 1996; and Lawrence RA: *Breastfeeding: a guide for the medical profession,* ed 5, St Louis, 1999, Mosby, with permission.

The interval between feedings will increase to every 3–4 hours with a longer night interval as the volume of feedings increases.

2. Infants should be cuddled and held during feedings, with head slightly above stomach to decrease reflux and choking and to allow swallowed air to collect at the top of the stomach for easy burping. Upright position minimizes fluid entering eustachian tubes, which may decrease the risk for otitis media.

3. Once infant is positioned, rub nipple along lower lip to encourage infant to open mouth; slip nipple into mouth on top of tongue to facilitate appropriate sucking; bottle angle should ensure constant filling of nipple neck to prevent air entry during sucking.

B. Formulas
1. Commercially prepared *iron-fortified* infant formula (Table 8-2) is the only acceptable alternative to breast-feeding the newborn infant.
   a. Unmodified whole cow's milk is unacceptable for the newborn because the iron is poorly absorbed and because it is an inferior source of vitamin C.
   b. Goat's milk and rice milk are unacceptable for the newborn because they have inadequate amounts of vitamins C and D, folic acid, and iron.
   c. Specialized formulas may be recommended for the infant with clinically suspected lactose intolerance or for the infant with persistent digestive problems.
   d. Long-term use of low-iron formulas places the infant at risk for anemia.

● TABLE 8-2
Human Milk and Commercial Formulas* Specifications

Formula (Manufacturer)	Protein Source	Carbo-hydrate Source	Fat Source	Indications for Use	Comments (Nutritional Considerations)
HUMAN AND COW'S MILK FORMULAS					
Human breast milk	Mature human milk; whey/casein ratio: 60:40	Lactose	Mature human milk	For all full-term infants except those with galactosemia; may be used with low-birth-weight infants	Recommended as sole form of feeding for first 5–6 months; nutritionally complete except for fluoride
Evaporated cow's milk formulas	Milk protein; whey/casein ratio: 18:82	Lactose, sucrose	Butterfat	For full-term infants with no special nutritional requirements; use of undiluted cow's milk after 12 months	Supplement with iron and vitamins C, A, and D if not fortified; give fluoride if fluoridated water is not used for formula preparation
COMMERCIAL INFANT FORMULAS					
Enfamil (Mead Johnson)	Nonfat cow's milk, demineralized whey; whey/casein ratio: 60:40	Lactose	Palm olein, soy, coconut, HOSun† oils	For full-term and premature infants with no special nutritional requirements	Available fortified with iron, 12 mg/L Also available in 24 kcal/oz
Similac (Ross)	Nonfat cow's milk; whey/casein ratio: 18:82	Lactose	Soy, coconut oils	For full-term and premature infants with no special nutritional requirements	Available fortified with iron, 12 mg/L
SMA (Wyeth)	Nonfat cow's milk, reduced-mineral whey; whey/casein ratio: 60:40	Lactose	Oleo, coconut, oleic (safflower), soy oils	For full-term and premature infants with no special nutritional requirements	Supplemented with iron, 12 mg/L
Baby Formula (Gerber)	Nonfat cow's milk; whey/casein ratio: 18:82	Lactose	Palm olein, soy, coconut, HOSun oils	For full-term and premature infants with no special nutritional requirements	Available fortified with iron, 11.5 mg/L

Product	Protein source	Carbohydrate source	Fat source	Indications	Comments
Good Start H.A. (Carnation)	Hydrolyzed whey	Lactose, malto-dextrin	Palm olein, soy, coconut, HOSun oils	For full-term infants	Manufacturer's claim regarding hypoallergenicity has been withdrawn
Good Nature (Carnation)	Nonfat cow's milk	Corn syrup solids	Palm, corn, oleic oils	For feeding older infants	Contains more protein and calcium than "starter" formulas
Similac Natural Care (Ross)	Nonfat cow's milk; whey protein concentrate	Hydrolyzed corn starch, lactose	MCT[†] coconut, soy oils	For low-birth-weight infants; fed mixed with human milk or fed alternately with human milk; improves vitamin/mineral content of human milk	Protein, 2.7g/100 mL; osmolality—24 cal/oz —300 mOsm/kg water
Enfamil Human Milk Fortifier (Mead Johnson)	Whey protein concentrate, casein	Corn syrup solids	Trace	For low-birth-weight infants; fed mixed with human milk; increases protein, calories, calcium, phosphorus, and other nutrients	Used only as human milk fortifier, not as separate formula; one pack of powder supplies 3.5 kcal/mL
FOR MILK PROTEIN–SENSITIVE INFANTS ("MILK ALLERGY"); LACTOSE-INTOLERANT INFANTS					
Prosobee (Mead Johnson)	Soy protein isolate	Corn syrup solids	Palm, soy, coconut, HOSun oils	With milk protein allergy, lactose intolerance, lactase deficiency, galactosemia	Hypoallergenic, zero band antigen; lactose- and sucrose-free
Isomil (Ross)	Soy protein isolate	Corn syrup, sucrose	Soy, coconut oils	With milk protein allergy, lactose intolerance, lactase deficiency, galactosemia	Hypoallergenic; lactose-free
Isomil OF (Ross)	Soy protein isolate	Hydrolyzed corn starch	Soy, coconut oils	For use during diarrhea	Lessens amount and duration of watery stools; contains fiber
Lactofree (Mead Johnson)	Milk protein isolate	Corn syrup solids	Palm olein, soy, HOSun oils	With lactose intolerance, lactase deficiency, galactosemia	Lactose-free
Nursoy (Wyeth)	Soy protein isolate	Sucrose (liquid formula) Corn syrup solids (powdered formula)	Oleo, coconut, soy, HOSun/safflower oils	With milk protein allergy, lactose intolerance, lactase deficiency, galactosemia	Lactose-free

(Continued)

Human Milk and Commercial Formulas* Specifications—cont'd

Formula (Manufacturer)	Protein Source	Carbo- hydrate Source	Fat Source	Indications for Use	Comments (Nutritional Considerations)
Soyalac (Loma Linda)	Soybean solids	Sucrose, corn syrup	Soy oil	With milk protein allergy, lactose intolerance, lactase deficiency, galactosemia	Lactose-free
I-Soyalac (Loma Linda)	Soy protein isolate	Sucrose, tapioca, dextrin	Soy oil	With milk protein allergy, lactose intolerance, lactase deficiency, galactosemia	Lactose- and corn-free
FOR INFANTS WITH MALABSORPTION SYNDROMES, MILK ALLERGY (HYDROLYSATE FORMULAS)					
RCF (Ross Carbohydrate-Free) (Ross)	Soy protein isolate		Soy, coconut oils	With carbohydrate intolerance	Carbohydrate added according to amount infant will tolerate
Portagen (Mead Johnson)	Sodium caseinate	Corn syrup solids, sucrose, lactose	MCT (coconut source), corn oil	For impaired fat absorption secondary to pancreatic insufficiency, bile acid deficiency, intestinal resection, lymphatic anomalies	Nutritionally complete
Nutramigen (Mead Johnson)	Casein hydrolysate, L-amino acids§	Corn syrup solids, modified corn starch	Corn, soy oils	For infants and children sensitive to food proteins; also used with galactosemic	Nutritionally complete; hypoallergenic formula; lactose- and sucrose-free
Pregestimil (Mead Johnson)	Casein hydrolysate, L-amino acids	Corn syrup solids, modified tapioca starch	MCT, soy, HOSun oils	Disaccharidase deficiencies, malabsorption syndromes, cystic fibrosis, intestinal resection	Nutritionally complete; easily digestible protein, carbohydrate, and fat; lactose- and sucrose-free

Product	Protein source	Carbohydrate source	Fat source	Indications	Comments
Alimentum (Ross)	Casein hydrolysate, L-amino acids	Sucrose, modified tapioca starch	MCT, oleic, soy oils	For infants and children sensitive to food proteins or with cystic fibrosis	Nutritionally complete; hypoallergenic formula; lactose-free
SPECIALTY FORMULAS					
Lonalac (Mead Johnson)	Casein	Lactose	Coconut	For children with congestive heart failure, who require reduced sodium intake	For long-term management, additional sodium must be given; supplement with vitamins C and D and iron; Na = 1 mEq/L
Similac PM 60/40	Whey and caseinate (60:40)	Lactose	Coconut, corn oils	For newborns predisposed to hypocalcemia and infants with impaired renal, digestive, and cardiovascular functions	Low calcium, potassium, and phosphorus; relatively low solute load; Na = 7 mEq/L
DIET MODIFIERS					
Polycose (Ross)		Glucose polymers (corn syrup solids)		Used to increase calorie intake, as for failure-to-thrive infants	Carbohydrate only; a powdered or liquid calorie supplement; powder, 23 kcal/tsp
Moducal (Mead Johnson)		Hydrolyzed corn starch		Used to increase carbohydrate intake	Carbohydrate only; a powdered calorie supplement, 30 kcal/tsp
Casec (Mead Johnson)	Calcium caseinate			Used to increase protein intake	Protein only; negligible fat and no carbohydrate
MCT Oil (Mead Johnson)			90% MCT (coconut sources)	Supplement in infants with fat malabsorption conditions	Fat only; 8.3 kcal/g, 115 kcal/tbsp

(Continued)

Human Milk and Commercial Formulas* Specifications—cont'd

Formula (Manufacturer)	Protein Source	Carbohydrate Source	Fat Source	Indications for Use	Comments (Nutritional Considerations)
FOR INFANTS WITH PHENYLKETONURIA‖					
Lofenalac (Mead Johnson)	Casein hydrolysate, L-amino acids	Corn syrup solids, modified tapioca starch	Corn oil	For infants and children	111 mg-phenylalanine per quart of formula (20 cal/qt); must be supplemented with other foods to provide minimal phenylalanine
Phenyl-Free (Mead Johnson)	L-amino acids	Sucrose, corn syrup solids, modified corn starch	Corn, coconut oils	For children over 1 year of age	Phenylalanine-free; permits increased supplementation with normal foods
Phenex-1 (Ross)	L-amino acids	Hydrolyzed corn starch	Soy, coconut, palm oils	For infants	Phenylalanine-free, fortified with L-tyrosine, L-glutamine, L-carnitine, and taurine; contains vitamins, minerals, and trace elements
Phenex-2 (Ross)	L-amino acids	Hydrolyzed corn starch	Soy, coconut, palm oils	For children and adults	Phenylalanine-free, fortified with L-tyrosine, L-glutamine, L-carnitine, and taurine; contains vitamins, minerals, and trace elements
Pro-Phree (Ross)	None	Hydrolyzed corn starch	Soy, coconut, palm oils	For infants and toddlers requiring reduced protein intake	Must be supplemented with protein; has vitamins, minerals, and trace elements

*All formulas provide 20 kcal/oz except as noted in product information from the manufacturers. For the most current information, consult product labels or package enclosures.
†HOSun, high-oleic sunflower.
‡MCT, medium-chain triglycerides.
§L-amino acids include L-cystine L-tyrosine, and L-tryptophan, which are reduced in hydrolyzed, charcoal-treated casein.
‖Ross Laboratories and Mead Johnson manufacture specialty formulas for metabolic disorders in infants.
From Wong DL: *Whaley & Wong's nursing care of infants and children*, St Louis, 1995, Mosby, pp 319-322.

2. Fluoride supplementation (0.25 mg/day) may be recommended at 6 months of age if the local water supply used to prepare the formula contains <0.3 ppm fluoride or if bottled water is used.
3. In most circumstances, clean technique is sufficient for formula preparation.
   a. Bottles, nipples, and all equipment should be washed with hot soapy water (in the top rack of the dishwasher, bottle sterilizer, or clean sink) and then thoroughly rinsed in hot water and allowed to air-dry.
   b. Before opening, the top of the formula can and can opener should be washed with hot soapy water and rinsed.
   c. Ready-to-feed formula should be used without dilution; powdered formula should be prepared according to the manufacturer's recommendations.
   d. Bottles should be prepared with volumes expected to be consumed at one feeding. This prevents reuse after a period of time, which might allow multiplication of bacteria introduced during a previous feeding.
   e. Bottles can be safely prepared and stored in the refrigerator for a 24-hour period.
   f. Formula can be warmed to room temperature before a feeding by placing the bottle in a pan of warm water; microwave heating is not recommended because of the possibility of hot spots in the formula, which might injure the infant, and the possibility of overheating, which can destroy vitamins. Temperature of warmed formula should be tested by shaking a few drops onto the sensitive inner aspect of the wrist.
   g. Ready-to-feed formula manufactured in sterile bottles can be stored at room temperature until the bottle seal is broken or until expiration date.
4. Sterile technique should be used in formula preparation if a clean water supply and refrigeration are not available or if the infant has an immature or deficient immune response.

BURPING AND REGURGITATION

A. **Burping**
   1. Should be attempted after every 0.5–1 oz of formula and at the end of the feeding to help remove swallowed air, which might cause distention and discomfort. Feeding the infant in an upright position favors spontaneous burping.
   2. Place infant in a sitting position on lap, supporting head and trunk with one hand; gently rub or pat from lower back upward. This position allows continuous observation of infant.
   3. Alternatively, infant may be held upright against mother's chest with back of the head supported and held above mother's shoulder, or infant may be placed prone across mother's lap while back is gently rubbed.
B. **Regurgitation**
   1. "Wet burps" containing small amounts of formula are physiologically normal in the first 6 weeks of life.

2. Forceful "projectile" vomiting, loss of the entire feeding, or bilious vomiting is abnormal. Infant should be evaluated for the possibility of esophageal abnormality or intestinal obstruction.

FEEDING DIFFICULTIES

A. **Establishing Pattern**: Occasionally an infant, particularly one who has experienced a difficult or prolonged delivery, may be slow to establish a regular, vigorous feeding pattern.
   1. Review risk factors, vital signs, and physical examination to evaluate for signs/symptoms of illness; evaluate infant's suck.
   2. In the absence of illness, feeding attempts should be limited to 15 minutes and the infant allowed to rest for 20–30 minutes before another attempt.
   3. With stable blood glucose, several feeding attempts can be made.
   4. If unsuccessful after a 3- to 6-hour interval, consider gavage feeding with a heightened suspicion of and close observation for signs or symptoms of illness.
   5. An experienced staff person may be able to encourage a difficult feeder with oral stimulation, chin support, or trial of different nipple types.
   6. The infant should not be discharged until fed successfully by a parent.
B. **Regurgitation**: For frequent regurgitation of curdled formula, mucus, or meconium/blood-stained amniotic fluid, consider lavage with 5–10 mL of normal saline; persistent regurgitation requires further evaluation for gastrointestinal abnormality.
C. **Low Blood Glucose:** Infants with borderline glucose levels require more frequent feedings.

POSITIONING AFTER FEEDING

For sleeping, according to the AAP, "infants should be placed down for sleep in a non-prone position. Supine (wholly on the back) confers the lowest risk and is preferred. The side is a reasonable alternative which also carries a significantly lower risk than prone" (AAP, 1996).

REFERENCES

American Academy of Pediatrics: Breastfeeding and the use of human milk, *Pediatrics* 100(6):1035-1039, 1997 (*www.aap.org/policy/re9729.html*).

American Academy of Pediatrics: The transfer of drugs and other chemicals into human milk, *Pediatrics* 108(3):776-789, 2001 (*www.aap.org/policy/0063.html*).

American Academy of Pediatrics: Prevention of rickets and vitamin D deficiency: new guidelines for vitamin D intake, *Pediatrics* 111(4):908-910, 2003 (*www.aap.org/policy/s010116.html*).

American Academy of Pediatrics, Committee on Nutrition: Fluoride supplementation in children: interim policy recommendations, *Pediatrics* 95:777, 1995.

American Academy of Pediatrics and American College of Obstetricians and Gynecologists: *Guidelines for perinatal care,* ed 5, Elk Grove Village, IL, 2002, American Academy of Pediatrics.

Berens PD. Prenatal, intrapartum, and postpartum support of the lactating mother, *Pediatr Clin North Am* 48(2):365-375, 2001.

Lawrence RA, Lawrence RM. *Breastfeeding: a guide for the medical profession,* ed 5, St Louis, 1999, Mosby.

Li R, Zhao Z, Mokdad A, et al: Prevalence of breast-feeding in the United States: the 2001 national immunization survey, *Pediatrics* 111(5):1198-1201, 2003.

Murray SS, McKinney ES, Gorrie TM: *Foundations of maternal newborn nursing,* Philadelphia, 2002, WB Saunders.

Neifert M: *Dr. Mom's guide to breastfeeding,* New York, 1998, Plenum Press.

Odaffer LL: Feeding with a bottle and burping. In Smith DP, editor: *Comprehensive child and family nursing skills,* St Louis, 1991a, Mosby, pp 379-383.

Odaffer LL: Supporting breast-feeding in special situations. In Smith DP, editor: *Comprehensive child and family nursing skills,* St Louis, 1991b, Mosby, pp 384-392.

Slusser W, Frantz K: High-technology breast-feeding, *Pediatr Clin North Am* 48(2):505-516, 2001.

Snowden HM, Renfrew MJ, Woodridge MW: Treatments for breast engorgement during lactation, *Cochrane Database Syst Rev* (2)CD000046, 2001.

Walker M: Breastfeeding and engorgement, *Breastfeeding Abstracts* 20(2):11-12, 2000.

Wight NE: Management of common breast-feeding issues, *Pediatr Clin North Am* 48(2):321-344, 2001.

Wong DL: *Whaley & Wong's nursing care of infants and children,* St Louis, 1999, Mosby.

9 Routine Care

Robyn E. Berryman, RNC, MS, NNP ▪ *Sharon M. Glass, RNC, MS, NNP*

CONTINUOUS OBSERVATION

A. Vital Signs: Obtained at a minimum frequency of every 8 hours when infant is quiet to ensure continued stable functioning

1. Temperature
   a. Three-minute axillary with glass thermometer or as needed to register with electronic thermometer (tympanic thermometers may give inaccurate readings).
   b. Normal axillary range: 36.5–37° C (97.9–98.3° F).
   c. Intervention and increased monitoring if temperature is outside normal range.
      (1) If <36.5° C, place infant skin-to-skin with parent (if possible) or under a radiant warmer; monitor temperature every 30 minutes until it returns to normal range. Review risk factors and evaluate infant for any other evidence of illness.
      (2) If >37° C, evaluate and remove environmental influences (high room temperature, overdressing/overwrapping); monitor temperature every 30 minutes until it returns to normal range. Review risk factors and evaluate infant for any other signs of illness.
   d. If infant is hypo- or hyperthermic, considerations include environmental factors, sepsis, postasphyxial insult, and decreased subcutaneous and brown fat stores.
2. Heart rate (HR)
   a. Auscultate apical pulse for 1 minute at the left lower sternal border.
   b. Normal range is 80–160 bpm; rate is slower during sleep and more rapid with crying.
   c. Assess heart sounds for rhythm, rate, murmurs.
      (1) S_1 ("lub"): Closure of tricuspid/mitral valves after atrial ejection of blood.
      (2) S_2 split ("dub"): Closure of aortic/pulmonic valves after ventricular ejection of blood.
         (a) Slight separation of valve sounds is evident after 24–48 hours of age, resulting in normal split sound.
         (b) Single S_2 with click and systolic blood pressure differential of >20 mm Hg between upper and lower extremities may indicate coarctation.
      (3) S_3: Produced by vibration during ventricular filling; can be normal in the newborn.

(4) S_4: Gallop rhythm; always abnormal and indicates congestive failure.

(5) Most murmurs in the newborn are benign and secondary to closing patent ductus arteriosus or patent foramen ovale. Most common cardiac lesion is ventricular septal defect, which may be associated with a high-pitched pansystolic murmur best heard at the lower left sternal border.

    (a) Evaluate infant for symptoms of cardiovascular compromise (tachycardia; increased, diminished, or unequal pulses; blood pressure differential; poor perfusion; increased precordial activity; hepatomegaly; respiratory distress; cyanosis).

    (b) If infant is asymptomatic without significant extremity blood pressure differential, communicate presence of murmur to parents and primary care provider for follow-up examination.

d. Abnormal rate

(1) Persistent bradycardia (HR <80 bpm) is abnormal and requires evaluation (can be associated with congenital heart block, sepsis, asphyxia, hypoxemia).

(2) Persistent tachycardia (HR >180 bpm) is abnormal and requires evaluation (can be associated with anemia, hypoxemia, hypovolemia, sepsis, hyperthermia).

e. Abnormal rhythm: Paroxysmal supraventricular tachycardia (SVT) is an electrical dysrhythmia that requires immediate treatment. Can be due to rapid ectopic pacemaker, direct muscular connection between atria and ventricle that allows signal reentry (Wolff-Parkinson-White [WPW] abnormality), cardiac malformation, tumors, and myocarditis (Flanagan, Yeager, Weindling, 1999).

(1) Presentation includes sudden onset of rapid regular rhythm (>230 bpm—does not slow when infant is quiet), irritability, poor nippling, vomiting, tachypnea, cyanosis or ashen gray color, cold extremities.

(2) Electrocardiogram (Figure 9-1) shows rapid regular rhythm originating in the atria, no P waves, normal or slightly widened QRS complex, normal or slightly depressed ST segments.

(3) Treatment (rapid conversion)

    (a) First, attempt vagal stimulation (gagging, ice compresses to the face, rectal stimulation).

    (b) Give IV adenosine (90% effective) (Rossi and Burton, 1989).

        (i) Rapid IV injection (half-life is 10 seconds, total clearance in 30 seconds).

        (ii) Begin with 75 µg/kg and give incremental doses of 150 µg/kg and 225 µg/kg at 2- to 3-minute intervals.

        (iii) Hazards include sinus bradycardia (aminophylline reverses atrioventricular block) and atrial/ventricular fibrillation (cardiopulmonary resuscitation/cardioversion).

    (c) Digoxin (70% effective) may require 12–24 hours for conversion (contraindicated in WPW syndrome).

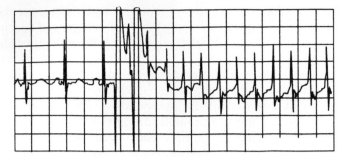

FIGURE 9-1 ● Supraventricular tachycardia (SVT). Note normal sinus rhythm (three PQRST complexes) on the left and the abrupt onset of a very fast rhythm (SVT) on the right. (From Wong DL: *Whaley & Wong's nursing care of infants and children,* St Louis, 1995, Mosby, p 1555, with permission.)

        (d) Cardioversion (2–4 J) is reserved for the infant with persistent SVT resulting in congestive failure.

      (4) Cardiac consult and follow-up are indicated because recurrence is common. Discuss with parents and primary care provider.

  3. Respirations

    a. Observe chest excursions for 1 minute for rate, rhythm, depth, retractions.

    b. Normal range is 30–60 breaths/minute.

    c. Auscultate lung lobes for wheezes, rales, rhonchi, stridor, or grunting, indicating pulmonary/cardiovascular disease.

    d. Apnea (cessation of breathing for >15 seconds) may be associated with prematurity, central nervous system (CNS) injury, CNS depression (sepsis, maternal drugs/medications), metabolic abnormalities (hypoglycemia, hypocalcemia, hypermagnesemia), anemia.

    e. Tachypnea (respiratory rate >60 breaths/minute) can be associated with pulmonary, cardiovascular, or metabolic disease; it is most commonly transient tachypnea of the newborn (see Chapter 6).

  4. Blood pressure (BP)

    a. Screening of well newborn infants is no longer recommended by the American Academy of Pediatrics and the American Academy of Obstetricians and Gynecologists (2002).

    b. Obtain four-extremity BP if indicated by cardiovascular symptomatology (persistent murmur, abnormal pulses, tachycardia, poor perfusion, abnormal precordial activity, hepatomegaly).

    c. Normal ranges for term newborn infants in the first 24 hours of life vary by method and birth weight (Figure 9-2). Accuracy of Doppler monitoring can be enhanced by performing only when the infant is quiet and ensuring an appropriately sized cuff (width 50%–67% of length) (Versmold, Kitterman, Phibbs et al., 1981).

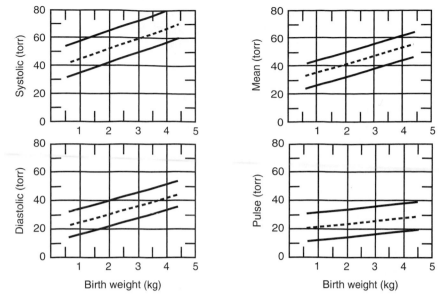

FIGURE 9-2 ● Average systolic, diastolic, and mean pressures during the first 12 hours of life in normal newborn infants according to birth weight. (From Versmold HT, Kitterman JA, Phibbs RH, et al: Aortic blood pressure during the first 12 hours of life in infants with birth weight 610 to 4220 grams, *Pediatrics* 67:611, 1981, with permission.)

B. Color
  1. Observe face, trunk, and extremities for cyanosis or differences in skin color.
  2. Observe for presence and level of jaundice (see Chapter 14).
C. Weight
  1. Minimum assessment: Admission and discharge weight; daily weight if >24-hour hospital stay.
  2. Expected weight loss <10% in the first 7–10 days of life.
  3. Considerations for evaluation of excessive weight loss include inadequate feeding volume, cold stress, excessive output (urine, water loss stools, regurgitation), measurement error.
  4. Primary care provider should be notified of discharge weight. Early follow-up (within the first week of life) should be recommended for breast-fed infants and infants with excessive weight loss.

CONTINUED SURVEILLANCE

  A. **Hypoglycemia** (see Chapter 16)
    1. Continue monitoring glucose before feedings until assured of stability for infants of diabetic mothers, infants who are large or small for gestational age, and preterm infants.
    2. Persistent hypoglycemia requires further evaluation for adequacy of feedings (volume and timing), signs of infection, hypoxemia, cold stress.

B. **Hyperbilirubinemia** (see Chapter 15)
  1. Continue to monitor infant for presence and level of jaundice.
  2. Infant's blood type, Rhesus status, and Coombs test results should be obtained and documented before discharge if mother's blood type is O or Rhesus status is negative.
  3. Early onset (<24 hours of age) or rapid progression (>1 mg/dL/hr) of jaundice requires evaluation of direct and indirect serum bilirubin levels, assessment of risk for hemolysis, and consideration of possible infection and hepatic dysfunction.
C. **Respiratory Distress** (see Chapter 6)
  1. Continue to observe for respiratory distress (grunting, flaring, retracting, cyanosis, tachypnea, apnea, oxygen requirement).
  2. Consider evaluation of chest radiograph if symptoms persist.
D. **Sepsis** (see Chapters 20 and 21)
  1. Review maternal history for risk factors.
  2. Continue observation for signs of infection, which might include subtle changes in vital signs, color, feeding patterns, activity, alertness, tone, thermoregulation.

NEUROLOGIC EXAMINATION

A. **Quality and Quantity of Spontaneous Movements:** These are the best indicators of adequacy of neuromuscular function (assess symmetry of movement and tone, range of motion).
B. **Reflexes:** Several primitive reflexes are present in the newborn and can be elicited to test symmetry and neuromuscular function—Moro, palmar/plantar grasps, tonic neck, stepping, placing, truncal incurvation (see Chapter 7).
C. **Reactivity**
  1. Two periods of heightened reactivity occur during the transitional period (see Chapter 5).
  2. Thereafter, spontaneous reactivity varies with the individual child and the adequacy of feedings; infants should be easily arousable with gentle handling and undressing.
  3. When necessary, infants should be brought slowly from a sleeping state to an aroused state by soft verbalizations and gentle handling.

HEARING SCREENING

A. Hearing loss is found in 1 to 3 per 1000 infants in the normal newborn population. The incidence is higher in the newborn intensive care population.
B. The AAP Task Force on Newborn and Infant Hearing endorses the Joint Committee on Infant Hearing recommendation of implementing universal newborn hearing screening in all hospitals providing obstetric services (AAP, 1999).
C. Current recommendation is for newborn screening to be completed before discharge from the hospital when possible.

D. Additionally, all infants who fail the newborn screen should be referred to qualified expert professionals by 3 months of age.

VOIDING

A. All newborn infants without abnormalities will void by the first 17–36 hours of life (ensure that delivery room staff document any voids at the time of delivery).

B. Urine should be pale yellow to colorless with one or two voids in the first 24 hours and five to eight voids/day by the second day of life.

C. Urate crystals can be a normal finding in the first 24 hours (thereafter, crystals could indicate dehydration).

D. Failure to void in the first 36 hours of life requires evaluation for obstructive uropathy, acute tubular necrosis (history of asphyxia), renal vein thrombosis (infant of a diabetic mother).

E. Inadequate output after initial voiding requires evaluation of adequacy of feeding volume.

STOOLING

A. Of newborn infants without abnormalities, 98.5% will pass a meconium stool in the first 24 hours; 100% will stool by 48 hours of life.

B. Delayed stooling requires evaluation for imperforate anus, intestinal obstruction, bowel infection, Hirschsprung disease, hypothyroidism, and meconium ileus.

C. Initial stools are sticky black (meconium), changing to soft brown-green (transitional—part meconium/part fecal) by day 2 or 3 with establishment of feedings; thereafter, stools differ with type of feeding (Color Plate 47).

1. Breast-fed stools are generally more frequent and more liquid, with very small yellow curds. May be passed as often as after every feeding or occasionally as infrequently as every 48 to 72 hours.

2. Formula-fed stools have larger green-brown curds, which make them more pasty in appearance. Average is one or two stools per day, but more infrequent stooling is considered normal if intake is adequate and stools are of normal consistency when passed.

D. The number of stools passed by healthy infants is extremely variable, ranging from as few as 1 every 4 to 5 days to as many as 10 per day.

1. Regardless of frequency, an infant is not constipated unless stools consist of hard, dry pellets that are passed with difficulty and distress (such pellets may be blood-streaked). Adequacy of fluid intake should be assessed. Laxatives are generally discouraged, but a sliver of glycerin suppository is often effective, especially in preterm infants who have a functional constipation that is probably related to weak muscular control.

2. Diarrhea (frequent, loose stools) is usually due to an intolerance to formula protein or to enteral infection. Infants often appear ill and may quickly

become dehydrated and acidotic (as compared with breast-fed infants, who may also have frequent, loose stools but appear well and thrive).

CORD CARE

A. Umbilical cord should be cleaned with each diaper change.

B. Apply alcohol to the base of the cord to encourage rapid drying, which helps to prevent infection.

C. Diaper should be folded and secured below the cord to avoid irritation and moisture.

D. Serous, purulent, or sanguineous drainage from the umbilicus or circumferential erythema at the base of the cord is abnormal and requires immediate evaluation for omphalitis, which can be life-threatening and requires parenteral antibiotic therapy.

E. Delayed cord separation (>2 weeks) requires evaluation for persistent urachus or deficient neutrophil function and chemotaxis.

F. Granulation tissue may form as a solid yellow mass and requires desiccation with silver nitrate (Color Plate 26). Inspect area to rule out the possibility of everted intestinal mucosa that would permit the entrance of a probe.

SLEEP PATTERNS

A. After the initial period of reactivity, infants should sleep for 2 to 4 hours between feedings.

B. There should be smooth transition between states (deep sleep to light sleep to fussy and then crying/quiet alert to drowsy to light sleep and then deep sleep).

C. In the first week of life, expect 20 to 22 hours of sleep per day.

PARENT-INFANT INTERACTION

A. Model appropriate behaviors any time the infant is handled in the parent's presence: affection, gentle handling, talking to the infant, consoling.

B. Observe parental interaction during holding, feeding, and changing; look for and comment on parent-infant interaction and responsiveness.

C. Verify any concerns through more intensive observation and, if needed, referral for social services evaluation before discharge.

REFERENCES

American Academy of Pediatrics: Newborn and infant hearing loss: detection and intervention, *Pediatrics* 103:527-530, 1999.

American Academy of Pediatrics and American College of Obstetricians and Gynecologists: Care of the neonate. In

Gilstrap LC, Oh W, editors: *Guidelines for perinatal care*, ed 5, Elk Grove Village, IL, 2002, American Academy of Pediatrics, pp 198-215.

Flanagan MF, Yeager SB, Weindling SN: Cardiac disease. In Avery GB, Fletcher MA, Macdonald MG, editors: *Neonatology:*

pathophysiology and management of the newborn, ed 5, Philadelphia, 1999, JB Lippincott, pp 577-646.

Hockenberry M, et al: *Wong's nursing care of infants and children,* ed 7, St Louis, 2003, Mosby.

Rossi AF, Burton DA: Adenosine in altering short- and long-term treatment of supraventricular tachycardia in infants, *Am J Cardiol* 64:685-686, 1989.

Versmold HT, Kitterman JA, Phibbs RH, et al: Aortic blood pressure during the first 12 hours of life in infants with birth weight 610 to 4200 grams, *Pediatrics* 67:611, 1981.

Genetic Screening

Sharon M. Glass, RNC, MS, NNP

NEWBORN GENETIC SCREEN (NBGS)

A. **Goals**
  1. To prevent serious morbidity or death from a *treatable disorder* by identifying affected infants prior to the onset of symptoms
  2. To obtain a specimen from *every* neonate before discharge or transfer regardless of age or feeding status
B. **Privacy and Insurance** (Latham et al., 1996; Rothenberg, 1995).
  1. All children who test positive for genetic diseases can now benefit from insurance coverage. Some have, in the past, been classified with a "preexisting" medical condition, which has excluded them from certain insurance policies or allowed an extra premium charge. These children are now protected from this type of discrimination by federal legislation enacted in 1996 through the Health Information Portability and Accountability Act (HIPAA). Although there are still some gaps, HIPAA affords a beginning mandate for privacy protections through restrictions against unauthorized access to genetic information included in medical records.
  2. Medicaid provides protection for eligible children by requiring state-funded programs to provide appropriate medical care for any child with a genetic diagnosis resulting from newborn screening.
  3. In addition, the State Child Health Insurance Plan (SCHIP) was established to meet the requirements of Title XXI of the Social Security Act in 1998 to provide insurance coverage for low-income children who are not eligible for Medicaid. Benefits under this plan vary according to state funding.
  4. Department of Health and Human Services website offers an in-depth discussion of health insurance implications at *www.nhgri.nih.gov/NEWS/Insurance/index.html.*
C. **Ethical Issues** (AAP, Committee on Genetics, 2000)
  1. Newborn genetic screening affords the opportunity not only to prevent the devastating effects of metabolic errors but also to develop an appropriate long-term plan for therapy, health supervision, counseling, and anticipatory guidance for the child and family. However, NBGS carries other implications for the entire family and can permanently alter family dynamics. Private family matters such as paternity and adoption may be exposed. Family members who carry an abnormal gene may experience anger; those who escape disease may experience feelings of guilt.

2. Genetic counseling is an essential component in ensuring that family members receive the assistance necessary to cope with positive test results. Counseling must be a priority of the primary care practitioner.

D. Diseases Included in NBGS

1. The number of tests included differs according to individual state health regulations. All 50 states and the District of Columbia screen for phenylketonuria (PKU) and congenital hypothyroidism.

2. A number of states have added additional tests to their newborn screening programs, depending on financial resources. Visit *http://www.ncsl.org/programs/health/screen.htm* for documentation regarding individual state regulations, laws, and accepted exemptions for newborn screening. Table 10-1 lists the mandated tests in each state (National Newborn Screening and Genetics Resource Center, 2003).

3. Molecular genetic testing is now available to test for a number of previously undetectable genetic diseases in which children appear normal at birth but can develop devastating symptoms at a later time (AAP, Committee on Genetics, 2000). Newspapers have reported that a variety of private labs are now offering supplemental newborn screening at an additional cost (usually $25–$60) to parents at the time of their infant's birth increasing the need for clinicians to be informed and aware of new technologies and issues involved in newborn screening. Supplemental screening, requiring only one heel puncture, can be performed at the time of the infant's routine newborn screen. Parents obtain a blood spot card for collection of the specimen and packaging to mail the card to the processing laboratory. Parents must supply a physician's name and phone number for return of test results. This allows appropriate notification of abnormal results and affords the opportunity for therapy, counseling, and follow-up. The March of Dimes advocates expanded newborn screening. Their website, *www.marchofdimes.com*, offers information on the newborn screening tests, screening labs, and a variety of educational materials regarding genetic diseases, treatment, and outcomes.

4. Government agencies, medical societies, and patient advocacy groups are currently debating whether a national screening program or national screening recommendations should be created (Elliott, 2002).

E. Testing Guidelines (AAP and ACOG, 2002; AAP, Committee on Genetics, 1996, 2000; AAP, Section on Endocrinology, 1993, Mountain States Genetic Network, 2001; Wallman, 1998).

1. Screen *every* neonate as late as possible (but not later than 72 hours) before discharge, transfer, or administration of blood transfusion or IV antibiotics, regardless of age or feeding status.

2. AAP recommends retesting at 1–2 weeks of age if initial specimen is obtained at <24 hours of age (some infants may not have ingested sufficient protein for amino acid elevation).

3. Cord blood is not a satisfactory sample because of placental clearance of abnormal metabolites before birth.

4. Documentation

● TABLE 10-1
Disorders for Which Newborns Were Screened in the United States (2000)

	State/Territory	Hyperphenyl-alaninemia	Hypo-thyroidism	Classical Galac-tosemia	Maple Syrup Urine Disease	Homo-cystin-uria	Biotin-idase	Congenital Adrenal Hyper-plasia	Cystic Fibrosis	Tyro-sinemia	Toxo-plasmo-sis	Hemo-globino-pathy	MCAD
1	Alabama	R	R	R								R	
2	Alaska	R	R	R	R			R				R	
3	Arizona	R	R	R	R	R	R					R	
4	Arkansas	R	R	R	R	R	R					R	
5	California	R	R	R								R	
6	Colorado	R	R	R	R	R	R	R^b	R			R	
7	Connecticut	R	R	R	R	R	R	R	V			R	
8	Delaware	R	R	R	R	R						R	
9	District of Columbia	R	R	R	R	R						R	
10	Florida	R	R	R	R	R		R				R	
11	Georgia	R	R	R	R	R	R	R		R		R	
12	Hawaii	R	R	R	R		R	R				R	
13	Idaho	R	R	R^a	R		R	R					
14	Illinois	R	R	R		R	R	R				R	
15	Indiana	R	R	R	R	R	R	R				R	
16	Iowa	R	R	R	R	R		R				R	P
17	Kansas	R	R	R		R		R				R	
18	Kentucky	R	R	R			R					V	
19	Louisiana	R	R				R	R				R	
20	Maine	R	R	R	R	R	R	R				V	R
21	Maryland^d	V	V	V	V	V	V	V		V		V	R
22	Massachusetts	R	R	R	R	R	R	R	P	P	R	R	R
23	Michigan	R	R	R	R	R	R	R				R	
24	Minnesota	R	R	R								R	
25	Mississippi	R	R	R								R	

#	State							
26	Missouri	R	R					R
27	Montana	R	R					P
28	Nebraska	R	R	R				R
29	Nevada	R	R	R				R
30	New Hampshire	R	R	R			R	V
31	New Jersey	R	R	R				R
32	New Mexico	R	R	R	R			R
33	New York[e]	R	R	R	R	R		R
34	North Carolina	R	R	R	R	R	R	R
35	North Dakota	R	R	R	R			V
36	Ohio	R	R	R	R			R
37	Oklahoma	R	R					R
38	Oregon	R	R	V^a	R	V^a		R
39	Pennsylvania	V, R^f	R	V^a	V^a	V, R^f	V^a	R
40	Rhode Island	R	R	R	R	R		R
41	South Carolina	R	R	R		R	R	R
42	South Dakota	R	R					
43	Tennessee	R	R	R		R^c		R
44	Texas	R	R	R		R		R
45	Utah	R						
46	Vermont	R	R	R	R	R		R
47	Virginia	R	R	R	R	R		R
48	Washington	R	R			R		
49	West Virginia	R	R					V
50	Wisconsin	R	R				R	V
51	Wyoming	R	R	R	R	R		R
52	Puerto Rico	P	R	R	R	R		R
53	Virgin Islands	R	R	R				R

R, required; V, voluntary; P, pilot

a, Supplemental newborn screening program through Neo Gen. Screening, Inc.; b, CAH testing since 8/00; c, started screening 10/00; d, Maryland law requires that hospitals or birthing centers offer testing, which can be refused without reason, so Maryland is listed as voluntary; e, other disorders screened HIV-1 antibodies; f, supplemental newborn screening program through Neo Gen. Screening, Inc. (voluntary 1/1/00 to 9/31/00 and part of PA state screening program 10/1/00 to 12/31/00).

Taken from National Newborn Screening and Genetics Resource Center: National newborn screening report—2000, Austin, TX, NNSGRC, February 2003.

      a. Nursery procedures should clearly identify time and personnel responsible for performing and documenting completion of NBGS and person responsible for later communication with primary care provider if hospital is notified of inadequacy of original specimen.

      b. Care provider coordinating discharge should again document performance of screen.

  5. Methodology

      a. Specimen should be obtained on standard filter paper manufactured for the collection of screening exams, which contains preprinted circles.

      b. Alcohol used to prepare the infant's heel should be allowed to dry before puncture.

      c. Wipe away the first drop of blood because it contains tissue fluids that might alter results.

      d. Blood should be dripped onto the paper from the infant's heel by touching the blood drop to the paper without touching the heel to the paper.

      e. The spot should be completely filled with blood (front and back of paper); care should be taken to avoid extra blood outside the circle.

      f. Blood should be obtained from a single session and not layered at a later time.

      g. Allow specimen to thoroughly air dry on a horizontal surface.

  6. Factors affecting results

      a. Antibiotics can interfere with some of the assays.

      b. Total parenteral nutrition can affect results because of the high circulating levels of amino acids.

      c. Transfusion may result in false-negative results for galactosemia and hemoglobinopathies or false-positive results for hemoglobinopathies secondary to circulating foreign red cells.

      d. Dialysis or transfusion may decrease concentration of abnormal metabolites and result in false-negative results.

      e. Normal intake of dietary substrate may be necessary to produce detectable levels of abnormal metabolites. Alterations in diet might affect the accuracy of screening.

  7. Positive results for galactosemia and maple syrup urine disease require immediate initiation of treatment. Otherwise, therapy should not be initiated until positive screen results are confirmed with specific diagnostic testing.

F. Testing Errors (Greene, 1998)

  1. Assuming that a normal screen excludes disease. Sensitivity and specificity of screens vary (Table 10-2). Inadequacy of a metabolic marker or laboratory error could cause affected infants to be missed. Any infant with specific symptomatology should be retested in spite of a normal NBGS.

  2. Assuming a negative test without notification. The primary care provider is responsible for ensuring that the test was performed and that the results are recorded.

● TABLE 10-2
Sensitivity/Specificity of Genetic Screens

Genetic Screening Tests*	Sensitivity False-Positive Errors	Specificity False-Negative Errors
Phenylketonuria	1.5%	0.6%
Hypothyroidism	1.2%	0.7%
Galactosemia	0.6%	0%
Congenital adrenal hyperplasia	1.7%	1.0%
Maple syrup urine disease	2.4%	0.7%
Homocystinuria	0%	3.3%
Biotinidase deficiency	0.4%	2.1%
Cystic fibrosis		

*For greater patient safety, screening programs are designed to minimize false-negative reports.

3. Samples containing illegible or incomplete information. All requested information is essential for accurate interpretation of results and proper identification of the newborn.
4. Prescribing treatment for PKU before confirming testing. Starting treatment might be harmful for the infant without PKU or might interfere with further diagnostic testing.
5. Failure to obtain a screen before transfusion, dialysis, or transfer to another institution.
6. Failure to collect an adequate sample. Inaccurate results may result from submission of a test with insufficient sample or contaminated sample.
7. Failure to provide a sample. Home births might result in failure to sample if the birth attendant or family member is uninformed about the requirements for and processing of the sample.

DISEASES SCREENED BY THE NBGS

A. **Phenylketonuria (PKU)**
   1. Inherited genetic defect (autosomal recessive): Deficiency or absence of phenylalanine hydroxylase, the enzyme required for conversion of phenylalanine to tyrosine. When this conversion is blocked, phenylalanine accumulates in body fluids and results in central nervous system (CNS) damage.
      a. Phenylalanine level may be within normal range for the first 12 hours (30% of infants with PKU) and for the first 24 hours (10% of infants with PKU). Testing before 48 hours must be repeated to ensure full detection (usually at 1–2 weeks of age).
      b. All infants with confirmed hyperphenylalanemia should be tested for disorders of tyrosine and biopterin metabolites because a low-phenylalanine diet will not alleviate metabolic defect in these disorders.

2. Incidence
    a. In United States: 1 in 10,000–25,000 live births
    b. Overall range: 1 in 4800 (Ireland) to 1 in 60,000 (Japan)
3. Presentation: Biochemical effects begin immediately, with symptoms apparent at about 3 months of age (vomiting, feeding difficulties, irritability, infantile eczema, hypopigmentation of skin and hair, urine with "musty odor" caused by excretion of phenylacetic acid).
4. Treatment
    a. Well-controlled phenylalanine-restricted diet for classical PKU (specialized formula, ongoing adjustments).
    b. Heterogeneity expressed in variation of disease severity and phenylalanine tolerance. Less stringent dietary control required in some PKU patients.
    c. Long-term studies of children allowed a normal diet after age 5–6 (after complete CNS myelination) show loss of intellectual function years later. Dietary restrictions to maintain phenylalanine concentrations <15–20 mg/dL are now recommended for life.
    d. Microcephaly, mental retardation, seizures, and congenital heart disease occur in offspring of women with PKU whose diets are not restricted; dietary restriction for several months before conception and during pregnancy can prevent adverse outcome.
5. Outcome
    a. Untreated: Profound mental retardation; 95% will have an IQ <50.
    b. Treated: Normal intelligence in children treated from the first few weeks of life.

B. **Galactosemia**
1. Inherited genetic defect (autosomal recessive): Heterogeneous disorder, most commonly a deficiency of galactose-1-phosphate uridyltransferase, an enzyme that mediates the conversion of galactose to glucose in the digestion of lactose; affected infants cannot digest lactose (milk sugar). Name derives from the abnormal presence of galactose in the blood and urine.
2. Incidence: 1 in 60,000–80,000 live births
3. Presentation
    a. Intrauterine growth retardation
    b. Vomiting and diarrhea occur during lactose feeds
    c. Hypoglycemia
    d. Gram-negative sepsis *(Escherichia coli)* precipitated by gastrointestinal mucosal damage from the galactose metabolite
    e. Hepatic damage with secondary hyperbilirubinemia, hepatomegaly, cirrhosis
    f. Urine positive for reducing substance
    g. Cataract development at approximately 3 months of age
4. Treatment
    a. Lifelong dietary restriction of lactose (difficult dietary management because of the common use of lactose as a food additive)
    b. Aggressive surveillance and treatment of sepsis

5. Outcome
   a. Untreated: Usually death; survivors will have severe mental retardation, cerebral palsy, cataracts, and liver disease.
   b. Treated: May have normal intellect with early diagnosis and treatment; many have developmental and learning disabilities despite treatment; high incidence of secondary ovarian failure in females.

C. **Maple Syrup Urine Disease**
   1. Inherited genetic defect: Branched-chain ketoacid decarboxylation disorder resulting in elevated serum levels of leucine, isoleucine, valine, and their corresponding ketoacids.
   2. Incidence: Rare autosomal recessive trait; 1 in 250,000–300,000 live births.
   3. Presentation
      a. Fulminant disease with severe ketoacidosis.
      b. Symptoms usually evident in the first 48–72 hours of life and include lethargy, poor feeding, vomiting, weight loss, abnormal tone, seizures, and loss of reflexes.
      c. Urine has characteristic odor of maple syrup.
      d. Some infants have milder variants and are asymptomatic in the newborn period.
   4. Treatment
      a. Peritoneal/hemodialysis to clear accumulated acids; discontinue protein intake.
      b. Chronic treatment is dietary, with limitation of branched-chain amino acids, especially leucine, titrated through use of special formula along with fruits, vegetables, low-protein foods.
      c. Thiamine might stimulate dehydrogenase activity.
   5. Outcome
      a. Untreated: Death ensues within the first weeks of life.
      b. Treated: May have normal outcome depending on timing of diagnosis/ treatment; many have residual neurologic defects with delay in diagnosis.

D. **Cystic Fibrosis (CF)**
   1. Inherited genetic defect: Gene defect on the long arm of the seventh chromosome results in disturbance of electrolyte composition of saliva, sweat, pulmonary, and pancreatic secretions as a result of diminished epithelial permeability to chloride; NBGS detects increased blood levels of immunoreactive trypsinogen (elevated trypsinogen resulting from obstructed pancreatic ducts).
   2. Incidence: 1 in 2000–2800 Caucasian births (most common disorder among whites).
   3. Presentation
      a. Approximately 35% of infants with meconium ileus at birth will have CF.
      b. Poor nutrition (decreased fat stores, poor weight gain).
      c. Pulmonary dysfunction (abnormal quantity and quality of pulmonary secretions).
      d. Increased susceptibility to infection (particularly *Pseudomonas* pneumonia).

4. Treatment and outcome
   a. Currently, CF is an incurable disease that leads to early pulmonary death. With early, aggressive therapy (replacement enzymes, antibiotics, fat-soluble vitamin supplements, predigested formula), most of those affected have an improved quality of life with mean life expectancy in the 20s.
   b. Lung transplants and the prospect of gene therapies offer hope for increased life span in the future.

E. **Hemoglobinopathies (Sickle Cell)**
   1. Diagnostic considerations
      a. Specimen is tested for hemoglobin abnormalities with major goal of identifying sickle cell disease before onset of pneumococcal infection.
      b. Infants with sickle cell anemia should be started on penicillin prophylaxis as soon as diagnosis is confirmed.
      c. Confirmatory testing is necessary to differentiate infants with the disease from those who are only carriers (sickle cell trait).
   2. Incidence
      a. The autosomal recessive sickle gene is carried by 10% of African-Americans in the United States.
      b. 1 in 400 African-American infants will have sickle cell anemia.
      c. Less severe forms occur in Arabs, East Indians, and those of Middle Eastern and southern European descent.
   3. Presentation (onset at approximately 4 months of age)
      a. Hand-foot syndrome (low-grade fever, painful swelling of hands and feet as a result of infarction of metacarpal and metatarsal bones).
      b. Splenic sequestration crisis (massive pooling of blood in the spleen can lead to vascular collapse; anemia, splenomegaly, hypotension).
      c. Frequent life-threatening infections.
   4. Treatment is symptomatic, with restoration of intravascular volume, red blood cell transfusions, splenectomy, prophylactic antibiotics, pneumococcal immunization.
   5. Outcome
      a. Untreated: Can be lethal in infancy; cerebral vascular accidents, aseptic bone necrosis, retinopathy, infections.
      b. Treated: Death from overwhelming sepsis can be prevented by heightened vigilance and penicillin prophylaxis; developmental and physical disabilities can be minimized.

F. **Hypothyroidism** (AAP, 1993)
   1. Conditions resulting in abnormally low serum T_4 concentrations: thyroid agenesis, heterotopic thyroid gland, and inherited disorders in thyroid hormone biosynthesis.
   2. Thyroid is an endocrine gland that concentrates iodide from the blood, then manufactures and secretes the iodothyronines (T_3, T_4), which enhance cellular protein and enzyme synthesis important for growth, development, and thermogenesis.

3. NBGS also measures thyroid stimulating hormone (TSH) which helps to distinguish false-positive results (low T_4, elevated TSH indicates primary hypothyroidism); 6%–12% will be detected only by the second screening. (See Table C-8 in Appendix C for normal laboratory thyroid values.)
4. Incidence: 1 in 3600–5000 screened infants
5. Presentation
   a. Of affected infants, 95% will be asymptomatic at birth.
   b. Infants with thyroid agenesis will have the classical findings of atypical facies, hypertelorism, exophthalmos, short nose, enlarged protruding tongue, large fontanelles, and umbilical hernias.
   c. Untreated hypothyroidism results in mental retardation, delayed development, constipation, feeding difficulties, poor growth, hypothermia, and hypoactivity.
6. Treatment
   a. Lifelong thyroid replacement with synthetic T_4.
   b. Intermittent monitoring/dosage adjustment to achieve normal serum thyroxin level for age.
7. Outcome
   a. The earlier the presentation, the poorer the outcome.
   b. Early diagnosis and treatment may prevent mental retardation.

G. Biotinidase Deficiency

1. Biotinidase is an enzyme responsible for sequestration of dietary biotin after bacterial synthesis in the intestine.
   a. Biotin is then available for use as a cofactor in biotin-dependent carboxylase enzymes.
   b. Carboxylases are important in fatty acid synthesis, amino acid digestion, and gluconeogenesis.
2. Biotinidase deficiency is an autosomal recessive disorder leading to multiple carboxylase deficiency.
3. Presentation
   a. Neurologic and cutaneous abnormalities include myoclonic seizures, hypotonia, dermatitis, alopecia, and conjunctivitis.
   b. Later findings include hearing loss, optic atrophy, developmental abnormalities, and immunologic abnormalities.
   c. Ketoacidosis and organic acidemia can lead to coma and death if untreated.
   d. Onset varies from 2 weeks to 3 years.
4. Incidence
   a. 1 in 72,000 to 126,000 live births in the United States.
   b. Deficiency can be profound (<10% enzyme activity) or partial (10%–30%).
5. Prevention
   a. Children identified by early diagnosis with newborn genetic screening are asymptomatic after treatment.
   b. Oldest child identified by screening and treated before becoming symptomatic is currently 15 years old.

6. Treatment
   a. Oral biotin replacement, 10 mg/day (some children have required higher doses).
   b. Inexpensive therapy, ~ $25–$100/year.
7. Outcome
   a. Marked improvement after treatment; long-term outcome unknown.
   b. Residual hearing loss, vision loss, and developmental delay have been seen after treatment in symptomatic children.

H. **Congenital Adrenal Hyperplasia (CAH)**
   1. Autosomal recessive genetic disorder of the adrenal glands in which there is a block in the production and manufacture of cortisol, the stress hormone. Both classic and nonclassic forms of the disease are caused by deficiencies in the adrenal enzymes used to synthesize glucocorticoids. The result is increased production of cortisol precursors and androgens from the adrenal gland. The resulting secretion of large quantities of androgens early in life leads to virilization of female fetuses. Some patients with CAH also lack aldosterone, which helps maintain sodium levels. Because aldosterone is necessary for normal retention of sodium by the kidneys, its absence leads to a "salt-wasting" disorder.
   2. Incidence: 1 in 10,000–16,000 live births
   3. Presentation
      a. Simple virilizing form—ambiguous genitalia
      b. Salt-wasting form—adrenal crisis between 1 to 4 weeks of age, presenting with poor appetite, vomiting, failure to grow, and potentially fatal electrolyte and water imbalance
   4. Treatment
      a. All patients with CAH, regardless of form, are treated with glucocorticoid replacement therapy.
      b. Patients with the salt-wasting form of deficiency must also receive mineralocorticoid therapy to normalize the abnormalities in sodium balance associated with aldosterone deficiency.
      c. Surgical procedures are used to correct the genital abnormalities of girls with the virilizing form of CAH.
   5. Outcome
      a. Early diagnosis through newborn screening may avert salt-losing crisis.
      b. Lifelong monitoring and treatment are required.

CHROMOSOME ANALYSIS

A. Suspect chromosome abnormality when three or more minor anomalies are present.
B. Review family history for comparable defects, consanguinity, frequent fetal loss.
C. Review prenatal history for maternal exposure to infection, illness, fever, medication, x-ray procedures, known teratogens, substance abuse.

D. If diagnosis is suspected, provide appropriate explanations to parents and primary care provider regarding abnormalities that indicate the possibility of a genetic or chromosomal problem. Proceed with work-up at the discretion of the primary care provider.

E. If diagnosis is obvious (e.g., some infants with Down syndrome), discuss management with the primary care provider and consider blood sample for chromosome analysis and/or genetic consult.

PARENTAL CARE WHEN THE CHILD HAS A CHROMOSOMAL ABNORMALITY

A. When appropriate, involve social services staff to begin grief counseling. (If prenatal diagnosis, consult with staff already involved with family.)

B. When appropriate, refer for genetic counseling, support groups.

C. Encourage verbalization of feelings, family involvement.

D. Relating "bad news" (Sharp et al., 1992).

  1. Parental desires at the first encounter

    a. Discuss suspected diagnosis within the first 24–48 hours, especially implications for mental retardation.

    b. Arrange for a private discussion with both parents present.

    c. Have child with parents when they are told.

    d. Informer should be caring and sympathetic and show feelings.

    e. Parents should be encouraged to show their feelings.

    f. Informer should be seated near and on the same level as parents, rather than standing remote from them.

    g. Follow up with an in-depth discussion later; details are usually not grasped the first time.

  2. Parental desires at a later time

    a. Practical information—discuss details of diagnosis and cause; what it means in terms of daily activities, child rearing; how parents can optimize their care; how to tell other family members.

    b. Talk about their feelings and ask questions in an "unhurried" atmosphere.

    c. Meet other families in the same situation.

    d. Provide referrals for community resources.

    e. Information about prognosis—express long-term, realistic expectations without eliminating all "hope."

  3. Supporting the grief process

    a. When given the diagnosis, parents lose their "perfect child" and must begin the process of accepting their "special child."

    b. Grief is a process that is ongoing and individualistic. Parents progress at different speeds, depending on their understanding, coping skills, and support systems.

    c. Community referral is essential because most of this process will take place after discharge.

REFERENCES

American Academy of Pediatrics, Committee on Genetics: Newborn screening fact sheets, *Pediatrics* 98(3):473-501, 1996 (*www.aap.org/policy/01565.html*).

American Academy of Pediatrics, Committee on Genetics: Molecular genetic testing in pediatric practice: a subject review, *Pediatrics* 106:1494-1497, 2000 (*www.aap.org/policy/re0023.html*).

American Academy of Pediatrics, Committee on Nutrition: Reimbursement for foods for special dietary use, *Pediatrics* 111(5): 1117-1119, 2003 (*www.aap.org/policy/s010102.html*).

American Academy of Pediatrics, Section on Endocrinology and Committee on Genetics: Technical report: congenital adrenal hyperplasia (RE0027), *Pediatrics* 106(6):1511-1518, 2000.

American Academy of Pediatrics, Section on Endocrinology and Committee on Genetics, and American Thyroid Association, Committee on Public Health: Newborn screening for congenital hypothyroidism: recommended guidelines, *Pediatrics* 91:1203-1209, 1993 (*www.aap.org/policy/04407.html*).

American Academy of Pediatrics and American College of Obstetricians and Gynecologists: Antepartum and intrapartum care. In Hauth JC, Merenstein GB, editors: *Guidelines for perinatal care,* ed 5, Elk Grove Village, IL, 2002, American Academy of Pediatrics; Washington DC, 2002, American College of Obstetricians and Gynecologists.

Elliott VS: *Should all newborns get the same tests? www.amednews.com,* February 4, 2002.

Greene C: Top ten pitfalls in newborn screening, *Genetic Drift* 15:1-4, 1998 (*www.mostgene.org/gd/gdvol15f.html*).

Latham EV et al: Genetic discrimination: perspectives of consumers, *Science* 274: 621-624, 1996.

Mountain States Genetic Network: *Newborn screening practitioner's manual,* ed 3, 2001 (*www.mostgene.org*).

National Committee for Clinical Laboratory Standards: *Blood collection on filter paper for neonatal screening program,* Wayne, PA, 1999, National Committee for Clinical Laboratory Standards. (Order filter paper [#LA4A3] from NCCLS, 940 West Valley Road, Suite 1400, Wayne, PA 19087 [phone: 510-688-0100])

National Newborn Screening and Genetics Resource Center: *National newborn screening report—2000,* Austin, TX, February 2003, NNSGRC (*http://genes-r-us.uthscsa.edu*).

Rothenberg KH: Genetic information and health insurance: state legislative approaches, *J Law Med Ethics* 23(4): 312-319, 1995.

Seashore MR: Neonatal screening for inborn errors of metabolism: update, *Semin Perinatal* 14:431-438, 1990.

Sharp MC, Strauss RP, Lorch SC: Communicating medical bad news: parents' experience and preferences, *J Pediatr* 121:539-546, 1992.

Wallman CM: Newborn genetic screening, *Neonatal Network* 17(3):55-60, 1998.

11 Circumcision

Sharon M. Glass, RNC, MS, NNP

Active debate about the benefits of circumcision is once again evident in the medical literature. The most recent policy statement by the American Academy of Pediatrics cites existing scientific evidence of potential circumcision benefits but does not recommend routine neonatal circumcision because of insufficient data. The AAP policy states "parents should determine what is in the best interest of the child" (AAP, 1999, p 686). Care providers are asked to provide accurate and unbiased information in discussions with parents to assist their decision. In a statement on circumcision, the American Medical Association reports that studies show parental decision regarding circumcision is based on father's circumcision status, opinions of significant others, and a desire for conformity rather than on a discussion of medical information of the potential advantages or disadvantages (AMA, 1999). Although numerous authors and organizations, including the American College of Obstetricians and Gynecologists support the AAP statement (ACOG, 2001), many others believe that the benefits of newborn circumcision as a preventive health measure far outweigh the minimal procedural risks. When parents choose circumcision, AAP strongly endorses the use of procedural analgesia or anesthesia to prevent pain and physiologic stress. Summary of currently available data is included to assist the health care provider with parental discussions.

INDICATIONS

A. **Prevention of Infection**
1. Balanoposthitis (inflammation of the glans and foreskin), balanitis (inflammation of the glans), and phimosis/paraphimosis (constriction of the glans by retraction and swelling of an inflamed foreskin) may necessitate eventual circumcision in 2%–5% of those not circumcised at birth. New medical management of phimosis with topical steroids might decrease the incidence of surgical intervention (Lerman and Liao, 2001; Monsour et al., 1999).
2. Urinary tract infection (UTI) (Schoen et al., 2000, Wiswell and Hachey, 1993).
   a. Predominance of UTI in males in the first year of life (~90% found in uncircumcised males), in contrast to higher incidence found in females later in life.
   b. Incidence of UTI is increased 12-fold among uncircumcised males in the first year of life, according to several retrospective studies.
   c. Uncircumcised males are more likely to require hospitalization for treatment, reflecting a 10-fold increase in the cost of therapy compared with circumcised males with UTI.

     d. Foreskin is thought to predispose to UTI because of higher periurethral bacterial colony counts. Uropathogens have been shown to preferentially bind to the foreskin mucosal surface as compared with the glans surface.

     e. Uncircumcised infants are more likely to be exposed to catheterization or bladder tap for diagnosis, increasing discomfort and associated morbidity.

     f. Renal scarring and sequelae is highest in infants with UTI in early life.

     g. Circumcision may benefit infants with anomalies of the urinary tract that predispose to UTI (such as hydronephrosis, ureteral reflux).

  3. Circumcision decreases the risk for sexually transmitted disease (STD), especially genital ulcerative disease (GUD) by 50% or more in high-risk populations (Bailey et al., 2001).

  4. Human immunodeficiency virus (HIV) (AAP, 1999; Bailey et al., 2001; Szabo and Short, 2000; Patterson et al., 2002)

     a. Protective effect of circumcision on HIV seroconversion may be due in part to the decreased risk for ulcerative disease. However, lack of circumcision has an association with HIV acquisition independent of GUD, which might be due to increased incidence of tears and abrasions during intercourse and moist environment conducive to viral replication and entry.

     b. Mucosal surface of the foreskin has a higher density of HIV target cells (CD4 T cells, Langerhans cells, macrophages) compared with the keritinized glans of the circumcised penis.

B. Prevention of Penile and Cervical Carcinoma

  1. Incidence of penile cancer in the United States is ~1 per 100,000 circumcised males and slightly more than twice that rate among uncircumcised males. This multifactorial disease is associated with numerous conditions in addition to lack of circumcision (e.g., poor hygienic practices, phimosis, human papilloma virus [HPV], genital warts, large number of sexual partners) (CDC, 2002).

  2. The uncircumcised male is four times more likely to develop penile HPV; in turn, HPV in the uncircumcised male increases the risk for cervical infection fourfold. HPV is strongly linked to >80% of cervical cancers and high-grade dysplasias (CDC, 2002; Castellsague et al., 2002).

CONTRAINDICATIONS

A. Anuria

B. Preterm, Sick, or Unstable Infants: Circumcision should be delayed.

C. Herpes Infection: Delay circumcision in those with risk factors for infection until cultures are proven negative (AAP, 2001).

D. Coagulopathy: Any infant with a family history of bleeding disorder.

E. Hypospadias, Epispadias, and Chordee: These abnormalities require evaluation and possible surgical correction before circumcision.

PROCEDURE RISKS

A. **Bleeding and Infection:** Risk associated with any surgical procedure; considered to be 0.2%–0.6% in routine newborn circumcision.

B. **Penile Injury:** Isolated reports of injury or partial amputation of glans, excessive skin removed from penile shaft, meatal ulceration, and meatal stenosis. Most complications are treatable with no long-term sequelae.

C. **Pain** (AAP, 1999; Taddio et al., 1997; Williamson and Williamson, 1983)

  1. Risks

    a. Anatomic and functional pathways of pain perception are present in newborn infants.

    b. Circumcision without anesthesia results in identifiable behavioral, physiologic, and biochemical manifestations of pain.

    c. Behavioral consequences of irritability, poor feeding, and disruption of normal sleep patterns can last 48 hours and disrupt parental-child interaction patterns.

    d. There is beginning evidence to indicate both short and long-term behavioral changes in infants circumcised without benefit of anesthesia.

  2. Anesthesia

    a. Dorsal penile nerve block (DPNB) (see "Circumcision Procedures" below)

     (1) Effective in reducing immediate behavioral, physiologic, and biochemical stress responses.

     (2) Subcutaneous injection of 1% lidocaine without epinephrine, 0.4 mL bilaterally at the dorsal penile root. Onset of action is 3–5 minutes, with duration of approximately 1–2 hours.

     (3) Buffered lidocaine solution is not recommended. The addition of bicarbonate may lessen the anesthetic effect of the lidocaine and did not show a difference in pain responses compared with the unbuffered solution in one study (Stang et al., 1997).

     (4) In a study of adults undergoing DPNB, significantly lower pain scores were achieved with very slow injection of lidocaine (Serour et al., 1998).

     (5) Risks are minimal when administered by the skilled practitioner and include mild bruising/edema at the injection site. There have been no reports of systemic toxicity with appropriate lidocaine use.

    b. Subcutaneous ring block

     (1) Attenuates all stress responses to circumcision. May be slightly more effective than DPNB in some stages of the procedure but does require more initial injections (AAP, 1999).

     (2) Circumferential local infiltration of the penile shaft below the prepuce approximately 1 cm above the root with 0.8 mL 1% Xylocaine without epinephrine.

    c. Eutectic mixture of local anesthetics

     (1) Topical anesthetic cream containing lidocaine and prilocaine.

   (2) Requires application of 1 g (0.5 mL) of the cream and occlusive covering for 1–2 hours before circumcision.

   (3) Modestly attenuates physiologic and behavioral pain responses when compared with placebo but is less effective than either DPNB or ring block (Taddio et al., 2000).

3. Supportive measures
   a. Sucrose pacifier has been shown to be a significant adjunct to anesthesia in soothing the infant and ameliorating the pain of the lidocaine injections. Its effectiveness is not thought to be exerted at a molecular level but the "sweet taste" stimulates the opioid pathway and release of endogenous pain relief chemicals (Kaufman et al., 2002).
   b. Use of 27- to 30-gauge needle diminishes the pain response to multiple injections.
   c. Acetaminophen, 15 mg/kg, has shown effect only 4–6 hours after the postoperative period.
   d. Padded restraint boards, upright positioning, use of only lower limb restraints and warm blankets add to the infant's comfort during the procedure.

D. **Urologic Consultation:** Should be obtained if abnormalities (glanular hypospadias) are encountered after the procedure is begun or if any complications occur.

INFORMED CONSENT

A. Parental written informed consent is required.
B. Explain procedure, risks, and proposed benefits.
C. Verbal explanations and written consents must be provided in the primary language of parents.

TYPES OF CIRCUMCISION

A. **Plastibell:** Prepuce is separated from glans; Plastibell (small plastic ring) is inserted between glans and prepuce; string is tied, securing the prepuce to the Plastibell and creating stasis prior to excision (see "Circumcision Procedures" below). Skin remnants under the string necrose, allowing the string and Plastibell to fall off in 6 to 8 days (Color Plate 7).

B. **Gomco:** Prepuce is separated from glans; Gomco clamp is positioned and tightened to crush nerve endings and vessels, promoting stasis prior to excision (see "Circumcision Procedures" below).

C. **Mogen:** Prepuce is stretched beyond the glans and pulled through a slit in the Mogen clamp before excision; penis is tightly wrapped to control bleeding.

CIRCUMCISION PROCEDURES (Kirya and Werthmann, 1978; Murray et al., 2002)

A. **Dorsal Penile Nerve Block for Circumcision**
   1. Outcome: To provide adequate analgesia for circumcision, in which pain and stress are definite side effects

2. General information
    a. Person doing the procedure should obtain consent for penile nerve block along with the consent for circumcision. Possible risks and benefits of this procedure should be discussed before obtaining consent.
    b. Subcutaneous edema at the injection site commonly occurs but should resolve within 24 hours.
    c. Complications are rare but can include local hematoma formation.
3. Equipment
    a. Two tuberculin syringes with 27- to 30-gauge needles.
    b. 1% lidocaine (without epinephrine).
    c. Antiseptic swabs.
    d. Equipment for circumcision procedure.
4. Procedure
    a. Ensure that consent has been obtained, all equipment is available, and infant is restrained.
    b. Observe Universal Precautions.
    c. Prepare each syringe with 0.4 mL of 1% lidocaine.
    d. Identify the 10 o'clock and 2 o'clock positions at the dorsal root of the penis and clean the sites with antiseptic swabs.
    e. Stabilize the penis with gentle downward traction at an angle of approximately 20–25 degrees. Pierce the skin at one of the dorsolateral positions (Figure 11-1) and advance the needle 0.25–0.50 cm so that the tip of the needle remains freely mobile in the subcutaneous tissue.
    f. Infiltrate with 0.4 mL of 1% lidocaine after aspirating with the syringe to ensure that a blood vessel has not been entered.
    g. Repeat procedure at the other site using the second syringe. Both infiltrations should produce a subcutaneous bleb spanning approximately 50% of the penile circumference.

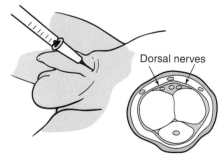

FIGURE 11-1 ● Dorsal penile nerve block injection. (From Spencer DM, Miller KA, O'Quinn M, et al: Dorsal penile nerve block in neonatal circumcision: chloroprocaine versus lidocaine, *Am J Perinatol* 9:216, 1992.)

      h. Wait 3 to 5 minutes after the injection of anesthesia before beginning the circumcision procedure.

    5. Documentation: Document dorsal penile nerve block procedure along with circumcision note in the medical record. Include amount and type of anesthesia used, patient tolerance, bleeding or edema at the injection site, and any complications.

B. Plastibell Circumcision (Figure 11-2)

    1. Outcome: Removal of the penile prepuce

    2. General information

      a. Consent for circumcision should be obtained by the person doing the procedure. Possible risks and benefits of this procedure should be discussed prior to obtaining consent.

      b. Resuscitation equipment must be immediately available.

      c. Ensure that the infant has voided at least once and has not been fed within 1 hour of the procedure.

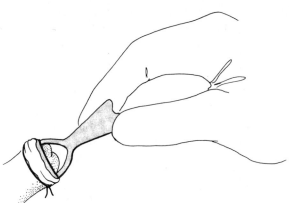

Bell is fitted over penis. Suture is tied around the rim of the bell, and excess prepuce is cut away

The plastic rim remains in place until healing occurs

FIGURE 11-2 ● Plastibell is fitted over the glans and the excess foreskin is pulled up over the plastic ring. A suture is tied around the rim to apply pressure to the blood vessels. The excess foreskin is removed. The plastic ring with the suture in place provides for hemostasis. As healing occurs, the plastic ring loosens and falls off. This process takes approximately 5 to 8 days. (From Murray SS, McKinney ES, Gorrie TM: *Foundations of maternal newborn nursing,* Philadelphia, 2002, WB Saunders, with permission.)

   d. Most complications are minor and include bleeding, local inflammation or minor infection, and urinary retention.

   e. Major complications that have occurred include excessive removal of preputial and penile skin, laceration of the urethra, formation of penile webs, adherence of prepuce to the glans, and penile loss or gangrene resulting from necrotizing infections.

   f. Close observation is necessary for any evidence of complications and to ensure that the infant voids following the procedure.

   g. Urologic consult should be obtained if complications occur.

3. Equipment

   a. Circumcision tray.

   b. Appropriate-sized Plastibell.

   c. Antiseptic solution.

4. Procedure

   a. Check the infant's identification band, restrain infant on circumcision board, offer the infant a sucrose pacifier, and wash the genital area with soap and water. Provide warmth.

   b. Observe Universal Precautions.

   c. With sterile procedure, open the circumcision tray and place the Plastibell on the tray. Prepare antiseptic solution and pour alcohol over the Plastibell string for easier manipulation.

   d. Prep the genital area with antiseptic on cotton swabs in a circular pattern three times. Drape with sterile drapes.

   e. Clamp the edge of the prepuce at the 10 o'clock and 2 o'clock positions with two curved hemostats.

   f. Carefully advance the straight clamp under the prepuce, opening it to break the adhesions at the 12 o'clock, 10 o'clock, and 2 o'clock positions. Then reinsert the clamp and rotate from the 10 o'clock to the 2 o'clock position to ensure that the adhesions are cleared.

   g. Advance one blade of the clamp to the root of the penis under the prepuce to measure the distance and clamp the foreskin at the midline approximately one third of the measured distance. Wait 45 seconds for stasis before proceeding.

   h. Place the string around the base of the penis and prepare a loose surgical knot.

   i. Unclamp the straight clamp and cut the foreskin down the center of the previously clamped area.

   j. Retract the foreskin and gently remove any remaining adhesions and smegma with the blunt probe. Check to see that the entire corona is visible.

   k. Pull the foreskin back into position and place the Plastibell over the tip of the penis, ensuring that the meatus is visible at the center.

   l. Pull the prepared string into position in the groove of the Plastibell and check to ensure that no scrotal skin is included.

   m. Pull gently on the opposite ends of the string to tighten. Again, check the string and when ensured that it is in appropriate position in the Plastibell groove, tighten securely and hold tight for 20 seconds. Tie two additional knots and cut the string ends, leaving short tails.

n. Unclamp the two curved hemostats and remove the excess foreskin with scissors following the ridge on the Plastibell.

o. Break off the Plastibell handle and gently clean the area inside the Plastibell ring with a dry cotton-tipped applicator.

p. Remove the sterile drapes and wash off any remaining antiseptic with warm water.

q. Give postoperative instructions to the caretaker/parents.

5. Documentation: Document the circumcision procedure in the medical record. Include any use of anesthesia (see "Penile Dorsal Nerve Block for Circumcision" above), size of Plastibell used, patient tolerance, complications, and condition of the infant at the conclusion of the procedure.

C. Gomco Circumcision (Figure 11-3)

1. Outcome: Removal of the penile prepuce

2. General information

    a. Consent for circumcision should be obtained by the person doing the procedure. Possible risks and benefits of this procedure should be discussed prior to obtaining consent.

    b. Resuscitation equipment must be immediately available.

    c. Ensure that the infant has voided at least once and has not been fed within 1 hour of the procedure.

    d. Circumcision should not be performed on infants with epispadias, hypospadias, chordee, herpes simplex virus risk, or bleeding disorders.

    e. Most complications are minor and include bleeding, local inflammation or minor infection, and urinary retention.

    f. Major complications that have occurred include excessive removal of preputial and penile skin, laceration of the urethra, formation of penile webs, adherence of prepuce to the glans, and penile loss or gangrene resulting from necrotizing infections.

    g. Close observation is necessary for any evidence of complications and to ensure that the infant voids following the procedure.

    h. Urologic consult should be obtained if complications occur.

3. Equipment

    a. Circumcision tray.

    b. Appropriate-sized Gomco clamp.

    c. Small sterile safety pin (optional).

    d. Antiseptic solution.

4. Procedure

    a. Check the infant's identification band, restrain the infant on circumcision board, offer the infant a sucrose pacifier, and wash the genital area with soap and water. Provide warmth.

    b. Observe Universal Precautions.

    c. With sterile procedure, open the circumcision tray and place the Gomco clamp and safety pin on the tray. Fill the cup with antiseptic solution.

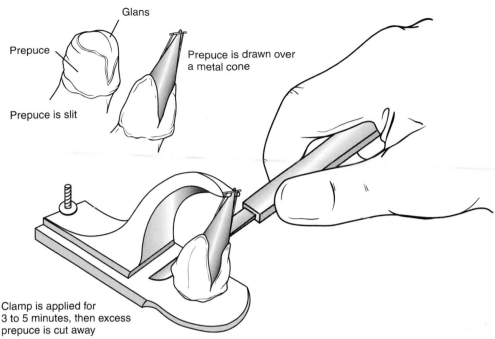

Glans

Prepuce

Prepuce is slit

Prepuce is drawn over a metal cone

Clamp is applied for 3 to 5 minutes, then excess prepuce is cut away

FIGURE 11-3 ● Gomco (Yellen) clamp. The physician pulls the prepuce over the metal cone-shaped device. The glans is protected by the metal cone. A clamp is applied around the cone and prepuce. The clamp is tightened to provide enough pressure to crush the blood vessels and provide for hemostasis. After 3 to 5 minutes, the excess foreskin is cut away. (From Murray SS, McKinney ES, Gorrie TM: *Foundations of maternal newborn nursing*, Philadelphia, 2002, WB Saunders, with permission.)

d. Prep the genital area with antiseptic on cotton swabs in a circular pattern three times. Drape with sterile drapes.

e. Clamp the edge of the prepuce at the 10 o'clock and 2 o'clock positions with the two curved hemostats.

f. Carefully advance the clamp under the prepuce, opening it to break the adhesions at the 12 o'clock, 10 o'clock, and 2 o'clock positions. Then reinsert the clamp and rotate from the 10 o'clock to the 2 o'clock position to ensure that the adhesions are cleared.

g. Advance one blade of the clamp to the root of the penis under the prepuce to measure the distance and clamp the foreskin at the midline approximately one half of the measured distance. Wait 45 seconds for stasis before proceeding.

h. Unclamp the straight clamp and cut the foreskin down the center of the previously clamped area.

     i. Retract the foreskin and gently remove any remaining adhesions and smegma with the blunt probe. Check to see that the entire corona is visible.

     j. Pull the foreskin back into position. Separate the Gomco bell from the clamp and place the bell over the tip of the penis. The small safety pin can be used to pin the top edges of the cut foreskin for easier manipulation of the foreskin through the Gomco clamp.

     k. Place the Gomco clamp over the bell, pulling the safety pin, and cut foreskin through the hole in the clamp. Check to ensure that no scrotal skin is included and secure the clamp against the bell. Tighten the Gomco screw as far as possible to achieve stasis.

     l. The Gomco clamp should remain in place for a full 5 minutes. The foreskin above the clamp is then carefully trimmed with a blade before the clamp is removed.

     m. Unscrew and remove the Gomco clamp. Very gently pry the remaining edge of foreskin from the Gomco bell with a wet 4×4.

     n. Remove the sterile drapes and wash off any remaining antiseptic with warm water.

     o. Give postoperative instructions to the caretaker/parents.

   5. Documentation: Document the circumcision procedure in the medical record. Include any use of anesthesia (see "Penile Dorsal Nerve Block for Circumcision" above), Gomco size, patient tolerance, complications, and condition of the infant at the conclusion of the procedure.

POSTCIRCUMCISION CARE

  A. If a Gomco clamp is used, petrolatum gauze dressing is loosely applied around the penis to prevent adherence of the diaper.

  B. No dressing is used with the Plastibell; petrolatum should be avoided because this could loosen the string.

  C. Avoid alcohol-containing wipes; the penis should be cleansed with clear water for the first few days until healing is evident.

  D. Position diapers loosely to avoid penile irritation.

  E. Document the first void following the circumcision or instruct parents that voiding should occur by 6–8 hours following the procedure.

  F. Instruct parents to observe and report unusual edema (swelling of entire penile shaft), erythema (entire length of penile shaft or on the abdomen at the penile base), bleeding (more than small spots on the diaper; bleeding that requires direct pressure), and drainage (serous or purulent).

  G. Describe the appearance of normal granulation tissue during the healing process.

  H. Reinforce the need for sponge baths until the circumcision is healed (usually about the same time required for umbilical cord separation).

REFERENCES

American Academy of Pediatrics: Circumcision policy statement, *Pediatrics* 103(3):686–693, 1999 *(www.aap.org/policy/RE9850.html)*.

American Academy of Pediatrics: Herpes simplex. In Peter G, editor: *Red book,* ed 24, Elk Grove Village, IL, 2001, American Academy of Pediatrics, p 275.

American Academy of Pediatrics, Committee on Infectious Diseases: In Pickering LK, editor: *Red book: report of the committee on infectious diseases,* ed 26, Elk Grove Village, IL, 2003, American Academy of Pediatrics, Committee on Infectious Diseases.

American College of Obstetricians and Gynecologists: ACOG Committee Opinion Number 260: Circumcision, *Obstet Gynecol* 98(4):707–708, 2001.

American Medical Association, Council on Scientific Affairs: *Neonatal circumcision,* Chicago, 1999, American Medical Association.

Bailey RC, Plummer FA, Moses S: Male circumcision and HIV prevention: current knowledge and future research directions, *Lancet Infec Dis* Nov 1(4): 223–231, 2001.

Castellsague et al: Male circumcision, penile human papillomavirus infection, and cervical cancer in female partners, *N Engl J Med* 346:1105–1112, 2002.

Centers for Disease Control and Prevention: Sexually transmitted diseases treatment guidelines—2002, *MMWR* 50(RR06): 1–80, 2002 *(www.cdc.gov/mmwr/preview/mmwrhtml/rr5106a1.htm)*.

Kaufman GE, Cimo S, Miller LW, Blass EM: An evaluation of the effects of sucrose on neonatal pain with two commonly used circumcision methods, *Am J Obstet Gynecol* 186(3):564–568, 2002.

Kirya C, Werthmann MW: Neonatal circumcision and penile dorsal nerve block—a painless procedure, *J Pediatr* 92:998-1000, 1978.

Lerman SE, Liao JC: Neonatal circumcision, *Pediatr Clin North Am* 48(6):1539–1557, 2001.

Monsour MA, Ribinovitch HH, Dean GE: Medical management of phimosis in children: our experience with topical steroids, *J Urology* 162:1162–1164, 1999.

Murray SS, McKinney ES, Gorrie TM: *Foundations of maternal newborn nursing,* Philadelphia, 2002, WB Saunders.

Patterson BK, Landay A, Siegel JN, et al: Susceptibility to human immunodeficiency virus-1 infection of human foreskin and cervical tissue grown in explant culture, *Am J Pathol* 161(3): 867–873, 2002.

Schoen EJ, Colby CJ, Ray GT: Newborn circumcision decreases incidence and costs of urinary tract infections during the first year of life, *Pediatrics* 105(4): 789–793, 2000.

Serour F, Mandelberg A, Mori J: Slow injection of local anaesthetic will decrease pain during dorsal penile nerve block, *Acta Anaesthesiol Scand* 48(2):926–928, 1998.

Stang HJ et al: Beyond dorsal penile nerve block: a more humane circumcision, *Pediatrics* 100(2):E3, 1997.

Szabo R, Short RV: How does male circumcision protect against HIV infection? *BMJ* 320(7249):1592–1594, 2000.

Taddio A, Katz J, Ilersich AL, Koren G. Effect of neonatal circumcision on pain response during subsequent routine vaccination, *Lancet* 349:599–603, 1997.

Taddio A, Ohlsson K, Ohlsson A: Lidocaine-prilocaine cream for analgesia during circumcision in newborn boys, *Cochrane Database Syst Rev* (2):CD000496, 2000.

Williamson PS, Williamson ML: Physiologic stress reduction by a local anesthetic during newborn circumcision, *Pediatrics* 71:36–40, 1983.

Wiswell TE, Hachey WE: Urinary tract infections and the uncircumcised state: an update, *Clin Pediatr* 32:130–134, 1993.

12 Immunizations

Sharon M. Glass, RNC, MS, NNP

A. **Hepatitis B Vaccine (HBV):** (American Academy of Pediatrics [AAP], 2000, 2003a, 2003b; Centers for Disease Control [CDC], 2003)
   1. Recommendations: CDC and AAP Committee on Infectious Diseases recommend universal immunization of all newborns and infants before hospital discharge regardless of mother's hepatitis B surface antigen (HBsAg) status (Figure 12-1).
      a. Dose depends on the product: Engerix-B dose is 10 μg; Recombivax (thiomerosal-free) dose is 5 μg. Both doses require administration of 0.5 mL IM and provide equally effective seroconversion.
      b. Immunization is recommended at birth, following the infant's bath, with two additional doses at 1–2 months after the first dose and at 6–18 months of age. Timing of additional doses depends on maternal HBsAg status (Table 12-1).
      c. Informed parental consent is required in some institutions.
      d. Hepatitis B virus has an external coat (hepatitis B surface antigen) and an internal core (hepatitis B core antigen). Core also contains hepatitis B e antigen. Maternal infection status can be identified by presence of antigens and/or antibodies (Table 12-2).
   2. Indications: Over 1.25 million people in the United States suffer chronic infection with hepatitis B, with 80,000 acute infections per year that can result in chronic liver disease and hepatocellular carcinoma. Chronic carriers are reservoirs of the infectious agent, which can be found in blood and body fluids, including saliva, urine, semen, cervical secretions, and wound exudates. Transmission via inanimate objects (towels, toothbrushes) may occur since the virus can survive at least 1 week in the environment. Risk for maternal hepatitis B infection resulting in acquired fetal/newborn infection is as follows:
      a. About 5% acquired by transplacental transfusion; highest risk occurs with birth exposure to maternal blood or secretions (90%).
      b. Breast-feeding does not influence the rate of transmission and should not be delayed until after the infant is immunized.
      c. Newborn treatment with HBV and hepatitis B immune globulin (HBIG) reduces the risk for viral transmission to ~5%. HBV provides

---

FIGURE 12-1 ● Recommended childhood immunization schedule, United States, 2004. (From the National Immunization Program, *www.cdc.gov/nip/*.)

Recommended Childhood and Adolescent Immunization Schedule—United States, January–June 2004

Vaccine ▼ / Age ►	Birth	1 mo	2 mos	4 mos	6 mos	12 mos	15 mos	18 mos	24 mos	4–6 yrs	11–12 yrs	13–18 yrs
Hepatitis B[1]	HepB #1 only if mother HBsAg (–)		HepB #2			HepB #3					HepB series	
Diphtheria, Tetanus, Pertussis[2]			DTaP	DTaP	DTaP		DTaP			DTaP	Td	Td
Haemophilus influenzae Type b[3]			Hib	Hib	Hib[3]	Hib						
Inactivated Poliovirus			IPV	IPV		IPV				IPV		
Measles, Mumps, Rubella[4]						MMR #1				MMR #2	MMR #2	
Varicella[5]						Varicella					Varicella	
Pneumococcal[6]			PCV	PCV	PCV	PCV				PCV	PPV	
Hepatitis A[7]											Hepatitis A series	
Influenza[8]						Influenza (yearly)						

Range of Recommended Ages　　Catch-up Immunization　　Preadolescent Assessment

Vaccines below this line are for selected populations

This schedule indicates the recommended ages for routine administration of currently licensed childhood vaccines, as of December 1, 2003, for children through age 18 years. Any dose not given at the recommended age should be given at any subsequent visit when indicated and feasible. ▨ Indicates age groups that warrant special effort to administer those vaccines not previously given. Additional vaccines may be licensed and recommended during the year. Licensed combination vaccines may be used whenever any components of the combination are indicated and the vaccine's other components are not contraindicated. Providers should consult the manufacturers' package inserts for detailed recommendations. Clinically significant adverse events that follow immunization should be reported to the Vaccine Adverse Event Reporting System (VAERS). Guidance about how to obtain and complete a VAERS form can be found on the Internet: http://www.vaers.org/ or by calling 1-800-822-7967.

1. Hepatitis B (HepB) vaccine. All infants should receive the first dose of hepatitis B vaccine soon after birth and before hospital discharge; the first dose may also be given by age 2 months if the infant's mother is hepatitis B surface antigen (HBsAg) negative. Only monovalent HepB can be used for the birth dose. Monovalent or combination vaccine containing HepB may be used to complete the series. Four doses of vaccine may be administered when a birth dose is given. The second dose should be given at least 4 weeks after the first dose, except for combination vaccines which cannot be administered before age 6 weeks. The third dose should be given at least 16 weeks after the first dose and at least 8 weeks after the second dose. The last dose in the vaccination series (third or fourth dose) should not be administered before age 24 weeks.

　　Infants born to HBsAg-positive mothers should receive HepB and 0.5 mL of Hepatitis B Immune Globulin (HBIG) within 12 hours of birth at separate sites. The second dose is recommended at age 1 to 2 months. The last dose in the immunization series should not be administered before age 24 weeks. These infants should be tested for HBsAg and antibody to HBsAg (anti-HBs) at age 9 to 15 months.

　　Infants born to mothers whose HBsAg status is unknown should receive the first dose of the HepB series within 12 hours of birth. Maternal blood should be drawn as soon as possible to determine the mother's HBsAg status; if the HBsAg test is positive, the infant should receive HBIG as soon as possible (no later than age 1 week). The second dose is recommended at age 1 to 2 months. The last dose in the immunization series should not be administered before age 24 weeks.

2. Diphtheria and tetanus toxoids and acellular pertussis (DTaP) vaccine. The fourth dose of DTaP may be administered as early as age 12 months, provided 6 months have elapsed since the third dose and the child is unlikely to return at age 15 to 18 months. The final dose in the series should be given at age ≥4 years. **Tetanus and diphtheria toxoids (Td)** is recommended at age 11 to 12 years if at least 5 years have elapsed since the last dose of tetanus and diphtheria toxoid-containing vaccine. Subsequent routine Td boosters are recommended every 10 years.

3. Haemophilus influenzae type b (Hib) conjugate vaccine. Three Hib conjugate vaccines are licensed for infant use. If PRP-OMP (PedvaxHIB or ComVax [Merck]) is administered at ages 2 and 4 months, a dose at age 6 months is not required. DTaP/Hib combination products should not be used for primary immunization in infants at ages 2, 4, or 6 months, but can be used as boosters following any Hib vaccine. The final dose in the series should be given ≥12 months.

4. Measles, mumps, and rubella vaccine (MMR). The second dose of MMR is recommended routinely at age 4 to 6 years but may be administered during any visit, provided at least 4 weeks have elapsed since the first dose and both doses are administered beginning at or after age 12 months. Those who have not previously received the second dose should complete the schedule by the 11- to 12-year-old visit.

5. Varicella vaccine. Varicella vaccine is recommended at any visit at or after age 12 months for susceptible children (i.e., those who lack a reliable history of chickenpox). Susceptible persons age ≥13 years should receive 2 doses, given at least 4 weeks apart.

6. Pneumococcal vaccine. The heptavalent **pneumococcal conjugate vaccine (PCV)** is recommended for all children age 2 to 23 months. It is also recommended for certain children age 24 to 59 months. The final dose in the series should be given at age ≥12 months. **Pneumococcal polysaccharide vaccine (PPV)** is recommended in addition to PCV for certain high-risk groups. See MMWR 2000;49(RR-9):1–38.

7. Hepatitis A vaccine. Hepatitis A vaccine is recommended for children and adolescents in selected states and regions, and for certain high-risk groups; consult your local public health authority. Children and adolescents in these states, regions, and high-risk groups who have not been immunized against hepatitis A can begin the hepatitis A immunization series during any visit. The 2 doses in the series should be administered at least 6 months apart. See MMWR 1999;48(RR-12):1–37.

8. Influenza vaccine. Influenza vaccine is recommended annually for children age ≥6 months with certain risk factors (including but not limited to asthma, cardiac disease, sickle cell disease, human immunodeficiency virus infection, and diabetes; and household members of persons in high risk groups [see MMWR 2003;52(RR-8):1–36]), and can be administered to all others wishing to obtain immunity. In addition, healthy children age 6 to 23 months are encouraged to receive influenza vaccine if feasible, because children in this age group are at substantially increased risk of influenza-related hospitalizations. For healthy persons age 5 to 49 years, the intranasally administered live-attenuated influenza vaccine (LAIV) is an acceptable alternative to the intramuscular trivalent inactivated influenza vaccine (TIV). See MMWR 2003;52(RR-13):1–8. Children receiving TIV should be administered a dosage appropriate for their age (0.25 mL if age 6 to 35 months or 0.5 mL if age ≥3 years). Children age ≤8 years who are receiving influenza vaccine for the first time should receive 2 doses (separated by at least 4 weeks for TIV and at least 6 weeks for LAIV).

For additional information about vaccines, including precautions and contraindications for immunization and vaccine shortages, please visit the National Immunization Program Website at www.cdc.gov/nip/ or call the National Immunization Information Hotline at 800-232-2522 (English) or 800-232-0233 (Spanish).

Approved by the Advisory Committee on Immunization Practices (www.cdc.gov/nip/acip), the American Academy of Pediatrics (www.aap.org), and the American Academy of Family Physicians (www.aafp.org).

● TABLE 12-1
Hepatitis B Immunoprophylaxis

Considerations	#1 HBV	HBIG	#2 HBV	#3 HBV
Maternal HBsAg negative	Before discharge	No	1–2 mo†	6–18 mo
Maternal HBsAg positive	Birth (within 12 hr)	Birth (within 12 hr)	1–2 mo†	6 mo
Maternal status unknown	Birth (within 12 hr)	Check maternal status; if positive, give before 7 days of age	1–2 mo†	6 mo
Preterm infant >2 kg Maternal HBsAg negative	Birth (within 12 hr)	No	1–2 mo†	6 mo
Preterm infant <2 kg Maternal HBsAg negative	1 month regardless of gestational age or weight	No	2 mo	6 mo
Preterm infant Maternal HBsAg positive	Birth (within 12 hr)	Birth (within 12 hr)	1–2 mo†	6 mo
Preterm infant <2 kg Maternal status unknown	Birth (within 12 hr)*	Within 12 hr if status is still unknown*		

*Poor immunogenicity achieved; should not be counted in required 3 doses to complete series.
†At least 1 month after the first dose.

● TABLE 12-2
Maternal Hepatitis Status

Hepatitis B Virus Antigens and Antibodies	Designation	Clinical Indication
Hepatitis B surface antigen	HBsAg	Acute or chronic infection. Appears 1 week to 2 months before onset of signs/symptoms.
Antibody to HBsAg	Anti-HBs	Resolved HBV infections or immunization immunity.
Hepatitis B e antigen	HBeAg	Infected, high risk for transmission. Indicates replicating virus. Detected at the same time as HBsAg; persists until anti-HBe rises.
Antibody to HBeAg	Anti-HBe	Infected, lower risk for transmission. Viral replication has stopped. Appears 5-6 weeks after onset; declines after 1-2 months.
Antibody to HBcAg	Anti-HBc	Acute, resolved, or chronic HBV infection. First antibody to be detected, present ≥1 week after onset, IgM lasts several months, IgG lasts for years.
IgM antibody to HBcAg	Anti-HBc IgM	Acute or recent HBV infection. HBsAg might not yet be positive; "window."

active immunization for long-term protection. HBIG provides passive protection for ~6 weeks.

    d. Monovalent vaccines are required for the birth dose; combination vaccines can be used to complete the series.

   3. Medication risks: Genetically engineered (synthetic) vaccine contains no blood products. No serious side effects have been documented.

B. Hepatitis B Immune Globulin (HBIG)

   1. Recommendations: CDC and AAP Committee on Infectious Diseases recommend administration to all newborns whose mother's HBsAg status is positive or unknown (AAP, 2003b).

    a. Prepared from plasma of donors with known high-titer anti-HBs.

    b. Dose: 0.5 mL of HBIG IM.

    c. If maternal HBsAg status is unknown, risk behaviors should be ascertained (history of IV substance abuse, hepatitis, unexplained jaundice, hemophilia/blood product exposure, sexually transmitted disease [STD]). If risk behaviors are present or if the infant is preterm with birth weight <2 kg and status cannot be determined in 12 hours, HBIG should be administered as soon as possible.

   2. Medication risks: HBIG is a pooled human blood product that has been purified and is therefore free from all antigens other than immunoglobulin G (IgG) antibody. Processing eliminates HIV and HCV.

C. Continuing Immunization Needs (AAP 2003a; 2003b)

   1. The National Childhood Vaccine Injury Act (1986) included requirements for notifying *all* patients and parents about vaccine benefits and risks. Vaccine Information Statements (VIS) are two-sided, one-page information sheets produced by the CDC that explain benefits and risks of each vaccine. VIS forms have been translated into a number of different languages and can be printed from the National Immunization Program website *(www.cdc.gov/nip)* or obtained from each state health department.

   2. AAP recommends that the following be documented in the medical record: date, site, and route of administration, vaccine manufacturer, lot number, expiration date, name and business address of the provider, VIS date, and date on which the VIS was provided to the caregiver.

   3. Predictors of poor immunization coverage (Wiecha and Gann, 1994)

    a. Ethnic and racial minority background.

    b. Lack of a regular source of health care.

    c. Lack of health insurance.

    d. Use of hospital emergency services for routine care.

    e. Low socioeconomic status/income.

    f. Large family size.

    g. Lack of knowledge and opinions about immunization.

    h. Missed opportunities to vaccinate due to illness.

    i. High proportion of missed prenatal visits.

   4. Timing (see Figure 12-1).

   5. Adverse events

      a. Common vaccine side effects such as local inflammation, fever, or rash are mild to moderate in severity and have no permanent sequelae. An adverse event occurring in timely association with vaccine administration in a single individual does not provide causal evidence. However, such events should be reported since multiple similar events might indicate an adverse reaction attributable to the vaccine components.

      b. The National Childhood Vaccine Injury Act of 1986 requires health care providers to report occurrences of adverse events via the Vaccine Adverse Event Reporting System (VAERS). Reporting information and forms can be found at *www.fda.gov/cber/vaers/vaers.htm* or 1-800-822-7967.

6. Vaccine risks and adverse effects (Ellenberg and Chen, 1997; AAP, 2003b)

      a. Poliomyelitis

          (1) The live-attenuated vaccine is associated with acute paralytic disease and is no longer recommended for use.

          (2) The inactivated vaccine (IPV) carries no risk for paralytic disease but requires injection and may be less efficacious. Contraindications include anaphylactic reactions to neomycin, streptomycin, or polymyxin B.

      b. Tetanus

          (1) Risks are associated with overuse.

          (2) Polyneuropathy incidence is ~0.4 in 1 million vaccine doses; onset is within 14 days of administration; complete recovery is the norm.

      c. Acellular pertussis

          (1) Whole-cell pertussis is associated with neurologic disease and is no longer recommended.

          (2) Acellular pertussis is less likely to produce adverse reactions because antigenic components are purified.

          (3) Vaccine efficacy of acellular pertussis is comparable to whole-cell pertussis.

          (4) No increased risk for Guillain-Barré syndrome has been documented with acellular preparations. Acute encephalopathy occurs rarely: 0–10 cases per 1 million doses administered. Contraindications include encephalopathy within 7 days of administration of a previous dose.

      d. Rubeola

          (1) Vaccine may produce clinical rubeola with the same complications (retinopathy, optic neuritis, encephalopathy, encephalomyelitis, meningitis) seen after naturally occurring infection. However, the incidence of complications from the vaccine compared with the natural infection is much reduced: ~1.1 in 1 million versus ~39 in 1 million.

          (2) Subacute sclerosing panencephalitis, a severe central nervous system (CNS) degenerative disease, occurs in 8.5 in 1 million with

naturally occurring viral infection and 0.7 in 1 million in vaccine recipients.

    (3) Contraindications include known immunodeficiency and anaphylactic reaction to neomycin or gelatin. Combination vaccines (MMR) are derived from chick embryos but hypersensitvity reactions in children with egg allergies are rare and do not contraindicate vaccination.

e. Hepatitis B

    (1) Anaphylaxis is rare, ~1 in 600 000. Guillain-Barré syndrome, rheumatoid arthritis, and demyelinating diseases of the CNS rarely have been reported; evidence for a causal link has not been found. Data show no association between vaccine and sudden infant death syndrome, multiple sclerosis, autoimmune disease, or chronic fatigue syndrome.

    (2) Contraindications include anaphylactic reaction to baker's yeast.

f. Haemophilus influenzae type b (HIB)

    (1) No significant adverse reactions or contraindications.

7. Immunization record should be initiated with HBV administration and given to the parents before discharge.

8. Parental teaching

a. Serious vaccine-preventable infectious diseases have shown a significant decline in incidence, morbidity, and mortality with the recommended immunization guidelines.

b. Risk from vaccination is small, as outlined above.

c. Preterm infants should be vaccinated at the recommended chronologic age with the full dose regardless of gestational age.

d. Contraindications

    (1) Use of live vaccines for children with congenital disorders of immune function, those receiving immunosuppressive therapy, and those with human immunodeficiency virus (HIV) or household contact with HIV-infected or immunodeficient persons.

    (2) Encephalopathy occurring within 5–15 days of a prior dose.

    (3) Anaphylactic reaction to a specific vaccine.

    (4) Anaphylactic reaction to a substance in a specific vaccine.

    (5) Mild upper respiratory infection and/or low-grade fever are not contraindications to vaccination; moderate to severe illness precludes immunization during the illness.

    (6) Evolving neurologic disease.

e. Retaining, updating, and keeping written immunization records available for physician visits and hospital admissions ensures immediate identification of deficiencies.

f. Completed immunizations are required before entry to school in the United States.

REFERENCES

American Academy of Pediatrics, Committee on Infectious Diseases: Hepatitis B. In Pickering LK, editor: *Red book: report of the committee on infectious diseases,* ed 25, Elk Grove Village, IL, 2000, American Academy of Pediatrics, pp 289-302.

American Academy of Pediatrics, Committee on Infectious Diseases: Recommended childhood and adolescent immunization schedule—United States, 2003, *Pediatrics* 111:212-216, 2003a *(www.aap. org/policy/0212.html).*

American Academy of Pediatrics, Committee on Infectious Diseases: In Pickering LK, editor: *Red book: report of the committee on infectious diseases,* ed 26, Elk Grove Village, IL, 2003b, American Academy of Pediatrics. *(http://aapredbook.aappublications.org).*

Centers for Disease Control: Recommended childhood immunization schedule—United States, 2003, *MMWR* 52(4):Q1-4, 2003 *(www.cdc.gov).*

Ellenberg SS, Chen RT: The complicated task of monitoring vaccine safety, *US Pub Health Serv Pub Health Reports* 112(1): 10-20, 1997.

Saari TN: AAP preference for birth dose of hepatitis B, *Section Infect Dis Newsletter* 6(1), 2003.

Wiecha JM, Gann P: Does maternal prenatal care use predict infant immunization delay? *Fam Med* 26:172-178, 1994.

13 Legal Issues

Sharon M. Glass, RNC, MS, NNP

ROUTINE CARE REFUSAL

A. Parental refusal for routine screen tests, immunizations, and prophylaxis should be documented in the permanent medical record by a letter or waiver of medical care signed by the parents and a note explaining short- and long-term risk factors that were discussed with the parents.

B. Care providers should ascertain parental understanding of the issues that have led to their decision. If their information is erroneous, frank discussions of specific concerns and provision of factual information can assist the parents in making an informed choice (AAP, Committee on Infectious Diseases, 2003).

C. Professionals who work with newborns must advocate for the health and safety of the newborn infant and seek judicial intervention if deemed essential for life preservation.

TESTING FOR DRUGS OF ABUSE (ACOG, 2003; Foubister, 2001; MCH Consultant, 2001)

A. Random checks without clinical suspicion are unethical and illegal.

B. Tests should be performed to direct immediate medical interventions.

C. Directions to Indian Health Services facilities under the direction of Maternal Child Health, U.S. Department of Health and Human Services, may serve as guidelines for development of hospital policies and procedures regarding testing for newborns:

1. Perform perinatal drug and alcohol tests as medically indicated (consistent with routine medical practice/treatment).

2. Explicit consent of the parent and/or guardian is not required, but the medical reason for testing should be documented in the patient's medical record when the order is written.

3. Refer patients into treatment.

4. Report positive test results in a newborn to the appropriate authority, as identified in the local policy.

5. Primary care providers are strongly encouraged to discuss the report and the significance of the positive test with the newborn's parent(s) and/or guardian.

6. If a drug or alcohol test is performed for a nonmedically indicated reason, such as local medical screening practices, the patient/parent must give consent.

237

    D. Figure 13-1 provides a sample information sheet that could be used to initiate discussion with parents regarding infant testing.

ADOPTION (AAP, Committee on Early Childhood, Adoption, and Dependent Care, 1991; Menard, 1997)

  A. Verify decision to place infant for adoption.

  B. Ascertain birth father's involvement and knowledge of adoption plan.

  C. Facilitate relinquishment through social services referral.

    1. Discuss adoption options or facilitate agency procedures if already in progress.

    2. Provide counseling or emotional support to birth mother, father, and family.

    3. Social worker may need to function as an intermediary between birth mother and father.

    4. Social worker needs to be knowledgeable of state laws regarding the father's rights.

  D. Birth Mother's Legal Rights

    1. May decide on the extent of infant viewing and her involvement with the care of the infant.

    2. Can consent to screening tests and procedures.

    3. Can authorize visitation by the adoptive family.

    4. Must legally authorize custody of the infant to an agency or individual before hospital discharge.

  E. Birth Father's Legal Rights

    1. Provision of legal rights afforded to the birth father varies considerably by state law.

    2. Father may have the right to custody over prospective adoptive parents if he is judged to be a fit parent and demonstrates full commitment to parental responsibilities.

    3. Some states require the father's written consent to adoption; others require only direct or indirect notification of adoption before termination of parental rights.

  F. Agency Adoption

    1. Infant is discharged to foster family to allow additional time for maternal decision for relinquishment if needed.

    2. Continued counseling is provided for the biologic mother.

  G. Private Adoption: Infant is discharged directly to the adoptive parents or representing attorney.

  H. Discharge Needs

    1. Provide agency or adoptive family with necessary medical instructions and routine care guidelines.

    2. Provide recommendations for pediatric follow-up care.

    3. There is no justification for keeping adoption a secret from a child and to do so may lead to mistrust, insecurity, and anger. The primary care provider can assist the adoptive family by guiding and supporting their

Special Testing of Your Infant

Due to the potential for long-term problems regarding your baby's health and the severity of symptoms of drug or alcohol withdrawal, which might include irritability, jitteriness, tremors, sneezing, breathing problems, unconsolable crying, poor sleep patterns, poor feeding, diarrhea, persistent weight loss, and seizures, it is necessary to document exposure to certain substances. This will allow the medical team to provide the appropriate observation for withdrawal behavior and appropriate medical care for your newborn.

Certain risk factors have been identified during your pregnancy that indicate the need for your infant to be tested for the possibility of drug or alcohol exposure. A urine or stool sample from the baby will be collected and tested. You will be given the results of the testing when available.

Report of positive test results will be sent to Social Services in the county of maternal residence and dealt with according to the protocols established in that county.

Please feel free to discuss this issue with your baby's doctor.

FIGURE 13-1 ● Sample parental information sheet regarding testing for drugs of abuse.

communications through an ongoing relationship (AAP, Committee on Early Childhood, Adoption, and Dependent Care, 1992; AAP, 2002).

CHILD PROTECTION

A. Protective Services

1. Primary care providers should be aware of the increasing number of families experiencing stress and should learn to recognize situations that interfere with safety of children and successful childrearing (AAP, Committee on Early Childhood, Adoption, and Dependent Care, 2001).
2. Institute multidisciplinary evaluation of any allegations of inappropriate care of the infant.
3. Involve community protective service staff before hospital discharge to ensure continued investigation, family counseling, and infant protection.
4. When necessary to ensure infant safety and protection, obtain court-ordered hold to maintain infant in custody of hospital staff until discharged to appropriate caretakers.
   a. Ensure that infant is attended by hospital staff at all times when out of the nursery. Infant should remain in the nursery if continuous observation is not practical.
   b. Ensure continuous close observation of the infant/family when visited in the nursery.
   c. Notify local police and hospital security personnel of infant hold and need for immediate response if called by staff to provide assistance.
5. Discharge against medical advice
   a. When parents insist on the discharge of their infant at a time considered inappropriate by the multidisciplinary team, the discharge is described as *against medical advice (AMA)*.
   b. Hospital procedure should be outlined to handle the situation and may include:
      (1) Presence of the attending physician, primary care nursing staff, and social service staff.
      (2) Documented proceedings of a conference with the parents to explain the risks of the discharge, to explain parental reasons for insisting on the discharge, and to explain any negotiations that were attempted to abort the situation.
      (3) AMA discharge form, which includes written explanation of the risks to the infant and acceptance by parents of full responsibility for the consequences of their actions with witnessed parental signatures.
      (4) Automatic referral to community protective services for surveillance and follow-up.

REFERENCES

American Academy of Pediatrics: *Adoption: guidelines for parents*, Elk Grove Village, IL, 2002, American Academy of Pediatrics. (Guide provides insight and advice for new adoptive parents, including when to tell children about their adoption, how to answer tough adoption questions, adopting older children, and learning about a child's medical history. Available online at the AAP Booksfare.)

American Academy of Pediatrics, Committee on Early Childhood, Adoption, and Dependent Care: Initial medical evaluation of an adopted child, *Pediatrics* 88: 642-664, 1991.

American Academy of Pediatrics, Committee on Early Childhood, Adoption, and Dependent Care: Families and adoption: the pediatrician's role in supporting communication, *AAP News* February, 1992.

American Academy of Pediatrics, Committee on Early Childhood, Adoption, and Dependent Care: The pediatrician's role in family support programs, *Pediatrics* 107:195-197, 2001.

American Academy of Pediatrics, Committee on Infectious Diseases: In Pickering LK, editor: *Red book: report of the committee on infectious diseases*, ed 26, Elk Grove Village, IL, 2003, American Academy of Pediatrics.

American College of Obstetricians and Gynecologists: *Illicit drug abuse and dependence in women*, 2003, *www.acog.org*. (This is a powerpoint educational program funded by the Physician Leadership on National Drug Policy at Brown University, Providence, Rhode Island, and the Physician Leadership on National Drug Policy project supported through contributions from individuals and foundations, primarily the Robert Wood Johnson Foundation and the John D. and Catherine T. MacArthur Foundation.)

Foubister V: *Drug testing of pregnant women quashed*. (Supreme Court rules hospital's policy is unconstitutional but leaves unanswered whether there are conditions under which medical privacy can be justifiably invaded, April 9, 2001 [*www.amednews.com*].)

MCH Consultant, PAIHS: *Perinatal maternal and neonatal drug and alcohol testing*, April 5, 2001, *www.ihs.gov*.

Menard BJ: A birth father and adoption in the perinatal setting, *Soc Work Health Care* 24:153-163, 1997.

Warning Signs of Common Problems of the Well Newborn

This section deals with the evaluation and treatment of common neonatal conditions and maternal problems that can affect the newborn. These include neonatal jaundice, plethora, pallor, problems commonly encountered with infants of mothers with diabetes, problems commonly seen in large- or small-for-gestational-age infants, and perinatal drug exposure issues.

14 Neonatal Jaundice

Elizabeth H. Thilo, MD

PHYSIOLOGY OF BILIRUBIN

A. **Metabolism of Bilirubin**
   1. Production of bilirubin
      a. Heme is the oxygen-carrying component of hemoglobin. Heme is broken down by the enzyme heme oxygenase to three components: iron (which is conserved by the body), carbon monoxide (which is exhaled), and biliverdin (which is further broken down to "unconjugated" bilirubin).
         (1) Breakdown of 1 g of hemoglobin produces 34 mg bilirubin.
         (2) Serum bilirubin conversions: 1 mg/dL (or mg%) = 17.2 μmol/mL.
         (3) Since carbon monoxide (CO) is produced as heme is degraded, measurement of CO in exhaled breath can be a measure of bilirubin production.
      b. Unconjugated bilirubin released into the bloodstream is rapidly bound to albumin and is then carried to the liver, where it is taken up by the hepatocyte and conjugated with glucuronide molecules by the enzyme glucuronyl transferase to make bilirubin glucuronide ("conjugated bilirubin").
      c. Conjugated bilirubin is then excreted via the bile to the intestine.
         (1) In the presence of gut flora, conjugated bilirubin is further metabolized and excreted in the stool; it is not absorbed from the intestine back into the blood.
         (2) In the absence of gut flora, or with prolonged time in the intestinal lumen, the glucuronide molecules are cleaved from conjugated bilirubin by β-glucuronidase in the intestinal lumen and mucosa, producing unconjugated bilirubin that can then be reabsorbed across the intestinal mucosa into the portal circulation and returned to the liver. This reabsorption path is referred to as the *enterohepatic circulation* (EHC).
B. **Definitions**
   1. **Unconjugated or indirect bilirubin:** Bilirubin not yet conjugated with glucuronide molecules but reversibly bound to albumin in blood (most of the unconjugated bilirubin in blood is bound to albumin). Unconjugated bilirubin builds up when glucuronyl transferase is deficient and conjugation is slow (as in the newborn).
   2. **Conjugated or direct bilirubin:** Bilirubin conjugated with glucuronide. It is water-soluble, which makes it readily excretable in bile and thus able to reach the intestine. Conjugated bilirubin builds up when obstruction to bile flow (cholestasis) occurs.

245

3. **Free bilirubin:** A very small amount of unconjugated bilirubin that is not bound to albumin and is therefore potentially available to cross the blood-brain barrier and cause damage to neurons.

C. **Laboratory Testing of Bilirubin**

1. Total serum bilirubin (TSB): Measures the sum of the unconjugated and conjugated bilirubin. TSB reflects the balance of bilirubin production and bilirubin clearance. Increased production and decreased clearance both lead to increased TSB levels. In general, jaundice in the first week of life is nearly all unconjugated bilirubin; thus TSB is commonly ordered for jaundiced infants in the first week of life.

2. Fractionated bilirubin: Provides the concentration of both the unconjugated and conjugated bilirubin.

3. Interlaboratory variability (the difference between two labs given the same specimen) is as high as 10% for unconjugated bilirubin measurements and even higher for conjugated bilirubin measurements.

4. Intralaboratory variability is lower than interlaboratory variability but is still as high as 5%. Therefore small changes in the value may be within lab error and not truly significant.

5. Whenever possible, all specimens from an individual infant should be sent to a single laboratory to facilitate comparisons and trending over time.

PHYSIOLOGIC JAUNDICE

A. **Incidence**

1. Visible jaundice (TSB >5 mg%–6 mg%) occurs in 60% or more of normal newborns.

2. Mean peak TSB is 5.5 mg% in Caucasian and African-American infants and 10 mg% in Asian infants by the third day of life.

3. TSB >5 mg% at 24 hours or >12 mg%–13 mg% by 48 hours should not be considered physiologic; a cause should be sought.

B. **Causes of Physiologic Jaundice**: Mechanisms contributing to physiologic jaundice may include any or all of the following:

1. Increased red cell mass in the neonate combined with shortened life span of fetal hemoglobin leads to greater daily production of bilirubin than is seen in the adult.

2. Decreased activity of UDP glucuronyl transferase (UDPGT) that correlates with gestational age, leading to decreased conjugation and excretion of bilirubin.

3. Increased enterohepatic circulation due to lack of intestinal flora, decreased gut motility, and small enteral intake, all of which are seen in the first days of life.

NONPHYSIOLOGIC JAUNDICE

A. **Definition:** In many cases it is difficult to differentiate between "physiologic hyperbilirubinemia" and "benign nonphysiologic hyperbilirubinemia."

In some instances, the bilirubin level is above the 95th percentile for gestational age and day of life (Figure 14-1), but the concentration of bilirubin poses no threat to the infant. On the other hand, there are relatively modestly increased bilirubin concentrations that result in significant brain damage because of other existing conditions that increase the risk for harm caused by a particular level of bilirubin. The goal of management of jaundice out of the "normal range" is to anticipate and treat bilirubin concentrations that might be potentially harmful to a particular patient (see "Kernicterus" below).

B. **Risk Factors for Significant Hyperbilirubinemia** (in decreasing order of importance)

   1. Early jaundice: Infants with clinical jaundice in the first 24–36 hours of life likely have increased production of bilirubin (e.g., hemolysis) or excessive blood cell breakdown from polycythemia or bruising.
   2. Significant jaundice in a previous infant.
   3. Exclusive breast-feeding: Infants who are breast-fed exclusively have little intake in the first few days, delayed institution of intestinal flora, and increased enterohepatic circulation of bilirubin (see below). Of the 90 cases of kernicterus reported from 1992 to 1999, breast-feeding was the only risk factor in about 50% of cases.

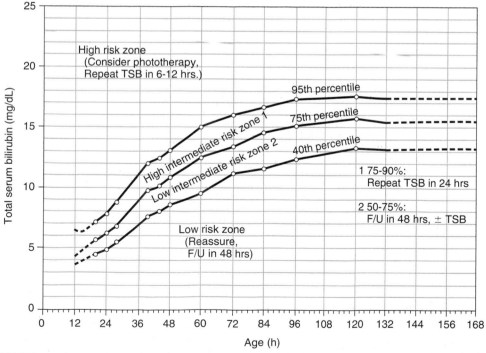

FIGURE 14-1 ● Bilirubin nomogram. (Adapted from Bhutani VK, Johnson L, Sivieri EM: Predictive ability of a predischarge hour-specific serum bilirubin for subsequent significant hyperbilirubinemia in healthy term and near-term newborns, *Pediatrics* 103:6-14, 1999.)

4. Gestational age <38 weeks: Mildly premature infants and borderline low-birth-weight infants are much more likely to have feeding difficulties and excessive jaundice than full-term, well-grown infants.
5. East Asian race: TSB >13 mg% occurs in approximately 20% of Asian infants as compared with 10% of Caucasian infants and 4% of African-American infants. This is due, at least in part, to prevalence of ABO incompatibilities and G6PD deficiency, and possibly also to racial variations in the Gilbert's syndrome variant of UDPGT (see below)
6. Cephalhematomas and bruising.
7. Maternal age ≥25 years.
8. Male sex.

CAUSES OF HYPERBILIRUBINEMIA

A. **Excessive Production of Bilirubin**
   1. Hemolysis leading to increased bilirubin production
      a. Antibody-mediated: Direct Coombs test– (also referred to as *direct antibody test*) or indirect Coombs test–positive
         (1) ABO incompatibility: Mother type O, baby type A or B
            (a) If antibody screen is negative (i.e., direct Coombs test– and indirect Coombs test–negative) on baby's blood, it is referred to as a "set-up." This occurs in 20% of mother-baby pairs. These infants are generally at no higher risk for jaundice than infants who are not a set-up.
            (b) If antibody screen is positive (i.e., direct Coombs test– or indirect Coombs test–positive) in infant's blood, it is called an "incompatibility." Although up to 33% of type A or B babies of type O mothers are antibody-positive, only about 20% of these infants develop severe jaundice.
         (2) Rh incompatibility: Mother Rh-negative, baby Rh-positive, baby's serum Rh antibody–positive.
            (a) Generally detected antenatally by maternal serum antibody screen and prevented by RhoGAM administration to Rh-negative women after miscarriage, abortion, or delivery of Rh-positive infant.
            (b) More predictable course of jaundice than with ABO incompatibility; increasing severity with each affected pregnancy.
         (3) Other incompatibilities due to so-called minor blood group antigens: e.g., Kell, Duffy, anti-E, anti-c, etc.
            (a) Uncommon, sometimes severe; similar pathogenesis to Rh disease.
      b. Nonantibody–mediated hemolysis: Direct Coombs test– or direct antibody test–negative
         (1) Red cell membrane defects: hereditary spherocytosis, elliptocytosis
            (a) Variable severity of hemolysis and jaundice but can require exchange transfusion.
            (b) Affected parent identified in only 70% of cases.

(c) May have mild to moderate splenomegaly on exam.

(d) Diagnosed by blood smear and osmotic fragility testing.

(2) Red cell enzyme defects: Glucose-6-phosphate dehydrogenase (G6PD) deficiency and pyruvate kinase deficiency

(a) G6PD deficiency is very common worldwide and may result in an accentuation of physiologic jaundice, occasionally severe, but rarely related to hemolysis alone (see Gilbert's syndrome below). It is an X-linked recessive disorder with highest prevalence in Southeast Asian, Mediterranean, and African individuals. As many as 11%–13% of African-Americans are affected.

(b) Diagnosis of these entities is by measurement of the enzyme in red cells.

2. Nonhemolytic causes of increased bilirubin production

   a. Bruising: On the head, face, or extremities, due to birth trauma; also includes cephalhematoma or other internal hemorrhages such as intracranial or adrenal bleeding.

   b. Polycythemia: Can be due to delayed cord clamping, twin-twin or maternal-fetal transfusions, or secondary to chronic intrauterine hypoxia, IUGR, or maternal diabetes.

B. **Decreased Bilirubin Clearance**

   1. Bowel obstruction: Delayed passage of meconium, increased enterohepatic circulation

   2. Inborn errors of metabolism

      a. Galactosemia: Jaundice with lethargy, hepatomegaly, and other signs of illness; frequently presents with infection, sepsis.

      b. Hypothyroidism: Excessive early or prolonged jaundice >2 weeks' duration in term infant; mechanism unknown.

      c. Glucuronyl transferase deficiency

         (1) Crigler-Najjar syndrome: Type I, the complete absence of glucuronyl transferase, is very severe and very rare and typically requires exchange transfusions in the first week. Type II, also rare, is less severe and responds to phenobarbital, which induces higher levels of the enzyme.

         (2) Gilbert syndrome: Mild deficiency of glucuronyl transferase and decreased hepatic uptake of bilirubin; frequently presents later in childhood or adolescence as mild persistent unconjugated hyperbilirubinemia, but now known to result in excessive levels of bilirubin in neonates who also have heterozygous or homozygous G6PD deficiency. Genetically prevalent (5% of most populations).

C. **Breast-Feeding–Associated Jaundice**

   1. Breast-feeding jaundice or "lack-of-breast-milk jaundice"

      a. Breast-fed infants have higher TSB in the first days of life than formula-fed infants, with 9% of breast-fed versus 2% of formula-fed infants having TSB of 13 mg%; 2% versus 0.3% having TSB of 15 mg%.

      b. Mechanism: Decreased enteral intake with increased enterohepatic circulation, analogous to starvation jaundice in adults. Note that jaundice may be an important indicator of inadequate breast milk supply or inadequate nursing and should prompt specific inquiries into this possibility.

2. Breast-milk jaundice syndrome
   a. Described in the 1960s; full-term breast-fed infants with persistent hyperbilirubinemia lasting 3-4 weeks after birth.
   b. Thought to be due to an inhibitory substance, perhaps β-glucuronidase, in the milk, although this has not been proven.
3. Breast-feeding jaundice and breast-milk jaundice syndrome may be the same entity because prolonged jaundice is common in breast-fed infants (20%–30%), and many of those with high bilirubin levels in the first days also have more persistent jaundice, suggesting a substantial overlap between the two syndromes.

TREATMENT OF HYPERBILIRUBINEMIA

A. **Treatment of Breast-Feeding–Associated Jaundice**
   1. Encourage frequent nursing, at least 8 to 10 times per day. Avoid pacifiers.
   2. Have mother pump her breasts after nursing with an electric breast pump to ensure adequate emptying of the breast and to bring in milk as quickly as possible.
   3. Avoid supplementation with water or glucose-water
      a. When studied, this has consistently produced an increase in maximal serum bilirubin.
      b. If supplementation is necessary for medical reasons (to support blood glucose or because of excessive weight loss), expressed breast milk or formula should be used, approximately 30 mL/feeding for term and near-term infants.
   4. Interruption of nursing is not necessary
      a. Study has shown that the most rapid decline in TSB occurs with phototherapy and adequate enteral intake of either breast milk or formula, as opposed to phototherapy without enteral intake or continued feeding without phototherapy.
      b. If formula supplementation is required, there may be a more rapid decline in TSB levels with casein-hydrolysate formula than with breast milk or standard cow milk–based formula
         (1) Human milk, but not formula, contains β-glucuronidase.
         (2) Casein-hydrolysate formula contains a β-glucuronidase inhibitor, which would suggest that the more rapid decline in TSB is due to decreased enterohepatic circulation.
      c. Therefore, continue breast-feeding or using expressed breast milk but supplement with formula (perhaps casein hydrolysate) to ensure adequate enteral intake during phototherapy.

B. **Phototherapy**
   1. Mechanism of action
      a. Light energy is absorbed by the bilirubin molecule and changes its stereochemical shape, creating configurational and structural isomers

that are more water-soluble and can be excreted in the bile without conjugation.

b. These processes occur as soon as the exposure to light occurs, making the bilirubin potentially less toxic long before the serum level falls.

2. Effectiveness

   a. Greatest impact occurs in the first 24–48 hours of therapy, with declining efficacy thereafter as the photo-isomers revert to natural unconjugated bilirubin in the intestine and are reabsorbed.

   b. Decreases the need for exchange transfusion in ABO and Rh hemolysis and in premature infants.

3. Factors affecting the efficiency of phototherapy: Wavelength, surface area of skin exposed, and irradiance

   a. Wavelength: 425–475 nm most effective (blue light)

   (1) Special blue lights (designated F20T12/BB) are the most effective, but these lights are the least tolerable to staff and make infants appear cyanotic.

   (2) Combination of special blue and white daylight lamps (four of each) works well and prevents staff discomfort.

   (3) Fiberoptic blankets using tungsten-halogen light are effective and portable; they also eliminate the need for eye patches and allow phototherapy to continue while the infant is held. However, because of the small surface area covered by a single blanket, they are less effective than standard daylight bulbs in term infants and should be combined with either standard phototherapy or with a second blanket on the infant's other side.

   b. Dose of light (irradiance)

   (1) Rapidity of bilirubin decline is directly related to irradiance ($\mu watt/cm^2$).

   (2) A minimum of 10-12 $\mu watt/cm^2$ is required; more is better.

   (3) Irradiance can be increased by bringing lights closer to the infant (reducing the distance from 30 cm to 15 cm, for example, increases irradiance from approximately 9 $\mu watt/cm^2$ to 15 $\mu watt/cm^2$). Providing more lights from several directions also increases irradiance.

4. Possible complications of phototherapy

   a. Retinal effects: Animal studies show some loss of rods and cones similar to premature aging. Eyes should be shielded from the light with commercially available eye protectors.

   b. Diarrhea: Frequent problem, possibly due to the high concentrations of bilirubin and bile salts excreted into the gut during phototherapy. Although the problem is not related to a lactase deficiency, as once suggested, feeding a lactose-free formula may help the diarrhea.

   c. Dehydration: Due to increased insensible losses of water through the skin and to increased water loss in the stool.

   d. Bronze-baby syndrome: Transient gray-bronze discoloration of infants with cholestatic jaundice treated with phototherapy.

(1) Probably due to accumulation of copper porphyrins.

(2) Not likely to be a problem in the absence of hepatosplenomegaly and light stools, but infants known or suspected to have cholestasis should not receive phototherapy.

(3) No known lasting adverse effects; eventually disappears after stopping phototherapy.

5. Guidelines for phototherapy in the term and near-term healthy infant (see Figure 14-1)

   a. Consider phototherapy if the screening TSB exceeds the 95th percentile on the hour-specific monogram. This is approximately:

   (1) TSB >8 mg% at 24 hours.

   (2) TSB >13 mg% at 48 hours.

   (3) TSB >16 mg% at 72 hours.

   (4) If phototherapy is not elected, follow-up TSB should be obtained in 12 hours.

   (5) Evaluation for excessive bilirubin production is indicated.

   b. In all cases, adequate feeding and elimination should be identified and ensured.

C. **Pharmacotherapy:** At the present time, there is no medication available for management of jaundice in the well-baby nursery. Future therapy for jaundice in these infants may include:

1. Heme oxygenase inhibitors (tin-protoporphyrin and tin-mesoporphyrin): These drugs suppress the formation of bilirubin and have been shown to decrease the severity of hyperbilirubinemia in term infants with ABO incompatibility and G6PD deficiency. A single dose injected shortly after birth may be all that is required; side effects appear to be limited to mild skin erythema if phototherapy is required. Not yet approved in the United States. The specifics of dosing, timing of dose, who should be treated, and possible side effects are still being defined, but this therapy may become much more common in the future.

2. Phenobarbital: When administered before birth to the mother of an infant with known severe hemolytic disease, phenobarbital will induce the infant's hepatic enzymes, as well as increase hepatic uptake of bilirubin and excretion of bilirubin into the bile. At least 10 days' prenatal therapy is required to reduce postnatal bilirubin on the fourth day by 50% and to reduce the need for exchange transfusion in infants with ABO incompatibility.

SYSTEM-BASED APPROACH TO JAUNDICE

A. A suggested system-based approach to the evaluation of jaundice and for prevention of bilirubin toxicity (Johnson et al., 2002)

1. Parental education regarding neonatal jaundice—prenatal and postnatal

2. Predischarge bilirubin management

   a. Visual evaluation for jaundice at the end of transition (6 hours) and at 12–24 hours with documentation in the chart and corroboration of perceived jaundice by transcutaneous (TcB) or serum bilirubin measurement per institutional policy. Some have advocated a universal hour-specific predischarge TcB or TSB at time of newborn genetic screen to identify infants at risk for potentially dangerous postdischarge hyperbilirubinemia (>75% on hour-specific bilirubin nomogram; see Figure 14-1).

   b. Evaluation of every infant for presence of known risk factors (hemolysis, birth trauma, inadequate nutrition, delayed stooling, etc.). In addition to TSB laboratory testing, this may include:

   (1) Blood type and Coombs testing.

   (2) CBC and smear.

   (3) Serial hematocrits if significant hemolysis is present. Hemolysis will continue even after the jaundice has resolved, and late anemia requiring intervention (3–6 weeks) can occur.

   (4) Fractionated bilirubin and urine for reducing substances if infant appears ill or septic, has hepatosplenomegaly, or produces light stools.

3. Postdischarge bilirubin management (follow-up)

   a. Mandatory evaluation by health care professional for jaundice and/or hyperbilirubinemia at 96 hours of age (range 84–108), or sooner if high risk by the hour-specific nomogram.

   b. Simultaneous evaluation of nutrition, elimination history, hydration, lactation issues, and cardiorespiratory stability. Specific inquiries and observations that need to be made at this early follow-up visit include:

   (1) Weight loss in excess of 8%–10%: Should be considered excessive and indicative of inadequate intake.

   (2) At least six noticeably wet diapers per day and at least 2–3 stools per day (no longer meconium).

   (3) Frequency and duration of nursing: Should be at least 8–10 times in a 24-hour period, for at least 10 minutes on each side each time. Swallowing should be audible.

   (4) Optional follow-up of high-risk babies at 7 days to assess for resolution of jaundice. Routine follow-up at 2 weeks to document complete resolution of jaundice.

BILIRUBIN TOXICITY (KERNICTERUS)

1. Pathology: At extreme levels, bilirubin causes brain damage; this is referred to as *bilirubin encephalopathy* or *kernicterus*, named for the yellow staining of brain nuclei ("kerns") seen at autopsy. With current management, bilirubin toxicity resulting in brain damage is rare. Bilirubin toxicity depends on many factors, and bilirubin level alone does not predict risk for toxicity. However, avoiding extreme levels of bilirubin is advisable.

2. Clinical features of bilirubin encephalopathy range from minimal encephalopathy with lethargy, hypotonia, and poor suck to severe, largely irreversible disease associated with coma and seizures (Bhutani et al., 1999).

3. Root cause analysis of the re-emergence of kernicterus shows the following fundamental causes (American Academy of Pediatrics, 2001):

   a. Early discharge (<48 hours) without early follow-up; particularly important in the near-term infant (35–37 weeks gestation).

   b. Failure to check the bilirubin level in an infant noted to be jaundiced before 24 hours of age.

   c. Failure to recognize the presence of risk factors for hyperbilirubinemia.

   d. Underestimating the severity of jaundice by clinical (e.g., visual) assessment.

   e. Lack of concern regarding the presence of jaundice.

   f. Delay in measuring serum bilirubin despite marked jaundice.

   g. Failure to respond to parental concerns regarding jaundice, poor feeding, or lethargy.

REFERENCES

American Academy of Pediatrics, Subcommittee on Neonatal Hyperbilirubinemia: Neonatal jaundice and kernicterus, *Pediatrics* 108:763-765, 2001.

Bhutani VK, Johnson LH: Kernicterus: lessons for the future from a current tragedy, *NeoReviews* 4(2):e30-32, 2003.

Bhutani VK, Johnson L, Sivieri EM: Predictive ability of a predischarge hour-specific serum bilirubin for subsequent significant hyperbilirubinemia in healthy term and near-term newborns, *Pediatrics* 103:6-14, 1999.

Brown AK: Kernicterus: past, present, and future, *NeoReviews* 4:e33-40, 2003.

Dennery PA, Seidman DS, Stevenson DK: Neonatal hyperbilirubinemia, *N Engl J Med* 344:581-590, 2001.

Gourley GR: Breastfeeding, diet, and neonatal hyperbilirubinemia, *NeoReviews* 1:e25-31, 2000.

Hammerman C, Kaplan M: Recent developments in the management of neonatal hyperbilirubinemia, *NeoReviews* 1:e19-24, 2000.

Johnson L, Brown AK: A pilot registry for acute and chronic kernicterus in term and near-term infants, *Pediatrics* 104:736, 1999.

Johnson LH, Bhutani VK, Brown AK: System-based approach to management of neonatal jaundice and prevention of kernicterus, *J Pediatr* 140:396-403, 2002.

Kaplan M, Hammerman C: Glucose-6-phosphate dehydrogenase deficiency: a worldwide potential cause of severe neonatal hyperbilirubinemia, *NeoReviews* 1:e32-38, 2000.

Kaplan M, Hammerman C, Feldman R, Brisk R: Predischarge bilirubin screening in glucose-6-phosphate dehydrogenase–deficient neonates, *Pediatrics* 105:533-537, 2000.

Kernicterus in full-term infants—United States, 1994-1998, *MMWR* 50(23):491-494, 2001.

Kernicterus threatens healthy newborns, *Sentinel Event Alert* 18, 2001 (*www.jcaho.org/edu*).

Neifert MR: Prevention of breastfeeding tragedies, *Pediatr Clin North Am* 48:273-297, 2001.

Newman TB, Xiong B, Gonzales VM, Escobar GJ: Prediction and prevention of extreme neonatal hyperbilirubinemia in a mature health maintenance organization, *Arch Pediatr Adolesc Med* 2000; 154:1140-7.

Poland RL: Preventing kernicterus: almost there, *J Pediatr* 140:385-386, 2002.

Plethora and Pallor

Janis J. Johnson, MD

PLETHORA AND POLYCYTHEMIA

Plethora is an excess of red blood cells leading to a ruddy appearance of the infant. Polycythemia is defined as a venous hematocrit >65%. Above 65% hematocrit, blood flow becomes increasingly hyperviscous, rising exponentially with the hematocrit. Since viscosity measurements generally are not available, hematocrit measurements are considered a good estimation of blood viscosity. Although polycythemia is the major cause of hyperviscosity, babies may also be hyperviscous because of the decreased red blood cell deformability, decreased plasma volume, increased plasma proteins, and hyperlipidemia. Decreased red cell deformability may be precipitated by hypoxia or acidosis.

A. **Infants at Risk for Polycythemia**
  1. Infants with intrauterine hypoxia, acute or chronic
     a. Infants of diabetic mothers (polycythemia may be secondary to other causes in these infants).
     b. Term and post-term infants who are small for gestational age.
     c. Newborns with perinatal asphyxia.
     d. Maternal smoking.
     e. Maternal preeclampsia.
  2. Neonates with placental transfusions.
     a. Recipient infant in twin-to-twin transfusion syndrome (e.g., monozygotic twins who share vascular connections).
     b. Maternal-fetal transfusion.
     c. Delayed cord clamping or "stripping" of the cord.
  3. Miscellaneous conditions with unknown causes.
     a. Chromosomal abnormalities (e.g., trisomies 13, 18, and 21).
     b. Beckwith-Wiedemann syndrome.

B. **Neonatal Evaluation**
  1. History: Information should be sought about conditions associated with chronic placental insufficiency, such as a history of maternal tobacco or drug use, chronic maternal illnesses, pre-eclampsia, or diabetes. Conditions associated with placental transfusions from delayed cord clamping include out-of-hospital or precipitous deliveries. In a study evaluating outcomes of unattended out-of-hospital births, the incidence of polycythemia was 14% (Bateman, 1994). Examination of the placenta of twins may reveal vascular connections responsible for a twin-to-twin transfusion.
  2. Examination: Clinical manifestations of polycythemia
     a. Plethora or ruddy appearance.

     b. Respiratory distress with grunting respirations, tachypnea, and/or nasal flaring.

     c. Cardiomegaly, congestive heart failure.

     d. Central nervous system signs, such as jitteriness, irritability, lethargy, seizures, or apnea.

     e. Hypoglycemia.

     f. Hypocalcemia.

     g. Feeding intolerance.

     h. Decreased urine output.

  3. Laboratory studies

     a. Screening candidates: The American Academy of Pediatrics (AAP) Committee on Fetus and Newborn does not recommend universal screening of all newborns, but rather screening of high-risk neonates only (AAP, 1993).

     b. Screening technique: Screening consists of a capillary hematocrit at 4–6 hours of age. The timing of the screening is important. In a study evaluating sequential hematocrits in full-term infants, it was found that the peripheral venous hematocrit was highest at 2 hours of age and dropped to cord blood levels by 18 hours of age. Only 38% of infants with hematocrits >64% at 2 hours of age continued to have a high level beyond 12 hours of age (Ramamurthy and Berlanga, 1987).

     c. Venous hematocrit

       (1) If the infant is found to have a capillary hematocrit >70%, a venous hematocrit is indicated. Venous hematocrits drawn from the antecubital fossa are often as much as 20% lower than the capillary hematocrit. Peripheral measurements are higher secondary to blood stasis.

       (2) If the venous hematocrit is >65%–70%, a partial exchange may be warranted. The use of partial exchange transfusion remains somewhat controversial. It is not clear whether the neurologic and developmental deficits found on long-term follow-up of polycythemic infant are secondary to the polycythemia or due to the underlying placental insufficiency that caused the polycythemia (Bada et al., 1992). However, most medical authorities continue to recommend partial exchange transfusion for infants with hematocrits >65% who have symptoms.

C. Treatment—Partial Exchange Transfusion

  1. Desired hematocrit: The partial exchange transfusion should be calculated to reduce the central hematocrit to a level between 50% and 55%.

  2. Volume calculation:

Volume of exchange in mL = (wt in kg) × (blood volume of 80 mL / kg)

$$\times \left(\frac{\text{observed Hct} \times \text{desired Hct}}{\text{observed Hct}} \right)$$

For example, the volume of blood to be exchanged in a 3.6-kg infant with hematocrit of 74% would be:

$$\text{Volume of exchange in mL} = (3.6 \text{ kg}) \times (80 \text{ mL} / \text{kg}) \times \left(\frac{74 - 50}{74}\right) = 93 \text{ mL}$$

3. Partial exchange transfusion technique: After insertion of an umbilical vein catheter, blood should be removed in 5- and 10-mL increments and replaced with an equal volume of normal saline or a colloid such as 5% albumin. An alternative method is an isovolumetric method, whereby blood is removed through an umbilical artery catheter as normal saline or colloid is infused via an umbilical vein catheter or peripheral intravenous line. The latter method is thought to result in fewer hemodynamic changes in the infant. We prefer to use normal saline rather than albumin because of the decreased cost and because saline does not expose the infant to a plasma product. There are no studies that compare the efficacy of crystalloid (e.g., normal saline) versus colloid (e.g., 5% albumin) in partial exchange transfusions.
4. Complications
   a. Thrombosis or phlebitis of the portal vein.
   b. Necrotizing enterocolitis. Because of the increased risk for necrotizing enterocolitis following exchange (Black et al., 1985), it may be advisable to give the infant's bowels a rest for 12–24 hours after exchange before resuming feedings.
5. Infants should be monitored for the development of hyperbilirubinemia, a known complication of polycythemia.
D. **Prognosis:** In the most severe form, polycythemia can be responsible for cerebral infarcts, heart failure, necrotizing enterocolitis, and acute tubular necrosis. It is hoped that partial exchange will prevent the likelihood of later neurologic delays. In a study of school-age children, comparing those who had a partial exchange for polycythemia with those who had not, researchers found that subtle neurologic signs persisted beyond early childhood (Delaney-Black et al., 1989).

PALLOR

A. **Signs of Anemia:** Pallor, or paleness, can be a sign of anemia, a disorder of an abnormally low red cell mass.
   1. The normal cord hemoglobin range of term infants is 16.7–17.9 g/dL; the normal cord hematocrit range is 48%–60%.
   2. Hemoglobin levels measured in capillary blood samples may be as much as 20% higher than venous samples.
   3. Serial measurements should be taken from the same source.
   4. Physiologic anemia
      a. The hemoglobin concentration of term infants decreases after the first week as a result of decreased red cell production coupled with shortened red cell survival as compared with adults (80–100 days).

      b. The nadir is reached between 2 and 3 months of age.

      c. Hemoglobin levels drop to as low as 11.4 g/dL.

      d. This is a normal drop in red blood cell mass and requires no treatment.

B. Causes of Anemia: Can be classified in three major categories:

  1. Blood loss (hemorrhage)

    a. Occult hemorrhage before birth

      (1) Fetal-maternal hemorrhage: The diagnosis of fetal-maternal hemorrhage can be made by the use of the Betke-Kleihauer test. This test, which should be performed within hours of delivery, looks for fetal cells in the maternal circulation. Acid elution destroys adult hemoglobin, whereas fetal cells stain red.

      (2) Twin-to-twin hemorrhage: Twin-to-twin transfusions occur only in monozygotic (identical), monochorionic pairs. When a significant hemorrhage has occurred, the hemoglobin difference between the twins exceeds 5 g/dL. Typically, if the transfusion has been chronic, there will be a marked difference in the weights of the twins. The donor twin may be small and have oligohydramnios, whereas the recipient twin will be much larger and plethoric. The anemic twin may develop signs of congestive heart failure. In contrast, the plethoric twin may have signs of polycythemia (see "Plethora," above).

    b. Obstetric accidents and malformation of placenta or cord

      (1) Rupture or hematoma of cord.

      (2) Incision of placenta during cesarean section.

      (3) Placenta previa.

      (4) Abruptio placentae.

    c. Internal hemorrhage

      (1) Cephalhematoma.

      (2) Subgaleal hemorrhage.

      (3) Adrenal hemorrhage.

      (4) Retroperitoneal hemorrhage.

      (5) Ruptured liver or spleen.

  2. Increased destruction (hemolysis) (see Chapter 14 for more details regarding evaluation and management).

    a. Hemolytic disease is common in the newborn period. It is often associated with indirect hyperbilirubinemia and is usually recognized because of the presenting jaundice. Signs of hemolytic disease include rapid fall in hemoglobin concentration, increased red cell production (reticulocytosis), and jaundice.

    b. Causes of hemolytic disease

      (1) Immunity: Immune-related anemias are by far the most common type of hemolytic anemia seen in the newborn period. Causes include Rh incompatibility, ABO incompatibility, and minor blood group incompatibilities.

      (2) Congenital defects of the red cell: These include glucose-6-phosphate dehydrogenase (G6PD) deficiency, pyruvate kinase deficiency,

hereditary spherocytosis, hereditary elliptocytosis, and alpha-thalassemia.

(3) Infection: Hemolysis may be induced by bacterial sepsis and a wide variety of congenital infections including those caused by syphilis, toxoplasmosis, cytomegalovirus (CMV), rubella, coxsackie B, and *Escherichia coli*.

(4) Macro- and microangiopathic hemolytic anemia.

(5) Disseminated intravascular coagulation.

c. Clinical findings may include jaundice, pallor, and enlargement of the liver and/or spleen.

d. Laboratory findings in hemolytic disease severe enough to cause anemia include falling hematocrit, increased reticulocyte count, blood smear with evidence of hemolysis, and a positive Coombs test.

3. Impaired red blood cell production: This is an unusual cause of anemia in the newborn period. The most common disorder is the Diamond-Blackfan anemia, also known as congenital hypoplastic anemia. Diagnosis is suspected by a decreased reticulocyte count in the face of anemia.

C. **Acute Versus Chronic Blood Loss**

1. Acute blood loss

   a. Infants with acute blood loss (20% of blood volume) will be pale with tachypnea, tachycardia, weak pulses, and low blood pressure. Hepatosplenomegaly is not present.

   b. Initial hematocrit may be normal.

   c. Repeat test 3–6 hours later will show a marked drop secondary to hemodilution.

2. Chronic blood loss (e.g., from maternal-fetal hemorrhage)

   a. May show minimal distress.

   b. Will only show severe distress when the hemorrhage has been so severe that the infant has signs of congestive heart failure as evidenced by cardiomegaly on chest x-ray and/or hepatomegaly.

D. **Treatment of Severe Anemia**

1. If the baby is in distress at birth, administer oxygen and secure the airway if necessary.

2. Insert umbilical venous line (peripheral access will be difficult if infant is profoundly hypertensive).

3. Obtain blood samples for hemoglobin and cross-match.

4. If hypovolemic shock is strongly suspected, administer volume in the form of 5% albumin. O-negative blood can also be given if available. If the infant suffered acute hemorrhage, dramatic improvement is often seen in perfusion and blood pressure after volume administration.

5. Warning: If the infant has been chronically anemic and shows signs of congestive heart failure, additional volume is contraindicated. In this instance, a partial exchange transfusion with packed red blood cells is more appropriate.

REFERENCES

American Academy of Pediatrics, Committee on Fetus and Newborn: Routine evaluation of blood pressure, hematocrit, and glucose in newborns, *Pediatrics* 92: 474-476, 1993.

American Academy of Pediatrics and American College of Obstetricians and Gynecologists: Perinatal infections. In *Guidelines for perinatal care*, ed 5, Elk Grove Village, IL, 2002, American Academy of Pediatrics and American College of Obstetricians and Gynecologists.

Bada HS, Korones SB, Pourcyrous M, et al: Asymptomatic syndrome of polycythemia hyperviscosity: effect of partial plasma exchange transfusion, *J Pediatr* 120:579-582, 1992.

Bateman DA, O'Bryan L, Nicholas SW, Heagarty MC: Outcome of unattended out-of-hospital births in Harlem, *Arch Pediatr Adolesc Med* 148:127-152, 1994.

Black VD, Rumack CM, Lubchenco LO, Koops BL: Gastrointestinal injury in polycythemic term infants, *Pediatrics* 76:225-231, 1985.

Delaney-Black V, Camp BW, Luchenco LO, et al: Neonatal hyperviscosity: association with lower achievement and IQ scores at school age, *Pediatrics* 83:662-667, 1989.

Ramamurthy RS, Berlanga M: Postnatal alteration in hematocrit and viscosity in normal and polycythemic infants, *J Pediatr* 110:929-934, 1987.

16 Approach to the Infant at Risk for Hypoglycemia

Susan F. Townsend, MD

IDENTIFICATION OF INFANTS AT RISK FOR HYPOGLYCEMIA

A. **Why Evaluate Newborns for Hypoglycemia?**

1. After birth, the continuous supply of glucose from the mother to the baby, via the placenta, is interrupted. The newborn must learn to regulate his or her blood glucose concentration and adjust to an intermittent feeding schedule. There can be many complications in this adjustment, including delayed metabolic adaptations, small volumes of food intake initially, and increased metabolic demands if the infant is stressed.

2. Prolonged, untreated, severe hypoglycemia has been associated with adverse neurodevelopment. We therefore evaluate infants at high risk or those with symptoms consistent with hypoglycemia in order to identify infants with low glucose concentrations and treat them to increase the blood glucose concentration to a physiologic range.

B. **Whom to Evaluate for Hypoglycemia?**

1. Definition: The definition of hypoglycemia varies depending on the population described—e.g., newborns with symptoms, newborns with risk factors, or healthy term newborns. Hypoglycemia is commonly defined as a blood glucose concentration less than 40 mg/dL (or 2.2 mmol/L) in asymptomatic term newborns. A higher level is commonly used for infants with abnormal clinical signs (45 mg/dL, 2.5 mmol/L).

2. Incidence: Although the reported incidence varies depending on the criteria used for the definition and the population studied, hypoglycemia is very common in the newborn, with an incidence of 2–10/1000 live births (AAP, 1993; Cornblath et al., 1993; Cornblath et al., 2000).

3. Which newborns do we screen? (Box 16-1)

   a. Because there is variability in the measurements obtained from reagent test strips compared with laboratory methods (AAP, 1993; Kaplan et al., 1989) and no evidence that treating asymptomatic infants will affect their outcome, the American Academy of Pediatrics (AAP) does *not* currently recommend universal screening of all newborns on admission (AAP, 1993). Instead, selective evaluation of infants at high risk or

---

---

infants with symptoms is recommended. In some nurseries, if the population of high-risk infants is the majority, screening of all infants may be warranted.

b. High-risk factors for hypoglycemia in infants include the following:
  (1) Birth weight <2500 g
  (2) Gestation <37 weeks
  (3) Small for gestational age (SGA) or large or gestational age (LGA)
  (4) Being the smaller of discordant twins (weight difference >25%)
  (5) Mother with diabetes
  (6) History of birth stress, as indicated by 5-minute Apgar score <5
  (7) Family history of neonate with hypoglycemia or unexplained infant death
  (8) Physical exam findings consistent with midline defects of the brain or with microphallus (at risk for panhypopituitary deficiencies)
  (9) Omphalocele, macroglossia, and/or hemihypertrophy (suggestive of a syndrome with increased risk for oversecretion of insulin)

c. Symptoms suggestive of hypoglycemia: The signs and symptoms of hypoglycemia in the newborn are nonspecific. They include the following:
  (1) Lethargy
  (2) Poor feeding
  (3) Irritability or jitteriness
  (4) Emesis
  (5) Tachycardia
  (6) Respiratory distress
  (7) Hypotonia
  (8) Temperature instability
  (9) Pallor or cyanosis
  (10) Apnea
  (11) Seizures

    d. Infants with symptoms of hypoglycemia should have a blood glucose concentration measured by a chemical determination in the laboratory, not solely by reagent test strip. If the blood glucose concentration is normal, other etiologies for these symptoms should be investigated.

  4. Hypoglycemia associated with other underlying diseases: Hypoglycemia can occur in isolation, or it may accompany other problems in the newborn. In particular, if infants are at risk for infection, polycythemia, congenital heart disease, or other congenital or metabolic diseases, these should be systematically investigated. Also, if symptoms fail to respond to appropriate treatment, other underlying conditions that could lead to hypoglycemia (especially treatable causes, such as bacterial infection) should be evaluated.

C. When to Evaluate for Hypoglycemia?

  1. In high-risk infants without symptoms, the initial routine screening should be obtained on admission to the nursery and no later than 2 hours of age. Repeated screening, every 2–3 hours or before feeds, is recommended in the first 8–12 hours of life in high-risk infants. SGA infants are more likely to have prolonged hypoglycemia and should have repeat screening at ~24 hours.

  2. Infants with symptoms suggesting hypoglycemia should be screened at the time symptoms are present, regardless of age.

D. How to Evaluate for Hypoglycemia: Initial screening may be done with a reagent test strip (e.g., Dextrostix or Chemstrip BG). However, these strips have been shown to be highly variable, especially at higher hematocrits (because of the lower plasma volumes) and at low blood glucose concentrations (AAP, 1993; Kaplan et al., 1989). Therefore all low values (<40–45 mg/dL) should be confirmed by a quantitative method in the laboratory, particularly in symptomatic infants or when considering treatment with intravenous glucose. Blood can be sampled by venipuncture, finger stick, or heel stick, using the appropriate technique. Although blood glucose concentrations will vary depending on whether a heel stick (capillary) or venous sample is obtained, these potential differences should not influence or delay treatment.

MANAGEMENT OF HYPOGLYCEMIA

A. The Vigorous Infant (Figure 16-1)

  1. Enteral feeds: Vigorous infants who are asymptomatic with a low blood glucose concentration should be fed promptly. Either glucose-water or formula can be used, with a minimum volume of 25 to 30 mL (a goal should be to provide about 10 mL/kg). Breast-feeding alone may not be adequate to correct the blood glucose concentration in the immediate hours after birth, because the breast milk supply is not developed. If the blood glucose concentration is >25 mg/dL, feeds alone may be adequate. A single gavage feed may be given if the infant is not interested in nippling. A repeat blood glucose concentration should be obtained 30 minutes to 1 hour after feeding, and feeds should be offered every 2 to 3 hours. The blood glucose should

LGA, SGA, IDM, <37 or >42 wks, history of birth stress*
Check glucose with test strip at 1–2 hours of age
CHECK STAT if there are SYMPTOMS**
SGA infants, recheck at 24 hours

Glucose test strip >40 (no symptoms)
Check glucose test strip x 2 or 3 before feeds
Check immediately if symptoms occur**

Glucose test strip 25–40 mg/dl: Feed Immediately
No symptoms present**; infant active, alert, vigorous
  Re-check glucose test strip in 1 hour
  Breast or formula feed, q 2–3 hours. No gavage
  Re-check glucose test strip x 3 ac and PRN
  If infant won't nipple feed, notify HO and prepare
    to transfer to NCU for IV glucose--can consider gavage
    feeds
Symptoms present**
  Confirm with whole blood glucose sent to lab
  Start IV, give 2 mL/kg bolus of D10W, and continue at
    100 mL/kg/day

**Glucose test strip 25–40 mg/dl, after 1 or 2 feeds,
or symptoms on any later checks**
  Confirm with whole blood glucose sent to lab
  Start IV, give 2 mL/kg bolus of D10W, and continue at
    100 mL/kg/day

Glucose test strip <25, with or without symptoms
  Confirm with whole blood glucose sent to lab
  Feed immediately if infant vigorous.
  Start IV, give 2 mL/kg bolus of D10W, and continue at
    100 mL/kg/day

*BIRTH STRESS
  5 minute Apgar <5
  Meconium noted
  Temp <36 on admission
  C/S for fetal distress
  Prolonged (>2 hr) 2nd stage
  Prolonged (>3) vacuum

**SYMPTOMS OF HYPOGLYCEMIA

Lethargy	Seizures
Poor feed	Respiratory distress
Irritability	Apnea
Emesis	Temp instability
Tachycardia	Tachypnea
Jitteriness	Pallor
Cyanosis	

FIGURE 16-1 ● Suggested guideline for management of hypoglycemia. All glucose values in mg/dL.

be rechecked before feeds until concentration is >50 mg/dL at least twice. Lack of interest in nipple feeds in a hypoglycemic infant should prompt treatment with intravenous glucose, rather than continued gavage feeding.

2. Intravenous glucose: A blood glucose concentration <25 mg/dL should prompt intravenous glucose infusion at 6 to 8 mg/kg/minute (about 100 mL/kg per day of a 10% dextrose solution in water), and monitoring of blood sugar should continue at 1- to 3-hour intervals until concentration is >50 mg/dL on two or more occasions. A bolus of 2 mL/kg of a 10% glucose solution can be given at the onset of treatment (McGowan et al., 2002). If the blood glucose concentrations remain low (<40–45 mg/dL), the infusion should be increased in 10%–15% increments. A blood glucose requirement of >12 mg/kg/min sustained over many hours should prompt concern for possible hyperinsulinism.

3. Feedings may be offered when infant is vigorous and blood glucose concentration has corrected. If the blood glucose concentration is >25 mg/dL but the infant is not interested in eating (does not appear hungry, will not suck and swallow), an intravenous glucose solution should be used to return the blood glucose concentration to the normal range.

B. **The Symptomatic, Lethargic, or Ill-Appearing Infant** (see Figure 16-1)

1. All infants with symptomatic hypoglycemia should have an IV placed if there is not immediate resolution of symptoms and correction of hypoglycemia after one nipple feed. If infant will not feed, an IV should be placed immediately and a bolus of 2 mL/kg 10% glucose should be given over several minutes followed by an infusion of 10% glucose to deliver 6–8 mg/kg/min (about 100 mL/kg/day). If blood glucose is <25 mg/dL, intravenous treatment should be started, regardless of whether infant will feed. The blood glucose concentration should be monitored at 3- to 4-hour intervals over the next 24 hours and glucose infusion increased or decreased to maintain blood glucose in a physiologic range (~50 mg/dL). Feeds should be offered as infant becomes more vigorous and symptoms diminish. Repeated gavage feeding should be avoided.

2. If symptoms persist or if the infant has other findings suggestive of underlying illness, other causes of hypoglycemia should be investigated. A white blood count can be obtained to screen for infection and a hematocrit to screen for polycythemia. Other conditions should be investigated depending on the character and duration of symptoms and any physical findings.

REFERENCES

American Academy of Pediatrics, Committee on Fetus and Newborn: Routine evaluation of blood pressure, hematocrit, and glucose in newborns, *Pediatrics* 92:474-476, 1993.

Cornblath M, Schwartz R: Hypoglycemia in the neonate, *J Pediatr Endocrinol* 6:113-129, 1993.

Cornblath M, Hawdon JM, Williams AF, Aynsley-Green A, Ward-Platt MP, Schwartz R, Kalhan SC: Controversies regarding definition of neonatal hypoglycemia: suggested operational thresholds, *Pediatrics* 105:1141-1145, 2000.

Kaplan M, Blondheim O, Alon I, Eylath U, Trestian S, Eidelman AI: Screening for hypoglycemia with plasma in neonatal blood of high hematocrit value, *Crit Care Med* 17:279-282, 1989.

McGowan JE, Hagedorn MI, Price WR, Hay WW Jr: Glucose homeostasis. In Merenstein GB, Gardner SL, editors: *Handbook of neonatal intensive care*, ed 5, St Louis, 2002, Mosby Year Book.

17 | The Large-for-Gestational-Age and the Small-for-Gestational-Age Infant

Susan F. Townsend, MD

THE LARGE-FOR-GESTATIONAL-AGE (LGA) INFANT AND THE INFANT OF THE DIABETIC MOTHER (IDM)

Background and Definitions

A. **Large-for-Gestational-Age (LGA) Infant**
   1. Fetal growth is influenced by maternal nutrition, genetics, placental function, environment, and other factors (Charlton V, 1991).
   2. Infants are considered "large for dates" or "large for gestational age" (LGA) if they weigh more than the 90th percentile for their gestational age.
   3. LGA infants can be the result of normal pregnancies or result from over stimulation of growth in utero.
   4. Infants of mothers with elevated blood sugars during pregnancy (i.e., diabetes mellitus or gestational diabetes) are exposed to high circulating blood sugars during fetal development and/or develop high circulating insulin levels and therefore may grow excessively.

B. **Infant of a Diabetic Mother (IDM)**
   1. A subpopulation of LGA infants consists of infants born to mothers with diabetes mellitus, which can be present before or develop during pregnancy. These infants are called infants of diabetic mothers, or IDMs.
   2. Some IDMs born to mothers with long-standing diabetes mellitus and vascular disease may be small for gestational age.

Neonatal Complications Related to LGA Infants and IDMs (Table 17-1)

A. **Traumatic Birth Injuries**
   1. Because of large fetal size, LGA infants are more likely to be delivered by cesarean section or to experience complications of vaginal delivery, such as shoulder or body dystocia.

● TABLE 17-1
● **Complications Frequently Seen in LGA Infants and IDMs in the Perinatal Period**

Complication	LGA	IDM
Birth trauma	X	X
Hypoglycemia	X	X
Polycythemia	X	X
Hyperbilirubinemia	X	X
Hypocalcemia		X
Respiratory distress		X
Major anomalies		X

2. LGA infants are therefore at greater risk for perinatal depression and/or birth injuries.
3. Common birth injuries include clavicle fractures, facial palsies, and brachial plexus injuries.

B. Hypoglycemia
1. All LGA infants, particularly IDMs, are at increased risk for hypoglycemia after birth. The risk is greatest in the first 6 hours of life; however, IDMs may experience earlier (at <1 hour of age) and more severe (<10 mg/dL) hypoglycemia.
2. Symptoms are nonspecific and may include jitteriness, cyanosis, lethargy, seizures, apnea, hypotonia, and poor feeding.
3. Many infants with hypoglycemia are asymptomatic. Table 17-2 is a guideline for normal and abnormal blood sugar values in term infants (see Figure 16-1 for an approach to hypoglycemia in LGA infants and IDMs).

C. Polycythemia
1. IDMs and LGA infants have higher hematocrits at birth and increased circulating red blood cell mass (see Chapter 15 for complications of polycythemia).
2. IDMs may be at additional risk for thrombosis because of relative hypercoagulability during the newborn period (Manco-Johnson et al., 1991).

● TABLE 17-2
● **Definition of Normal and Abnormal Blood Sugar Values (mg/dL) in Term Infants**

Age	Hypoglycemia	Normoglycemia	Hyperglycemia
0–6 hours	<25 mg/dL	40–100 mg/dL	>125 mg/dL
6–24 hours	<30 mg/dL	45–100 mg/dL	>125 mg/dL
>24 hours	<40 mg/dL	50–100 mg/dL	>125 mg/dL

Adapted from Schwartz R: Neonatal hypoglycemia: back to basics in diagnosis and treatment, *Diabetes* 40(suppl 2): 71-73, 1991.

D. Jaundice: Hyperbilirubinemia occurs with greater frequency in both IDMs and LGA infants. This may in part be related to polycythemia.

E. Hypocalcemia: IDMs have an increased incidence of hypocalcemia in the first days of life because maternal diabetes causes immaturity of parathyroid function in the newborn. Symptoms are similar to those seen with hypoglycemia (jitteriness, twitching, seizures).

F. Respiratory Distress: IDMs have an increased incidence of respiratory distress syndrome (even when born near term) secondary to a delay in the maturation of fetal surfactant production.

G. Congenital Anomalies (Table 17-3)

1. IDMs have a higher incidence of congenital anomalies due to the teratogenic effects of an abnormal maternal metabolic state early in embryogenesis.
2. The incidence of major anomalies in IDMs is about 6%–9% overall but increases substantially with poor maternal metabolic control (Green, 1993).
3. The most common defects are cardiovascular, including ventricular septal defects, transposition of the great vessels, hypoplastic left ventricle, and lesions associated with situs inversus.
4. Central nervous system, genitourinary, and gastrointestinal anomalies also occur with increased frequency in IDMs.
5. Some malformations, such as caudal regression syndrome, are almost uniquely associated with diabetes mellitus.
6. LGA infants who are the result of pregnancies not complicated by diabetes mellitus have no higher incidence of major congenital anomalies than the general population.

● TABLE 17-3
Anomalies That Occur With Greater Frequency in Infants of Diabetic Mothers (IDMs)

Anomaly	Estimated Relative Risk* (–fold increase over normal)	Prevalence in IDMs
Cardiac	4–5	4%–8%
Caudal regression/ sacral dysgenesis	200–400	1%–2%
Central nervous system	10	<1%
Holoprosencephaly	40–400	<1%
Situs inversus	80	<1%
Renal	5–20	<1%
Total (all anomalies)	5	5%–10%

*Risk is relative to a population of normal term infants.
Adapted from Greene M: Prevention and diagnosis of congenital anomalies in diabetic pregnancies, *Clin Perinatol* 20:533-547, 1993; Ballard R: Diabetes mellitus. In Taeusch H, Ballard RA, Avery M, editors: *Shaffer and Avery's diseases of the newborn*, ed 6, Philadelphia, 1991, WB Saunders, pp 66-71; Mills J: Congenital malformations in diabetes. In Gabbe S, Oh W, editors: *Infant of the diabetic mother, Report of the 93rd Ross Conference on Pediatric Research*, Columbus, OH, 1987, Ross Laboratories, pp 12-25.

Approach to the LGA Infant and IDM in the Perinatal Period

A. Physical Examination: This should focus on detection of traumatic injuries, including a careful neurologic evaluation to detect any nerve palsies.

    1. Most facial palsies will resolve without intervention, but brachial plexus injuries may not resolve completely and require careful neurologic follow up.

    2. A complete cardiac examination on admission and discharge should be directed at detection of murmurs, abnormal pulses, or cyanosis. A significant cardiac murmur or persistent cyanosis without respiratory distress in an IDM should generally prompt a consultation by a pediatric cardiologist and be evaluated by a chest radiograph and possibly an echocardiogram.

    3. The abdominal examination should be directed at the detection of any mass or renal enlargement. Many IDMs will have a slight increase in liver size detected by increased glycogen deposition in utero. If a single umbilical artery is present in an IDM, a renal ultrasound should be performed to seek anomalies.

    4. Other malformations should be clinically apparent or present with symptoms (i.e., feeding intolerance with hypoplastic left colon).

    5. Central nervous system signs, such as jitteriness or altered tone, are an indication to investigate for hypoglycemia by obtaining a blood glucose level.

B. Monitoring and Feeding During the First Hours of Life

    1. Glucose

        a. Within the first 1 to 2 hours of life, obtain a blood sugar measurement by reagent strip (such as Chemstrip bG or Dextrostix).

        b. If less than 40 mg/dL, consult flow chart (see Figure 16-1). If blood sugar >40 mg/dL and the infant remains asymptomatic, repeat measurement at 4 to 6 hours with hematocrit.

        c. Early feedings should be encouraged in LGA infants and IDMs who are vigorous at birth to prevent the development of hypoglycemia. In the presence of asymptomatic borderline hypoglycemia (25–40 mg/dL), use 20 cal/oz formula for the initial feed.

        d. If the mother wishes to exclusively breast-feed and the blood sugar remains <40 mg/dL 30 minutes after breast feeding, intravenous glucose supplementation should be given until her milk flow is established.

    2. Hematocrit: A hematocrit should be measured at 4 to 6 hours of life (with a repeat blood sugar reading in asymptomatic and vigorous infants). If obtained by a heel stick, a hematocrit >70% should be repeated by obtaining blood from a free-flowing venipuncture.

C. Specific Therapy

    1. Hypoglycemia (see Figure 16-1).

        a. LGA infants with any low blood glucose value obtained by reagent strip should be confirmed by an enzymatic laboratory method.

        b. IDMs and LGA infants should continue to be carefully observed for signs and symptoms of hypoglycemia during the first 24 hours of life.

  c. If symptoms consistent with hypoglycemia occur and the reagent strip indicates a normal blood sugar (>40 mg/dL), a confirmation should be done by laboratory testing since this is more accurate (Kliegman, 1993).

  d. A blood sugar <25 mg/dL requires *immediate* treatment with intravenous glucose, regardless of symptoms. Note that IDMs (and some LGA infants) have a very reactive insulin response to glucose infusion. Although it is important to increase a low glucose concentration quickly with a bolus of intravenous glucose, it should be anticipated that the baby will respond to the bolus with a rapid and often marked increase in insulin secretion, which in turn often results in the infant becoming hypoglycemic again in a short period of time. Thus the strategy with these infants is to give an acute bolus of glucose to increase the blood glucose concentration quickly, but this is to be followed by a constant glucose infusion in order to prevent "rebound" hypoglycemia. If the initial glucose is only mildly low (e.g., 30–35 mg/dL) and the decision is made to give IV glucose, a "slow" glucose bolus over 10–15 minutes is indicated as a measure to avoid rebound hypoglycemia. If any glucose bolus is given, a repeat glucose concentration should be checked 15–20 minutes later (even if a concurrent continuous glucose infusion is being given) in order in make certain that there is not significant rebound hypoglycemia. Repeated slow glucose boluses and/or increases in the continuous glucose infusion rate may be required to maintain stable and normal glucose concentrations. In infants who have fluctuating glucose levels, continue checking glucose concentrations until they are stable for 2 or 3 consecutive evaluations.

  e. Feeds should be introduced only gradually as tolerated in infants requiring intravenous glucose—and only after correction of the hypoglycemia. Many of these infants require gradual increases in enteral feeds with simultaneous decreases in intravenous glucose infusion rates in order to avoid rebound hypoglycemia. The rate at which an IDM with a history of significant hypoglycemia can be advanced to full enteral feedings without recurrences of hypoglycemia is unpredictable. Each infant should be managed individually without strict adherence to a single protocol.

2. Jaundice: The approach to jaundice in the LGA infant or IDM does not differ from the approach to jaundice in other term infants (Provisional Committee for Quality Improvement, 1994) (see Chapter 14).

3. Polycythemia: Although polycythemia is more common in LGA infants and IDMs than in other term infants, it is treated no differently (see Chapter 15).

  a. A venous hematocrit may be checked at 4 to 6 hours of age, or if the infant has any signs or symptoms possibly related to polycythemia such as acrocyanosis, poor circulation, tachypnea, hypoglycemia, irritability, or poor feeding.

     b. Many of the signs and symptoms of polycythemia are similar to those of hypoglycemia. Therefore, practically speaking, blood sugar and venous hematocrit values should be obtained from most LGA infants and IDMs who have these symptoms.

     c. A higher incidence of polycythemia is seen in infants with necrotizing enterocolitis; therefore, IDMs with polycythemia (especially with concurrent hypoglycemia) should be fed cautiously.

4. Hypocalcemia: IDMs are at greatest risk during the first few days of life.

     a. If the infant has symptoms of hypocalcemia (jitteriness, seizures) an *ionized* calcium should be checked.

     b. Hypocalcemia associated with symptoms should be treated with intravenous calcium as a slow infusion (over 15 to 30 minutes), preferably through a *central* venous line to avoid the possibility of a "burn" secondary to calcium extravasation. The recommended dose is 100 mg/kg of a 10% calcium gluconate solution (1 mL/kg).

     c. If symptoms are mild and hypocalcemia is detected early, enteral supplementation at twice the dosage (200 mg/kg 10% calcium gluconate) can be provided in divided doses over 24 hours.

     d. If hypocalcemia is severe or protracted, the infant's magnesium level should be checked since this is frequently low in IDMs and can interfere with parathyroid responsiveness. Hypomagnesemia can be corrected by 25–50 mg/kg of elemental Mg given intravenously.

5. Respiratory distress: IDMs born only slightly prematurely (i.e., 36–37 weeks gestation) may have classic hyaline membrane disease from delayed maturation of surfactant production.

     a. Any IDM with tachypnea, grunting, or cyanosis in the first hours of life should therefore have a chest radiograph done.

     b. If respiratory distress is severe and/or the oxygen requirement is >40% by hood in the first hours of life, an arterial blood gas should be obtained to check for any respiratory acidosis.

     c. Because most radiologists will not distinguish between HMD and congenital pneumonia, an abnormal chest radiograph in the presence of respiratory distress is considered an indication to treat with antibiotics while awaiting confirmation of infection by other testing (blood culture, complete blood count, etc.). Occasionally, if the infant is improving and the chest radiograph is not markedly abnormal, the infant can be observed without antibiotic treatment.

6. Follow-up of LGA infants and IDMs should be based on any complications occurring in the nursery, varying according to the organ system involved and the degree of abnormality. For example, heart murmurs can be followed clinically if there are normal upper and lower body blood pressures, no cyanosis, and no respiratory distress. Nerve palsies may recover, or they may require physical therapy to avoid development of contractures. Renal anomalies may require urologic consultation. Infants with neurologic signs or symptoms during the neonatal period or those experiencing more than one episode of severe hypoglycemia should have careful neurodevelopmental follow-up.

Long-Term Outcome of IDMs and LGA Infants

A. Neurodevelopment

1. Long-term neurodevelopmental outcome is normal for infants with good maternal metabolic control and without major congenital anomalies (Silverman et al., 1991; Sells et al., 1994).

2. IDMs whose mothers had poor control of diabetes during pregnancy or with major anomalies may have "less optimal" development.

3. A good correlation exists with outcome and head growth in infancy.

4. Repeated episodes of hypoglycemia may have an adverse outcome, but this is not clear (Lucas et al., 1988; Schwartz, 1991).

B. Obesity: Some evidence suggests that IDMs who are LGA at birth will be more likely to be obese during late childhood (Silverman et al., 1991; Vohr, 1987). No specific recommendations regarding nutritional counseling during childhood can be made at this time.

C. Insulin-Dependent Diabetes Mellitus (IDDM): IDDM occurs with no greater frequency in IDMs than in the general population. In fact, the incidence of IDDM is slightly increased in infants born to fathers with IDDM (Ballard, 1991).

THE SMALL-FOR-GESTATIONAL-AGE (SGA) INFANT
Background and Definitions

A. Definition of SGA

1. Infants are considered "small for dates" or "small for gestational age" (SGA) if they weigh less than the 10th percentile for their gestational age.

2. Some infants weigh more than the 10th percentile but still are considered "wasted" or thin relative to their length. Thus the usual definitions of SGA may exclude some infants who have not grown appropriately in utero and may be at risk for perinatal complications.

B. Symmetric Versus Asymmetric SGA Infants

1. Symmetric growth: SGA infants are considered "symmetric" if there are proportionate decreases in weight, length, and head circumference.

2. Asymmetric growth: SGA infants are considered "asymmetric" if the weight is reduced to a greater extent than the length while the head size is relatively normal. Most SGA infants are asymmetrically grown; this may represent a decrease in growth occurring later in gestation after an initial period of normal growth.

C. Etiologies: Many factors can reduce fetal growth (Charlton, 1991). Either maternal or fetal factors can be important, and placental disease often plays an important role. Common causes of decreased fetal growth resulting in SGA infants include the following:

1. Maternal smoking, alcoholism, or drug use.

2. Maternal chronic illness such as diabetes or lupus.

3. Complications of pregnancy such as pre-eclampsia or hypertension.

4. High altitude (because of hypoxia).

5. Intrauterine infection.

6. Genetic disorders in the fetus, such as trisomies.
7. Multiple gestation pregnancies secondary to restricted intrauterine space.

Complications in the Newborn Period (Leake, 1991)

A. **Perinatal Depression:** Because of decreased placental function, SGA infants are more likely to be acidotic and hypoxic at birth, even after an uncomplicated delivery. Therefore they are at greater risk for perinatal depression and frequently have low Apgar scores.

B. **Hypothermia**
   1. SGA infants are at increased risk for hypothermia because of decreased body fat, particularly brown fat stores.
   2. Hypothermia can produce a metabolic stress on the SGA infant, leading to increased risk for acidosis and hypoglycemia.

C. **Hypoglycemia**
   1. All SGA infants are at increased risk for hypoglycemia after birth.
   2. The risk is greatest in the first hours of life; however, hypoglycemia can be sustained over days as a result of many factors (Hay, 1984).
   3. Major determinants of hypoglycemia include decreased stores of glycogen in the liver, decreased ability to synthesize glucose, and increased brain size relative to body weight (the brain uses the majority of circulating glucose) (Leake, 1991; DiGiacomo, 1991).
   4. Cold stress can also lead to hypoglycemia in SGA infants.
   5. A useful guide to normal and abnormal blood sugars in term infants is shown in Figure 16-1.

D. **Polycythemia:** In SGA infants, polycythemia is thought to be secondary to chronic hypoxia in utero with resulting increased erythropoietin production (Leake, 1991). Complications of polycythemia are related to the increased viscosity of blood interfering with organ microcirculation.

E. **Hypocalcemia:** Low serum calcium levels may occur in SGA infants in association with perinatal asphyxia and treatment with sodium bicarbonate (Leake, 1991).

F. **Hypermetabolism:** SGA infants have an increased "basal" metabolic rate compared with appropriate-for-gestational-age (AGA) infants. This hypermetabolic state may be due to increased brain to body weight ratio and possibly a faster rate of growth (Bronstein, 1991). Caloric needs may be increased by cold stress as well.

G. **Respiratory Problems**
   1. SGA infants in general have *less* respiratory distress after birth compared with infants who are AGA at the same gestation, presumably because in utero stress induces maturation of the surfactant system (Leake, 1991; Hack et al., 1989).
   2. SGA infants are at increased risk for meconium aspiration related to perinatal depression.

H. **Congenital Anomalies:** There is an increased incidence of major anomalies in SGA infants, although no particular congenital anomaly predominates.

Approach to the SGA Infant in the Perinatal Period

A. Physical Examination

1. This should focus on detection of any malformations and include careful measurements of head circumference and length. A ponderal index (weight in grams × 100 ÷ length in centimeters) can identify significant growth abnormalities as well.

2. Central nervous system signs, such as jitteriness or altered tone, may indicate hypoglycemia, hypothermia, hypocalcemia, or polycythemia.

3. If symptoms suggestive of these complications are present at initial examination, blood sugar, ionized calcium, and hematocrit measurements should be obtained.

4. If there is suspicion of congenital infection as the cause of small size (e.g., presence of characteristic skin lesions, hepatosplenomegaly), appropriate work-up should be undertaken.

5. If there are dysmorphic features present, genetic evaluation should be considered.

B. Monitoring and Feeding During the First Hours of Life: Initial evaluation and stabilization of SGA infants should include preventing cold stress and the above complications. These infants require close evaluation and monitoring.

1. Temperature: The infant's temperature should be monitored every 30 minutes until stable × 2 (>36.5° C), then at least every 4 hours. Care should be taken to keep the infant warm with bundling and especially a hat to avoid hypothermia.

2. Blood glucose: Within the first 1–2 hours of life, obtain a capillary blood sugar measurement by reagent strip (such as Chemstrip bG or Dextrostix), even if asymptomatic.

3. Early feeding: Early feedings should be encouraged in SGA infants who are vigorous at birth to prevent the development of hypoglycemia. The approach to early feeds and hypoglycemia can be the same as in the LGA infant and IDM. However, SGA infants frequently are hypermetabolic, have increased nutritional requirements, and feed "voraciously" if healthy.

4. Hematocrit: Hematocrit should be measured at 4–6 hours of life (with a repeat blood sugar in asymptomatic and vigorous infants). If obtained by a heel stick, a hematocrit value >70% should be repeated by obtaining blood from a free-flowing venipuncture.

C. Therapy

1. Hypoglycemia

   a. Any low blood glucose value (i.e., <40 mg/dL) obtained by reagent strip should be confirmed by an enzymatic laboratory method.

   b. Values <25 mg/dL in an asymptomatic infant or less than <40 mg/dL in a symptomatic infant require immediate treatment with intravenous glucose, even while awaiting confirmation. Note that the SGA infant usually responds well to glucose infusion with a rise in the blood glucose concentration, as opposed to the IDM, who commonly has fluctuating glucose concentrations secondary to rapid and variable insulin secretion in response to glucose infusion. Hypoglycemia in the SGA infant is due to low energy stores rather than hyperinsulinemia, the cause in the IDM. Thus, even though the flow chart in Figure 16-1 can be used for both SGA infants and for IDMs and LGA infants, the amount of glucose required and pattern of long-term monitoring may be different for these groups of infants.

    c. In some cases, a more liberal intravenous glucose bolus (4 mL/kg $D_{10}W$ or 400 mg/kg dextrose) can be used, particularly if the blood glucose concentration does not respond to an initial, lower-glucose bolus.

    d. Carefully observe for signs and symptoms of hypoglycemia during the first 24 hours of life.

2. Polycythemia

    a. A venous hematocrit measurement should be obtained at 4–6 hours of age (AAP, 1993) or earlier if the infant has any signs or symptoms possibly related to polycythemia (i.e., acrocyanosis, poor circulation, tachypnea, hypoglycemia, irritability, or poor feeding).

    b. Many of the signs and symptoms of polycythemia are similar to those of hypoglycemia. Therefore, most SGA infants should have their blood sugar and venous hematocrit values checked when these symptoms occur.

    c. Hematocrit values <65% should not contribute to symptoms of hyperviscosity; values between 65%–70% may be of concern and treatment should be considered; values >70% should be treated by dilutional exchange transfusion if associated with symptoms (see Chapter 15).

3. Hypocalcemia: SGA infants who are exhibiting symptoms associated with hypocalcemia (i.e., jitteriness, hyperreflexia, increased extensor tone, stridor, apnea) should have an *ionized* calcium measurement. Treatment is the same as for hypocalcemia in the LGA infant and the IDM.

4. Follow-up

    a. SGA infant follow-up should be based on any complications occurring in the nursery, as well as the etiology of the restricted growth. For example, infants with congenital viral infections such as CMV are at greater risk for developing sensorineural hearing loss and should have their hearing evaluated regularly during the first year of life.

    b. Growth in length, weight, and head circumference and feeding patterns/caloric intake should be monitored carefully in the first year of life because there may be substantial "catch up" growth during this period.

Long-Term Outcome of SGA Infants

A. Neurodevelopment

1. Long-term neurodevelopmental outcome depends largely on the cause of the infant being SGA and whether the growth retardation is symmetric or asymmetric.

2. In general there is an increased risk for abnormal neurodevelopment in SGA infants, particularly if superimposed complications occur in the neonatal period (Leake, 1991; Hack et al., 1989).

B. Cardiovascular Disease in Adulthood

1. Epidemiologic data have demonstrated an increased rate of cardiovascular disease and non-insulin–dependent diabetes mellitus in adulthood after being SGA at birth (Barker et al., 1993).
2. It is speculated that undernutrition during pregnancy somehow changes the programming of metabolic signaling pathways.
3. Whether this association will be supported in all populations and whether interventions in childhood can alter this adverse long-term outcome remain to be discovered.

REFERENCES

American Academy of Pediatrics, Committee on the Fetus and Newborn: Routine evaluation of blood pressure, hematocrit, and glucose in newborns, *Pediatrics* 92:474-476, 1993.

Ballard R: Diabetes mellitus. In Taeusch H, Ballard RA, Avery M, editors: *Shaffer and Avery's diseases of the newborn*, ed 6, Philadelphia, 1991, WB Saunders, pp 66-71.

Barker D, Gluckman P, Godfrey K, Harding J, et al: Fetal nutrition and cardiovascular disease in adult life, *Lancet* 341:938-941, 1993.

Bronstein M: Energy requirements and protein energy balance in preterm and term infants. In Hay WW Jr, editor: *Neonatal nutrition and metabolism,* St Louis, 1991, Mosby–Year Book, pp 42-70.

Charlton V: Fetal growth: nutritional issues. In Taeusch H, Ballard RA, Avery M, editors: *Shaffer and Avery's diseases of the newborn*, ed 6, Philadelphia, 1991, WB Saunders, pp 58-65.

DiGiacomo J: Carbohydrates: metabolism and disorders. In Hay WW Jr, editor: *Neonatal nutrition and metabolism,* St Louis, 1991, Mosby-Year Book, pp 93-109.

Greene M: Prevention and diagnosis of congenital anomalies in diabetic pregnancies, *Clin Perinatol* 20:533-547, 1993.

Hack M, Breslau N, Fanaroff A: Differential effects of intrauterine and postnatal brain growth failure in infants of very low birth weight, *Am J Dis Child* 143:63-68, 1989.

Hay WW Jr: Fetal and neonatal glucose homeostasis and their relation to the small for gestational age infant, *Sem Perinatol* 8:101-116, 1984.

Kliegman R: Problems in metabolic adaptation: glucose, calcium, and magnesium. In Klaus M, Fanaroff A, editors: *Care of the high-risk neonate*, ed 4, Philadelphia, 1993, WB Saunders, pp 282-302.

Leake R: Growth disorders. In Taeusch H, Ballard RA, Avery M, editors: *Shaffer and Avery's diseases of the newborn*, ed 6, Philadelphia, 1991, WB Saunders, pp 236-242.

Lucas A, Morley R, Cole T: Adverse neurodevelopmental outcome of moderate neonatal hypoglycemia, *Br Med J* 297:1304-1308, 1988.

Manco-Johnson M, Abshire T, Jacobson L, Marlar R: Severe neonatal protein C deficiency: prevalence and thrombotic risk, *J Pediatr* 119:793-798, 1991.

Mills J: Congenital malformations in diabetes. In Gabbe S, Oh W, editors: *Infant of the diabetic mother, Report of the 93rd Ross Conference on Pediatric Research*, Columbus, OH, 1987, Ross Laboratories, pp 12-25.

Provisional Committee for Quality Improvement and Subcommittee on Hyperbilirubinemia: American Academy of Pediatrics practice parameter:

management of hyperbilirubinemia in the healthy term newborn, *Pediatrics* 94:558-565, 1994.

Schwartz R: Neonatal hypoglycemia: back to basics in diagnosis and treatment, *Diabetes* 40(suppl 2):71-73, 1991.

Sells C, Robinson N, Brown Z, Knopp R: Long-term developmental follow-up of infants of diabetic mothers, *J Pediatr* 125:S9-S17, 1994.

Silverman B, Rizzo T, Green O, Cho N, et al: Long-term prospective evaluation of offspring of diabetic mothers, *Diabetes* 40(suppl 2):121-125, 1991.

Vohr B: Long-term follow-up of the infant of the diabetic mother. In Gabbe S, Oh W, editors: *Infant of the diabetic mother, Report of the 93rd Ross Conference on Pediatric Research*, Columbus, OH, 1987, Ross Laboratories, pp 159-167, 1987.

18 Perinatal Drug Exposure

Sharon Langendoerfer, MD ▪ Janis J. Johnson, MD ▪ Patti J. Thureen, MD

Research has demonstrated that alcohol is the most dangerous of the common substances of abuse for exposed fetuses and accounts for the most serious permanent impairment. Tobacco use, the most common cause of low birth weight, is more prevalent and also appears to cause behavior problems in prenatally exposed children (Williams et al., 1998).

Abuse of illicit substances has declined modestly during the past 5 years. The effects on the fetus of specific drugs are difficult to assess, since they are commonly used in various combinations, along with alcohol and tobacco ("polysubstance abuse"). Furthermore, substance-abusing mothers are likely to have a number of other health, lifestyle, and even genetic risk factors that affect their babies. Despite the difficulties in determining cause and effect, the best available research indicates that most of these illegal drugs are less dangerous than previously thought (Chavkin, 2001). Nevertheless, their use results in an increased risk for adverse outcomes among the exposed offspring—because of the prenatal exposure, the associated neonatal complications, continued postnatal exposure, and environmental and parenting issues that are harmful to these already vulnerable children.

To minimize the long-term negative impact of these hazards, drug- and alcohol-exposed children should have the benefit of close follow-up and prompt intervention when medical conditions or developmental delays are detected because they are unlikely to "outgrow" their problems without help. These children also are at increased risk for physical, sexual, and emotional abuse (American Academy of Pediatrics [AAP], 1995).

While abuse of both legal and illegal substances is more common among mothers in lower socioeconomic groups, this problem occurs throughout our society.

MATERNAL DRUG USE

A. **Consideration of Drug or Alcohol Abuse in the Following Situations**
  1. Physical evidence of intravenous drug use
     a. Intoxication.
     b. Needle "tracks," scars from previous cellulitis or venous thrombosis.
     c. Nasal hyperemia or septal defects from snorting.
     d. Foreign body emboli in eye grounds.
  2. High-risk historical or social factors
     a. No prenatal care.

       b. Denial of pregnancy.

       c. Family history of drug or alcohol problems.

       d. History of "previous" drug or alcohol problem or intentional periods of abstinence.

       e. Previous child abuse or neglect.

       f. Minimal support system.

       g. History of serious psychiatric problems.

       h. History of domestic violence.

       i. History of legal problems or driving under the influence.

    3. Obstetric complications in previous or current pregnancy

       a. History of "spontaneous" abortion.

       b. Abruption.

       c. Unexplained preterm labor.

       d. Uterine trauma secondary to domestic violence.

       e. Intrauterine growth retardation.

       f. Previous poor birth outcome.

B. Maternal Complications Associated with Substance Abuse

    1. Neurologic

       a. Cocaine: seizures, postpartum intracerebral hemorrhage.

       b. Amphetamines, LSD: psychosis.

       c. Alcohol: delirium tremens, seizures.

       d. Heroin: abstinence syndrome, mononeuritis, polyneuritis, transverse myelitis.

    2. Cardiovascular

       a. Cocaine, amphetamines: hypertension, infarction, cardiomyopathy, arrhythmias, sudden death.

       b. Intravenous drugs: bacterial endocarditis.

    3. Infectious

       a. Intravenous drugs: hepatitis B and C, HIV, cellulitis.

       b. All drugs: pneumonia, urinary tract infection, sexually transmitted diseases (e.g., gonorrhea, chlamydia, syphilis, herpes).

    4. Gastrointestinal

       a. Cocaine: intestinal infarction.

       b. Intravenous drugs: acute and chronic hepatitis.

    5. Nutrition: poor nutrition common with alcohol and drug abuse.

C. Guidelines for Obtaining History of Substance Abuse: Most often the interview will reveal that the mother uses a combination of drugs, which has implications for the symptoms of the affected newborn (Dixon et al., 1990). Despite excellent interviewing skills, reliance on self-reporting will miss many affected pregnancies (Zuckerman et al., 1989).

    1. Obtain history verbally (not by self-administered written questionnaire) in a private setting away from family members and friends.

    2. Maintain a nonjudgmental attitude and make clear the primary interest is the child's welfare, not punishing the mother.

    3. Be direct with your questions.

    4. Collect data about habits of other household members as well as those of the patient.

5. If mother admits to drug or alcohol use, obtain information on routes, dose, and duration of use and history of drug treatment. Assess mother's perception of how the drug use has affected her life.

DRUG SCREENING TESTS

A. Principles of Testing

1. A recent U.S. Supreme Court decision (Ferguson, 2001) prohibits hospitals from testing women for illegal drug use without their consent and then reporting positive test results to law enforcement. Although laws vary from state to state, it is prudent to obtain consent for testing urine samples. However, if a neonate presents with unexplained neurologic symptoms, such as severe apnea or seizures, a drug test of the infant may be included in the medical evaluation without parental consent.

2. A history of alcohol or other substance abuse is one of many risk factors for inability to parent. Therefore it is appropriate to consult Child Protective Services regarding possible prior reports about the family and to request a home/family evaluation. Also, the baby's medical care provider should be alerted to carefully monitor the baby's health and development (AAP, 1995).

B. Urine Toxicology

1. Detects only recent use. Typical time periods for positive urine test after last use are as follows:
   a. Alcohol: hours.
   b. Amphetamines and cocaine: 1–3 days.
   c. Opiates: 2–4 days.
   d. LSD: 2–3 days.
   e. Marijuana: 7–30 days.

2. Maternal versus infant sampling: For the purpose of identifying infants exposed, it makes no difference if the positive urine sample was obtained from mother or newborn. (Either one or the other may be negative immediately after delivery.)

3. Urine tests for narcotics will be negative at the time the baby develops symptoms of narcotic withdrawal.

4. False-positive urine screens: Not all positive screens indicate substance abuse. If a drug screen is positive, review mother's medical record for narcotics or sedatives ordered and administered during labor.

C. Nonurine Drug Screening

1. Meconium and hair have been used to detect in utero drug and alcohol exposure during the second half of pregnancy (Callahan et al., 1992).

2. To improve sensitivity of meconium screening, collect the entire stool output from the first 48 hours of life. (False positives do occur.)

3. Hair sampling from babies is not practical.

FETAL AND NEONATAL EFFECTS OF SPECIFIC DRUGS

A. Alcohol: Exposure in pregnancy is associated with birth defects, mental retardation, and often lifelong disabling behavioral problems, even in the

absence of physical features of fetal alcohol syndrome (FAS). It is estimated that up to 5% of all congenital anomalies may be attributed to prenatal alcohol exposure. Initial recognition of the effects of alcohol on the fetus was made in 1968. Delineation of the full syndrome was made in 1973 (Jones, 1997).

1. Effects on fetus (Pietrantoni and Knuppel, 1991)
   a. Intrauterine growth retardation.
   b. Increased rates of malformation.
   c. Chronic fetal hypoxia.
2. Fetal alcohol syndrome (FAS) and alcohol-related effects (AAP, 2000)
   a. Incidence: One of the most common identifiable causes of mental retardation, with a worldwide incidence of 1.9 per 1000. The combined incidence of FAS plus alcohol-related neurodevelopmental disorders (ARND) is estimated to be at least 9.1 per 1000 live births (Sampson et al., 1997).
   b. Diagnostic criteria.
      (1) The 4-Digit Diagnostic Code (Astley and Clarren, 1991), published by the University of Washington's FAS Diagnostic & Prevention Network, is a user-friendly, comprehensive, reproducible method for diagnosing the full spectrum of outcomes of patients with prenatal alcohol exposure.
      (2) Box 18-1 describes fetal alcohol spectrum disorders, as reported by a National Academy of Sciences task force (Stratton et al., 1996).
   c. Neonatal identification: Recognition of FAS may be difficult in the immediate newborn period. Suspected cases should be followed closely to clarify the mother's alcohol use pattern and assist her in obtaining treatment, as well as to monitor the baby for growth deficiency, the emergence of typical facial features, and developmental or behavioral problems.
   d. Long-term effects: The 4-Digit Diagnostic Code (Astley and Clarren, 1991) may be used to reassess children periodically for early evidence of developing physical, mental, and behavioral disabilities seen in fetal alcohol spectrum disorders (Streissguth et al., 1991). Alcohol-affected children need prompt diagnosis and referral to appropriate services as soon as developmental or behavioral problems are recognized, since they will not outgrow their difficulties without intervention. The four categories of the 4-Digit Diagnostic Code are:
      (1) *Growth deficiency,* including both prenatal (IUGR) and postnatal growth problems despite adequate nutrition.
      (2) Characteristic FAS *facial features,* including shortened palpebral fissures, thin upper lip, flattened philtrum and flat midface.
      (3) Evidence of *brain dysfunction,* including microcephaly, structural abnormalities of the brain, neurologic conditions such as seizures, and varying degrees of behavioral and/or cognitive problems.
      (4) The fourth digit in the score reflects the most accurate estimate of the *amount of mother's alcohol consumption* during pregnancy. (More information may become available over time.)
3. Maternal consumption: There is no established "safe dose" of alcohol for pregnant women. A study of nonhuman primates showed that binge

● BOX 18-1
DIAGNOSTIC CRITERIA FOR FETAL ALCOHOL SYNDROME (FAS) AND ALCOHOL-RELATED EFFECTS

Fetal Alcohol Syndrome

1. FAS with confirmed maternal alcohol exposure[a]
   A. Confirmed maternal alcohol exposure[a]
   B. Evidence of a characteristic pattern of facial anomalies, including features such as short palpebral fissures and abnormalities in the premaxillary zone (e.g., flat upper lip, flattened philtrum, and flat midface)
   C. Evidence of growth retardation, as in at least one of the following:
      • Low birth weight for gestational age
      • Decelerating weight over time, not due to nutrition
      • Disproportionally low weight to height
   D. Evidence of CNS neurodevelopmental abnormalities, as in at least one of the following:
      • Decreased cranial size at birth
      • Structural brain abnormalities (e.g., microcephaly, partial or complete agenesis of the corpus callosum, cerebellar hypoplasia)
      • Neurologic hard or soft signs (as age-appropriate), such as impaired fine motor skills, neurosensory hearing loss, poor tandem gait, poor eye-hand coordination

2. FAS without confirmed maternal alcohol exposure
   B, C, and D as above

3. Partial FAS with confirmed maternal alcohol exposure
   A. Confirmed maternal alcohol exposure[a]
   B. Evidence of some components of the pattern of characteristic facial anomalies. Either C or D or E
   C. Evidence of growth retardation, as in at least one of the following:
      • Low birth weight for gestational age
      • Decelerating weight over time not due to nutrition
      • Disproportionally low weight to height
   D. Evidence of CNS neurodevelopmental abnormalities, as in:
      • Decreased cranial size at birth
      • Structural brain abnormalities (e.g., microcephaly, partial or complete agenesis of the corpus callosum, cerebellar hypoplasia)
      • Neurologic hard or soft signs (as age-appropriate) such as impaired fine motor skills, neurosensory hearing loss, poor tandem gait, poor eye-hand coordination
   E. Evidence of a complex pattern of behavioral or cognitive abnormalities that are inconsistent with developmental level and cannot be explained by familial background or environment alone—e.g., learning difficulties; deficits in school performance; poor impulse control; problems in social perception; deficits in higher level receptive and expressive language; poor capacity for abstraction or metacognition; specific deficits in mathematical skills; or problems in memory, attention, or judgment

Alcohol-Related Effects

Clinical conditions in which there is a history of maternal alcohol exposure, [a, b] and where clinical or animal research has linked maternal alcohol ingestion to an observed outcome. There are two categories, which may co-occur. If both diagnoses are present, both diagnoses should be rendered:

(Continued)

● BOX 18-1
● DIAGNOSTIC CRITERIA FOR FETAL ALCOHOL SYNDROME (FAS)
AND ALCOHOL-RELATED EFFECTS—cont'd

4. Alcohol-related birth defects (ARBD)
List of congenital anomalies, including malformations and dysplasias:

Cardiac	Atrial septal defects	Aberrant great vessels
	Ventricular septal defects	Tetralogy of Fallot
Skeletal	Hypoplastic nails	Clinodactyly
	Shortened fifth digits	Pectus excavatum and carinatum
	Radioulnar synostosis	Klippel-Feil syndrome
	Flexion contractures	Hemivertebrae
	Camptodactyly	Scoliosis
Renal	Ureteral duplications	Aplastic, dysplastic, hypoplastic kidneys
	Horseshoe kidneys	Hydronephrosis
Ocular	Strabismus	Refractive problems secondary to small globes
	Retinal vascular anomalies	
Auditory	Conductive hearing loss	Neurosensory hearing loss
Other	Virtually every malformation has been described in some patient with FAS.The etiologic specificity of most of these anomalies to alcohol teratogenesis remains uncertain.	

5. Alcohol-related neurodevelopmental disorder (ARND)
Presence of:
A. Evidence of CNS neurodevelopmental abnormalities, as in any one of the following:
- Decreased cranial size at birth
- Structural brain abnormalities (e.g., microcephaly, partial or complete agenesis of the corpus callosum, cerebellar hypoplasia)
- Neurologic hard or soft signs (as age-appropriate), such as impaired fine motor skills, neurosensory hearing loss, poor tandem gait, poor eye-hand coordination

and/or:
B. Evidence of a complex pattern of behavior or cognitive abnormalities that are inconsistent with developmental level and cannot be explained by familial background or environment alone, such as learning difficulties; deficits in school performance; poor impulse control; problems in social perception; deficits in higher level receptive and expressive language; poor capacity for abstraction or metacognition; specific deficits in mathematical skills; or problems in memory, attention, or judgment

Stratton K, Howe C, Battaglia F, editors: *Fetal alcohol syndrome: diagnosis, epidemiology, prevention and treatment,* Washington, DC, 1996, National Academy Press, 1996, pp 4-21. Copyright 1996 by the National Academy of Sciences. Courtesy of the National Academy Press.
ᵃA pattern of excessive intake characterized by substantial, regular intake or heavy episodic drinking. Evidence of this pattern may include frequent episodes of intoxication, development of tolerance or withdrawal, social problems related to drinking, legal problems related to drinking, engaging in physically hazardous behavior while drinking, or alcohol-related medical problems such as hepatic disease.
ᵇAs further research is completed and as, or if, lower quantities or variable patterns of alcohol use are associated with ARBD or ARND, these patterns of alcohol use should be incorporated into the diagnostic criteria.

drinking in the first few weeks of pregnancy followed by abstinence later in gestation was as dangerous to the fetus as exposure throughout pregnancy (Clarren et al., 1992).

   4. Breast-feeding: Alcohol passes into breast milk. Concerns for the infant include sedation, irritability, weak sucking, decreased milk supply, and increased milk odor. Breast-feeding should be avoided during and for 2–3 hours after drinking alcohol. Chronic and heavy consumers of alcohol should not breast-feed (Hale, 2002).

B. **Narcotics** (Hoegerman and Scholl, 1991): Opiates are derived from the opium-producing poppy, *Papaver somniferum.*

   1. Specific narcotics
      a. Naturally occurring opiates: codeine, morphine, and opium.
      b. Synthetic and semisynthetic narcotics: fentanyl, heroin, hydromorphone (Dilaudid), methadone, meperidine (Demerol), oxycodone (present in Percodan and Percocet), and propoxyphene (Darvon).

   2. Narcotic abuse
      a. Can be used by any route (i.e., intravenous, intramuscular, oral, smoking) and can be used sporadically, without addiction or dependence.
      b. Narcotic dependence is characterized by simultaneous tolerance to narcotics of any type (cross-tolerance), with symptoms of withdrawal upon discontinuation of use.

   3. Effects on fetus
      a. Increased rate of spontaneous abortion and stillbirths, some caused by withdrawal syndrome.
      b. Intrauterine growth restriction may be a direct effect on growth and/or related to poor nutrition and stressed lifestyle common among addicted women.

   4. Effects on newborn: Neonatal abstinence syndrome
      a. Signs and symptoms: High-pitched cry, tremulousness, sleeplessness, difficulty feeding, sweating, nasal stuffiness, sneezing, vomiting, cramping, and diarrhea. Seizures and EEG abnormalities may also occur. Symptoms are less common in premature infants, probably because of immaturity of the nervous system.
      b. Differential diagnosis: It is very important to rule out other causes of symptoms, such as sepsis, hypoglycemia, hypocalcemia, hypomagnesemia, central nervous system hemorrhage or infection, hypoxic-ischemic encephalopathy, respiratory disorders, and hyperthyroidism.
      c. Onset.
         (1) Symptoms of withdrawal in exposed infants usually develop within 48 hours of birth, 96% by 4 days (Finnegan, 1990). Age at onset may vary with the half-life of the specific drug and size and time of mother's last dose (Shaw and McIvor, 1994). Methadone withdrawal usually begins later than heroin withdrawal, but both typically occur before 48 hours of age.
         (2) Babies asymptomatic at 48 hours are usually discharged from the hospital after mother and/or other caretakers have been educated

about possible symptoms and a plan for close follow-up has been established.

d. Severity of the symptoms generally varies with mother's dose (Dashe et al., 2002).

e. Subacute symptoms of withdrawal can persist for 4–6 months after birth.

f. Management: Figure 18-1 is a Neonatal Abstinence Scoring System used to guide treatment (Finnegan, 1990).

(1) Scoring technique (see Figure 18-1)

(a) Assess the infant initially 2 hours after birth and then every 4 hours.

(b) Total the points for signs and symptoms seen during that interval. If score >8, change to every-2-hour evaluations and continue every 2 hours until 24 hours after the last total score >8; then resume every-4-hour evaluations. Use a new sheet for each day.

(c) Mother should be included in assessments of baby in preparation for monitoring symptoms at home.

(2) Therapy: The approach used at our hospital is as follows:

(a) Abstinence score <8: Offer supportive care, which includes swaddling, low light, quiet, swinging, and frequent feeding with high-calorie formula.

(b) Abstinence score >8, unresponsive to supportive measures: Start phenobarbital at 2.5 mg/kg/dose every 6–12 hours (no loading dose). The goal of treatment is for baby to be calm but not sedated in the first 2 hours after the dose, with only minimal recurrence of symptoms before the next dose. Using this strategy, abstinence scores above 10 are rarely observed and virtually every infant can be discharged by 48 hours after beginning medication.

(c) Treatment with phenobarbital usually lasts from 2–8 weeks. Mother is instructed to decrease the dose by 0.1 mL or lengthen the interval between doses as tolerated. The medical care provider should be contacted if the daily dose must be increased. Otherwise, the weaning schedule can be reviewed at regular outpatient visits (every 1–2 weeks until the infant is off medication).

(d) Note that symptoms of gut hypermotility (cramping, diarrhea, and vomiting) are *not* treated by phenobarbital and require change to a narcotic or chlorpromazine (see below.)

(e) Other medication options: The American Academy of Pediatrics (AAP, 1998) recommends *replacement* with a narcotic. However, in our experience, the gradual weaning of the narcotic dose requires *months* of medication, rather than weeks, to treat withdrawal symptoms with phenobarbital or chlorpromazine. Consider the following therapies:

(i) Tincture of opium (DDTO): Begin with 0.04 mg/kg/dose every 4 hours (must be diluted by pharmacy from 10 mg/mL to 0.4 mg/mL).

System	Signs and Symptoms	Score	Time (Hour of the Day at which Interval Began/Interval Duration) [2 hours or 4 hours]										
Central Nervous System	Excessive high-pitched or other cry	2											
	Continuous high-pitched or other cry	3											
	Sleeps <1 hour after feeding	3											
	Sleeps <2 hour after feeding	2											
	Sleeps <3 hour after feeding	1											
	Hyperactive Moro reflex	2											
	Markedly hyperactive Moro reflex	3											
	Mild tremors disturbed	1											
	Moderate-severe tremors disturbed	2											
	Mild tremors undisturbed	3											
	Moderate-severe tremors undisturbed	4											
	Increased muscle tone	2											
	Excoriation (specific area)	1											
	Myoclonic jerks	3											
	Generalized convulsions	5											
Metabolic/ Vasomotor/ Respiratory	Sweating	1											
	Fever <38.4°C (37.2° −38.2°)	1											
	Fever >38.4°C												
	Frequent yawning (>3–4 times)	1											
	Mottling	1											
	Nasal stuffiness	1											
	Sneezing (>3–4 times)	1											
	Nasal flaring	2											
	Respiratory rate >60/min	1											
	Respiratory rate >60/min + retractions	2											
Gastrointestinal	Excessive sucking	1											
	Poor feeding	2											
	Regurgitation	2											
	Projectile vomiting	3											
	Loose stools	2											
	Watery stools	3											
	Total score												
	Initials of scorer												

FIGURE 18-1 ● Neonatal Abstinence Scoring System. (Adapted from Finnegan LP: Neonatal abstinence. In Nelson NM, editor: *Current therapy in neonatal-perinatal medicine,* Philadelphia, 1990, BC Decker, pp 314-320.)

       (ii) Methadone: Begin with 0.05–0.1 mg/kg/dose every 6 hours; adjust to a dosing schedule of every 12–24 hours (oral solution contains 8% ethanol.)

      (iii) Chlorpromazine: 0.7–0.9 mg/kg/dose every 8 hours. Effective for all symptoms, including intestinal hypermotility. Side effects include tardive dyskinesia.

      (iv) Do *NOT* give paregoric: Contains multiple toxic compounds.

      (v) Breast-feeding while on methadone maintenance is approved by the AAP (AAP, 2001). Additional oral medication for abstinence syndrome may be required. Mother should watch for abstinence symptoms and for lethargy (extremely uncommon).

  5. Long-term effects: Children prenatally exposed to narcotics are at increased risk for learning and behavioral problems. However, because of all the associated risk factors, it is difficult to determine cause and effect.

C. Marijuana: One of most commonly used illicit drugs in the United States. Estimates of use are imprecise. As with other illicit substances, polydrug use is common.

  1. Active ingredient: Delta-9-tetrahydrocannabinol (THC), which freely crosses the placenta and accumulates in the fetus.

  2. Effects on fetus: No clear effect on fetal growth or the incidence of prematurity; no significant increase in the rate of either minor or major anomalies (Day and Richardson, 1991).

  3. Effects on newborn

    a. Decreased visual responsiveness.

    b. Increased tremors and startles.

    c. Management: Usually involves only supportive care (swaddling, swinging, frequent feeding with high-calorie formula, low lighting). Breast-feeding is not contraindicated since there is no evidence of effects on the infant. Marijuana use by breast-feeding mothers should be discouraged (AAP, 2001).

  4. Long-term effects: Increased incidence of learning deficits and behavioral problems is seen in children with multiple risk factors; therefore cause and effect is difficult to establish.

D. Cocaine

  1. Action: Classified as a stimulant

    a. Prevents dopamine and norepinephrine reuptake at the presynaptic nerve terminals. The stimulant effect includes enhanced alertness, reduced anxiety and social inhibitions, heightened energy, and improved self-esteem. These effects wear off and are replaced by anxiety, exhaustion, and depression.

    b. With chronic use, paranoid psychosis and mood disorders may result.

    c. Autonomic effects include vasoconstriction, tachycardia, hypertension, and uterine contractions.

2. Cocaine abuse
   a. Cocaine can be administered by smoking freebase cocaine (crack), inhaling (snorting), or using intravenous route.
   b. Cocaine may contain diluents and other impurities (talc, arsenic, lidocaine), which also can be toxic to mother and fetus.
3. Effects on fetus: Somewhat difficult to assess because of confounding variables, including other drug exposures and poor maternal nutrition
   a. Increased incidence of growth restriction.
   b. Increase in spontaneous abortions, stillbirths, and preterm births.
   c. No defined "fetal cocaine syndrome."
   d. Slightly increased incidence of congenital malformations caused by disruptive vascular events, including:
      (1) Placental abruption.
      (2) Intracranial hemorrhage and cerebral infarction.
      (3) Intestinal atresia or infarction.
      (4) Necrotizing enterocolitis.
      (5) Limb reduction defects.
      (6) Urinary tract anomalies.
4. Effects on newborn
   a. Slight increase in meconium staining.
   b. Problems associated with IUGR and prematurity.
   c. Increased incidence of irritability and poor organizational response to stimuli (as measured by the Brazelton Neonatal Behavioral Assessment Scale).
5. Management
   a. Pharmacologic therapy is rarely needed.
   b. Careful physical examination with emphasis on above mentioned congenital defects. Signs may include abdominal masses, vomiting, abnormal stooling or urination patterns, focal neurologic signs.
   c. Follow-up on maternal laboratory tests for syphilis, hepatitis B and C, and HIV because of increased risk associated with IV drug use and prostitution. All babies should receive hepatitis B vaccine before 12 hours after birth. If mother's HbsAg status cannot be determined, she should undergo blood testing as soon as possible. If mother is HbsAg-positive, the infant should receive hepatitis B immune globulin (HBIG) as soon as possible, at least within 7 days of birth (see Chapter 20).
   d. Referral to Child Protective Services to evaluate home environment and to arrange for appropriate support services.
   e. Breast-feeding: Acute cocaine intoxication from breast-feeding has been documented. Mothers should be warned of the dangers, and breast-feeding should be strongly discouraged in women who are likely to continue using cocaine.
6. Long-term effects: These children show an increased incidence of learning deficits and behavioral problems. However, because they have multiple risk factors, it is difficult to establish cause and effect (Frank et al., 2001).

E. Amphetamines (Plessinger, 1998)
  1. Action: Stimulant
     a. Stimulate release of stored norepinephrine, producing subjective central and autonomic effects similar to cocaine. However, amphetamines are more hallucinogenic at higher doses because of serotonin release.
     b. More slowly metabolized, hence longer-acting than cocaine.
     c. Multiple compounds, with minor differences in effect: amphetamines, methamphetamines, and "designer drugs" (modified amphetamines).
     d. Risks of living in or near a clandestine "meth lab," with multiple toxic compounds and vapors, remains largely unexplored.
  2. Amphetamine abuse
     a. Routes: Smoking, oral, and intravenous.
  3. Effects on fetus
     a. Intrauterine growth restriction, premature birth, fetal losses and anomalies caused by vascular accidents (similar to cocaine).
     b. Data suggesting anomalies different from cocaine exposure, including cleft lip and palate and higher incidence of cardiac anomalies (Plessinger, 1998).
  4. Effects on newborn (similar to cocaine)
     a. Problems associated with IUGR and prematurity.
     b. Increased incidence of irritability and poor organizational response to stimuli.
  5. Management: See under Cocaine, above.
  6. Long-term effects: As with other illicit drug exposure, children exposed to amphetamine abuse show an increased incidence of learning deficits and behavioral problems. However, because they have multiple risk factors, it is difficult to establish cause and effect.
F. Tobacco (Aranda et al., 2002; Kliegman and Das, 2002)
  1. Effects on fetus
     a. Growth restriction: Birth weight is decreased an average of 170 g with 10 cigarettes/day, and 300 g if >15 cigarettes/day. Smoking cessation in early pregnancy can eliminate growth-restricting effects.
     b. 30%–35% increased mortality risk secondary to abruption, placenta previa, prematurity, and respiratory disease. May also increase the risk for spontaneous abortion.
  2. Effects on newborn: Though nicotine does pass in breast milk, no neonatal effects have been described.
  3. Long-term effects: Somewhat easier to study than effects of illicit drugs, since cigarette smoking without use of other drugs is common.
     a. Increased risk for sudden infant death syndrome (SIDS) (Taylor and Sanderson, 1995).
     b. Behavioral problems, aggressive type (Williams, 1998).

REFERENCES

American Academy of Pediatrics: Hepatitis B. In Pickering LK, editor: *Red book: 2003 report of the committee on infectious diseases,* ed 26, Elk Grove Village, IL, 2003, American Academy of Pediatrics, pp 318-336.

American Academy of Pediatrics, Committee on Drugs: Neonatal drug withdrawal, *Pediatrics* 101:1079-1088, 1998.

American Academy of Pediatrics, Committee on Drugs: The transfer of drugs and other chemicals into human milk, *Pediatrics* 108:776-789, 2001.

American Academy of Pediatrics, Committee on Substance Abuse: Drug-exposed infants, *Pediatrics* 96:364-367, 1995.

American Academy of Pediatrics, Committee on Substance Abuse and Committee on Children With Disabilities: Fetal alcohol syndrome and alcohol-related neurodevelopmental disorders, *Pediatrics* 106:358-361, 2000.

Aranda JV, Edwards DJ, Hales BF, Rieder MF: Developmental pharmacology. In Fanaroff AA, Martin RJ, editors: *Neonatal-perinatal medicine,* ed 7, St Louis, 2002, Mosby, pp 144-166.

Astley SJ, Clarren SK: *Diagnostic guide for fetal alcohol syndrome and related conditions: the 4-digit diagnostic code,* ed 2, Seattle, 1991, University of Washington Publication Services.

Brown ER, Zuckerman B: The infant of the drug-abusing mother, *Pediatr Annals* 20:555-563, 1991.

Callahan CM, Grant TM, Phipps P, et al: Measurement of gestational cocaine exposure: sensitivity of infant's hair, meconium and urine, *J Pediatr* 120:763-768, 1992.

Chavkin W: Cocaine and pregnancy—time to look at the evidence, *JAMA* 285(12):1626-1628, 2001.

Clarren SK, Astley SJ, Gunderson VM, Spellman D: Cognitive and behavioral deficits in nonhuman primates associated with very early embryonic binge exposures to ethanol, *J Pediatr* 121:789-796, 1992.

Dashe JS, Sheffield JS, Olscher DA, et al: Relationship between maternal methadone dosage and neonatal withdrawal, *Obstet Gynecol* 100:1244-49, 2002.

Day NL, Richardson GA: Prenatal marijuana use: epidemiology, methodologic issues, and infant outcome, *Clin Perinatol* 18:77-91, 1991.

Dixon SD, Bresnahan K, Zuckerman B: Cocaine babies: meeting the challenge of management, *Contemp Pediatr* 7:70-92, 1990.

Ferguson v. City of Charleston, 121 S. Ct. 1281 (2001).

Finnegan LP: Neonatal abstinence. In Nelson NM, editor: *Current therapy in neonatal-perinatal medicine,* Philadelphia, 1990, BC Decker, pp 314-320.

Frank DA, Augustyn M, Knight WG, et al: Growth, development, and behavior in early childhood following prenatal cocaine exposure: a systematic review, *JAMA* 285(12):1613-1625, 2001.

Hale, Thomas W: Methadone in mothers' milk. In *Medications and mothers' milk,* ed 10, Amarillo, TX, 2002, Pharmasoft Pub, pp 462-464.

Hoegerman G, Scholl S: Narcotic use in pregnancy, *Clin Perinatol* 18:51-76, 1991.

Jones KL: Fetal alcohol syndrome, *Pediatr Rev* 8:122-126, 1986.

Jones KL: Developmental pathogenesis of defects associated with prenatal cocaine exposure: fetal vascular disruption, *Clin Perinatol* 18:139-146, 1991.

Jones KL: Fetal alcohol syndrome. In Jones KL, editor: *Smith's recognizable patterns of human malformation,* ed 5, Philadelphia, 1997, WB Saunders, pp 555-558.

Kliegman RM, Das UG: Intrauterine growth retardation: maternal contributions to aberrant fetal growth. In Fanaroff AA, Martin RJ, editors: *Neonatal-perinatal medicine,* ed 7, St Louis, 2002, Mosby, pp 228-262.

Pietrantoni M, Knuppel RA: Alcohol use in pregnancy, *Clin Perinatol* 18:93-111, 1991.

Plessinger MA: Prenatal exposure to amphetamines, *Obstet Gynecol Clin North Am* 25(1):119-138, 1998.

Sampson PD, Streissguth AP, Bookstein FL, et al: Incidence of fetal alcohol syndrome and prevalence of alcohol-related neurodevelopmental disorder, *Teratology* 56:317-326, 1997.

Shaw NJ, McIvor L: Neonatal abstinence syndrome after maternal methadone treatment, *Arch Dis Child Fetal Neonatal Ed* 71(3):F203-205, 1994.

Stratton K, Howe C, Battaglia F, editors: *Fetal alcohol syndrome: diagnosis, epidemiology, prevention and treatment*, Washington, DC, 1996, National Academy Press, 1996, pp 4-21.

Streissguth AP, Aase JM, Clarren SK, et al: Fetal alcohol syndrome in adolescents and adults, *JAMA* 265:1961-1967, 1991.

Taylor JA, Sanderson M: A reexamination of the risk factors for the sudden infant death syndrome, *J Pediatr* 126:887-891, 1995.

Williams GM, O'Callaghan MB, Najman JM, et al: Maternal cigarette smoking and child psychiatric morbidity: a longitudinal study, *Pediatrics* 102(e11):133-134, 1998.

Zuckerman B, Frank DA, Hingson R, et al: Effects of maternal marijuana and cocaine use on fetal growth, *N Engl J Med* 320:762-768, 1989.

Management of the Infant at Risk for Perinatal Infections

In this section, the major bacterial and viral infections that may be encountered in the Level I nursery will be discussed. Initial management of these infections will be reviewed, although many of these infants may be transferred to a Level II or III nursery for further evaluation and therapy. In addition, general principles of isolation will be outlined, with disease-specific isolation usually mentioned within the discussion of each particular infection.

19 Bacterial Infections

Daniel M. Hall, MD ■ *Patti J. Thureen, MD* ■ *Mark J. Abzug, MD*

SEPSIS AND MENINGITIS

A. **Background and Epidemiology:** Culture-proven sepsis in the newborn is relatively rare, occurring in approximately 2 of 1000 live births (Freedman et al., 1981; Kushner and Feldman, 1978; Pyati et al., 1981). Since undiagnosed and untreated infection carries a mortality as high at 50% (Kushner and Feldman, 1978; Placzek and Whitelaw, 1983; Pyati et al., 1981; Rabalais et al., 1987), it is imperative to identify who is and who is not infected. Because the early signs of sepsis can be protean and nonspecific and mortality is high, clinicians frequently err on the side of excessive septic work-ups. In fact, as many as 15% (Escobar et al., 2000; American Academy of Pediatrics [AAP], 2003a) of all inborn babies receive such evaluations, yet only 3%–8% (Gerdes, 1987; Hammerschlag et al., 1977; Placzek and Whitelaw, 1983) of these prove positive for infection. Furthermore, one third of nursery antibiotic courses have been judged to be too long (Hammerschlag et al., 1977), creating undue medical, financial, and social morbidities for babies and families. This antibiotic overexposure can result in the emergence of resistant, difficult-to-treat infections.

B. **Risk Factors for Infection:** Being familiar with risk factors for infection can direct caregivers in deciding for which patients an infection work-up is indicated and justified. Table 19-1 lists some commonly encountered risk factors and associated likelihood of proven or highly suspected sepsis.

C. **Maternal Antibiotic Therapy**
  1. Although maternal antibiotic treatment in labor reduces the risk for neonatal colonization and invasive disease, it also commonly results in bactericidal levels in cord blood, which may render neonatal blood cultures negative, falsely reassuring caregivers in the case of partially treated sepsis or pneumonia. This is most common following intrapartum chemoprophylaxis for group B streptococcus (GBS). The newest guidelines call for universal screening with maternal vaginal and rectal cultures at 35–37 weeks gestation (Centers for Disease Control and Prevention [CDC], 2002). The screening approach is preferred over risk factor–based approaches because of population-based data that suggest that the former method prevents more early-onset GBS disease (Hammerschlag et al., 1989). In addition to providing chemoprophylaxis to those who are culture-positive, chemoprophylaxis is provided in the following situations:
  a. Previous infant with GBS disease.
  b. GBS bacteriuria during the current pregnancy.

● TABLE 19-1
● **Risk Factors for Sepsis**

Risk Factor	Likelihood of Sepsis
Maternal group B streptococcus (GBS) colonization	0.5%–2%
Untreated in labor	5%
Treated	<1%
PROM	1%–2%
PROM plus GBS-positive	4%–10%
PROM plus Apgar score <6 at 1 or 5 minutes	3%–10%
PROM plus chorioamnionitis	3%–10%
PROM, prematurity, and intra-amniotic infection	5%–20%

PROM, prolonged rupture of membranes (refers to membranes ruptured >18 hours).
Centers for Disease Control and Prevention: Prevention of perinatal group B streptococcal disease: revised guidelines from CDC, *MMWR* 51(RR-11):1-22, 2002.

    c. Unknown GBS status with (1) delivery <37 weeks, or (2) rupture of membranes ≥18 hours, or (3) intrapartum temperature ≥100.4° F (≥38.0° C).
  2. Although maternal prophylaxis based on culturing with risk factor backup can dramatically reduce neonatal GBS disease, such situations as late or no prenatal care, inadequate culturing, or unavailable results create some failures, as well as confusion as to what to do with the newborn. The MMWR 2002 guidelines for management of a newborn whose mother received intrapartum antibiotics (IAP) are shown in Figure 19-1. It is important to note that these guidelines should not be used to direct the management of infants whose mothers did not receive IAP. These are fairly general guidelines, and it is recognized that individual practitioners or nurseries may vary from this algorithm based on their unit practices and clinical judgment. Though not identical to the MMWR guidelines (Hammerschlag et al., 1989), in general, we believe that the well-appearing term infant (whether or not the infant's mother received IAP) can be managed as discussed below under "Approach to the Infant with Possible Infection" (see also Box 19-1). In the setting of GBS, if the mother has received adequate chemoprophylaxis and reliable follow-up and communication can be ensured, infant discharge may occur as early as 24 hours. If follow-up is uncertain, the stay should be extended to 48 hours. The hospital observation should be done regularly by skilled health care professionals and should not be totally reliant on mother-baby surveillance (CDC, 2002; Nelson, 1993; Rabalais et al., 1987; Visser and Hall 1979).
 D. **Clinical Manifestations:** Although culture-proven sepsis in the newborn is relatively rare, many more infants present with signs suggestive of infection. These include the following:
  1. Apnea.
  2. Diminished activity.
  3. Poor feeding.

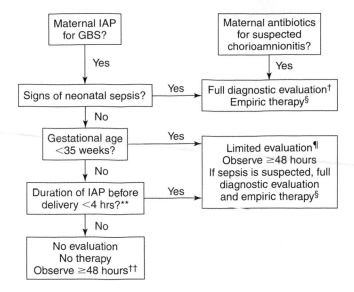

* If no maternal intrapartum prophylaxis for GBS was administered despite an indication being present, data are insufficient on which to recommend a single management strategy.

† Includes complete blood cell count and differential, blood culture, and chest radiograph if respiratory abnormalities are present. When signs of sepsis are present, a lumbar puncture, if feasible, should be performed.

§ Duration of therapy varies depending on results of blood culture, cerebrospinal fluid findings, if obtained, and the clinical course of the infant. If laboratory results and clinical course do not indicate bacterial infection, duration may be as short as 48 hours.

¶ CBC with differential and blood culture.

** Applies only to penicillin, ampicillin, or cefazolin and assumes recommended dosing regimens (Box 2).

†† A healthy-appearing infant who was ≥38 weeks' gestation at delivery and whose mother received ≥4 hours of intrapartum prophylaxis before delivery may be discharged home after 24 hours if other discharge criteria have been met and a person able to comply fully with instructions for home observation will be present. If any one of these conditions is not met, the infant should be observed in the hospital for at least 48 hours and until criteria for discharge are achieved.

FIGURE 19-1 ● MMWR 2002 guidelines for management of a newborn whose mother received intrapartum antibiotics (IAP).*

    4. Temperature instability.
    5. Respiratory distress.
    6. Poor color.
  E. Laboratory Tests: Because many uninfected newborns present with signs suggestive of infection, one must be able to select laboratory tests that can accurately identify those who are not infected, that is, a high negative predictive value, at a reasonable cost.

1. White blood cell count (WBC): A white count and manual differential are readily available, as well as easily and reliably performed, and can provide reassurance of no infection if done serially on days 1 and 2 (Gerdes and Polin, 1987; Luginbuhl et al., 1987; Mathers and Polhandt, 1987; Placzek and Whitelaw, 1983; Rodwell et al., 1988). The normal newborn WBC can range from 5000 to 30,000 cells/mm^3 (see Appendix C for normal WBC values over the first days of life). Table 19-2 indicates ways in which the WBC can be used to evaluate for sepsis in the neonate. Though a variety of other conditions can cause neutropenia in the neonate (e.g., asphyxia, maternal hypertension), 83% of noninfectious neutropenia normalizes within 48 hours (Freedman et al., 1981).

2. C-reactive protein (CRP): CRP is a nonspecific acute phase reactant synthesized by the liver in response to interleukin 6. It is useful in assessing infection with many bacterial pathogens. Because of a latency period of 6–8 hours and a stabilization time of 1–2 days after starting therapy, this test is best performed on the second day of life. A value of <1.0 mg/dL has a negative predictive value of 92%–99% (Liu et al., 1984; Matorras et al., 1991; Philip and Hewitt, 1980).

3. Blood culture: A blood culture should be obtained but may be affected if the mother received antibiotics in labor. Sample volume should be 1–2 mL because 23% will be falsely negative if less than 1 mL is drawn (Velaphi et al., 2003). Neonatal pneumonia will have negative blood cultures 50% of the time regardless of the above precautions (Sherman et al., 1980). Consequently, a clinical or radiographic diagnosis of pneumonia should be treated with a full course of antibiotics regardless of blood culture results. Given the above considerations, 96% of blood cultures are reliably negative at 48 hours and antibiotic therapy can be discontinued (Escobar et al., 2000; Placzek and Whitelaw, 1983; Visser and Hall 1979). This does not change if maternal antibiotics have been given before delivery.

4. Urine culture: Urine cultures in the first 72 hours of life are not routinely indicated because early bacteriuria is secondary to bacteremia (Weiss et al., 1991). If urine is to be cultured, the sample should be obtained by sterile

● TABLE 19-2
Negative Predictive Values of the WBC for Sepsis

WBC Component	Negative Predictive Value
WBC >5000	91%–96%
Absolute neutrophil count (ANC) >1750, where ANC = WBC × % total neutrophil count*	96%–99%
I/T ratio <0.3, where I/T = immature neutrophils† ÷ total neutrophil count	99%–100%

*Total neutrophil count = segmented neutrophils + band forms + myelocytes + metamyelocytes.
†Immature neutrophils = band forms + myelocytes + metamyelocytes.

catheterization or suprapubic needle aspiration to avoid contamination and falsely positive results.

5. Lumbar puncture (LP): The place of routine LP in the early neonatal septic work-up remains controversial. It is often unsuccessful (15%–30%) or bloody (30%) (Schwersenski et al., 1991) and may further compromise an already unstable infant. Meningitis in the absence of bacteremia is very uncommon, especially in neonates presenting with respiratory disease, occurring 1 in 1500 taps (Sanchy et al., 1990). It is therefore recommended that lumbar puncture be reserved for infants with central nervous system signs, proven bacteremia, or clinical sepsis (CDC, 2002).

6. Latex agglutination for GBS: A commonly used nonspecific laboratory test is the urine latex agglutination for group B streptococcal antigen. It may be a useful adjunctive test in a symptomatic infant if the mother is GBS-positive and treated in labor or in the presence of pneumonia with negative blood cultures. Complicating (confounding) factors include the following (Harris et al., 1989):

   a. The test only detects GBS, and only 45%–55% of neonatal sepsis is due to GBS.

   b. Positive latex agglutination and negative culture may occur with:

      (1) Low titer bacteremia.
      (2) Partial treatment.
      (3) Pneumonia.

   c. The test is not recommended as a routine screen for neonatal sepsis.

F. **Approach to the Infant With Possible Infection:** The above information can be used to formulate a sound, safe clinical approach for those newborns at risk. The intent is to readily identify those who are not infected, minimizing prolonged, costly, and unnecessary treatment, thus reserving therapy for those most likely infected. Box 19-1 summarizes the clinical approach for assessing possible sepsis in both well-appearing infants with risk factors for infection (e.g., maternal history) or one of the protean signs or symptoms of infection (e.g., a single episode of temperature instability), as well as infants with clinical courses more suggestive of infection. Note that this approach may preclude early hospital discharge.

G. **Therapy**

1. The appropriate initial choice of antibiotics depends on the likely organisms, pharmacokinetics, efficacy, and potential toxicities of the antimicrobial agents used. The most common organisms include group B streptococcus, *Escherichia coli, Klebsiella pneumoniae,* and *Enterococcus.* Ampicillin provides inexpensive, safe, and effective coverage for GBS, *Enterococcus, Listeria monocytogenes,* and some gram-negative organisms at a recommended dose of 50–75 mg/kg/dose every 8–12 hours. Gentamicin remains an inexpensive choice for gram-negative coverage and also offers synergy with ampicillin against GBS, *Enterococcus,* and *Listeria monocytogenes.* While some practitioners choose cefotaxime, it is more expensive and cephalosporin usage has been associated with nursery outbreaks of enterococcal and *Enterobacter* disease (Bryan et al., 1985; Manroe et al., 1979). Cefotaxime has a theoretical

● BOX 19-1
APPROACH TO EVALUATING INFANTS FOR POSSIBLE SEPSIS

Well-appearing term (≥37 weeks) infant
- Careful exam
- If mother has intrapartum fever or chorioamnionitis, check WBC
- If neutropenia or elevated I/T, treat as if sick
- Observe 24–48 hours

Well-appearing preterm (<37 weeks infant)
- Careful exam
- Observe 24–48 hours
- WBC—If neutropenia or elevated I/T, treat as if sick

Any age infant with signs or symptoms suggestive of infection
- Careful exam
- WBC days 1 and 2
- CRP day 2
- Blood culture (1–2 mL)
- Chest x-ray if respiratory symptoms present
- Antibiotics at least 48 hours
- Lumbar puncture if central nervous system signs present or if blood culture positive (if the infant has already received antibiotics, the glucose, protein, and cell count may indicate infection even if the CSF culture is negative)

advantage compared with gentamicin in central nervous system infections because of enhanced penetration across the blood-brain barrier. While published guidelines for gentamicin dosing call for intervals ranging from every 8 to 24 hours depending on age and weight (Philip, 1980), our experience suggests that with normal renal function it can be safely and effectively administered as follows for 48–72 hours without obtaining blood levels:

   a. Gestational age >34 weeks: 4 mg/kg/dose every 24 hours.

   b. Gestational age <34 weeks: 3.5 mg/kg/dose every 18 hours.

2. If suspected sepsis becomes proven, antibiotic therapy should be tailored based on the organisms, sensitivities, and clinical response. Therapy for uncomplicated sepsis should be a minimum of 10–14 days and for meningitis a minimum of 14–21 days. Most experts recommend use of the longer portion of these ranges for gram-negative enteric infection. The management of multiple organ dysfunction that frequently accompanies neonatal sepsis is beyond the intent and scope of this chapter.

NEONATAL CONJUNCTIVITIS

   A. Background and Epidemiology: *Ophthalmia neonatorum* refers to conjunctivitis occurring within the first 3–4 weeks of life. The etiologic distribution depends on the patient population, but in general, the most common causes are due to chemical irritation, *S. aureus*, *N. gonorrhoeae*, and *Chlamydia trachomatis*. Herpes simplex virus can also be a cause of neonatal keratoconjunctivitis. *Pseudomonas aeruginosa* is an occasional cause of severe conjunctivitis. Chemical conjunctivitis is usually due to instillation of prophylactic silver nitrate but may occur with topical antibiotics. Gonococcal and chlamydial conjunctivitis usually occur perinatally with infant exposure to infected maternal secretions, and 30%–40% of infants exposed to gonococcus or chlamydia at delivery will develop conjunctivitis (Schachter, 1989). Other bacterial infections are usually acquired postnatally from caretakers at home or in the nursery. Table 19-3 summarizes the etiologic agents, clinical findings, and therapy for the most common types of neonatal conjunctivitis.

B. **Diagnosis** (see Table 19-3): Any infant with a red eye and/or significant ocular discharge after 48 hours of age should undergo a diagnostic work-up, particularly a rapid assessment for herpes, *N. gonorrhoeae*, and chlamydia. If silver nitrate was not used and these symptoms are present before 48 hours of age, work-up should also be considered. All possible etiologies should be sought regardless of maternal history since mixed infections are common. Time of onset of symptoms is rarely of diagnostic use except for presentation within hours after use of silver nitrate. Prophylaxis may delay the onset of symptoms with infectious etiologies. The following work-up is suggested:
  1. Gram stain of the exudate (particularly to evaluate for *N. gonorrhoeae* and *Pseudomonas aeruginosa*).
  2. Prompt blood agar culture of the exudate, plus culture on chocolate agar, if Gram stain or maternal history suggests gonococcus or in areas of high rates of maternal gonococcal infection.
  3. Palpebral conjunctival scrapings with a blunt spatula or wire loop (cotton swabs are not adequate) for Giemsa stain and for *C. trachomatis* fluorescent antibody test and/or enzyme immunoassay.
  4. If herpes is suspected, fluorescent antibody test of a conjunctival swab confirmed by culture.

C. **Therapy** (see Table 19-3): Confirmation of conjunctivitis due to gonococcus or herpes simplex requires hospital admission, evaluation for systemic disease, and parenteral therapy. Since *Pseudomonas aeruginosa* can cause rapidly progressive disease, which may result in blindness, Gram stain demonstrating gram-negative rods requires prompt initiation of both topical and systemic antipseudomonal therapy pending culture results. Chlamydial conjunctivitis should be treated with an oral, rather than topical, antibiotic.

D. **Prophylaxis**
  1. Prophylaxis against neonatal eye infections is required by most states. Prophylaxis is most effective if given within 1 hour of delivery. The American Academy of Pediatrics has concluded that silver nitrate 1% solution, erythromycin 0.5% ointment, and tetracycline 1% ointment are all acceptable and equivalent prophylaxis for neonatal conjunctivitis (AAP, 2003a). In a prospective comparison of prophylactic agents, Hammerschlag et al. (1989) showed all three agents were equally effective

● TABLE 19-3
Neonatal Conjunctivitis

Etiologic Agent	Clinical Findings	Sequelae	Diagnosis	Therapy
Chemical	Usually occurs several hours after instillation of $AgNO_3$ drops, occasionally after topical antibiotic therapy. Conjunctival and lid erythema and edema; watery discharge. Resolves within 1–2 days.	None if properly administered.	Gram stain: PMNs and no organisms. Culture negative.	None. Rinsing the eye after instillation does not lessen symptoms or duration (Mathieu, 1958).
Neisseria gonorrhoeae	Usually presents within the first week (range, 2–3 days to 2–3 weeks of age) with bilateral copious, mucopurulent discharge (sometimes bloody). Lid and conjunctival edema and erythema.	Rare, but permanent visual impairment and/or systemic infection may occur. May be self-limited even without therapy.	Gram stain: gram-negative diplococci. Confirmed with positive identification on chocolate agar culture. Note: Evaluate for sepsis and meningitis.	Ceftriaxone 25–50 mg/kg/day IV or IM × 1 dose (in neonates with jaundice), cefotaxime 100 mg/kg/day IV or IM ×1 dose. Saline eye irrigation until discharge clears. Rule out systemic disease.
Chlamydia trachomatis	Usually presents 5–14 days of age, though may be delayed with prophylaxis (Laga et al., 1988). May have minimal symptoms but copious mucopurulent exudates with frequent pseudomembrane formation.	If untreated, may rarely lead to scarring with impaired vision.	Conjunctival scrapings; Giemsa stain-basophilic, intracytoplasmic, epithelial inclusion bodies, direct fluorescent antibody test, enzyme immunoassay, or culture.	Erythromycin ethylsuccinate 50 mg/kg/day PO divided qid × 14 days. Topical therapy is insufficient to eradicate nasopharyngeal colonization.

Other bacteria (*Staphylococcus* spp., *Streptococcus* spp., *Haemophilus* spp., gram-negative bacteria)	Mild, self-limited, mucopurulent discharge, conjunctival hyperemia, lid edema.	Rare systemic or cutaneous spread.	Gram stain suggests organism, confirmed by culture of the discharge.	Saline eye irrigation followed by topical antibiotic ophthalmic ointment or drops containing various combinations of bacitracin, neomycin, and polymyxin q6h × 7–10 days.
Pseudomonas aeruginosa	Onset 5–18 days of age. May begin as mild conjunctivitis but can rapidly progress over 12–24 hours. Prompt diagnosis essential.	May result in virulent necrotizing endophthalmitis and blindness.	Gram stain: gram-negative rods are highly suggestive. Need to confirm with culture.	Parenteral aminoglycoside plus antipseudomonal penicillin or cephalosporin (i.e., ceftazidime), plus topical aminoglycoside therapy × 7–10 days; start as soon as diagnosis suspected.
Herpes simplex virus	Onset 2–14 days after birth, no distinctive findings.	May cause conjunctivitis, cataracts, keratitis, chorioretinitis, optic neuritis. Frequent systemic spread if untreated.	Early diagnosis with positive fluorescent antibody test or Papanicolaou smear of conjunctival scrapings showing multinucleated giant cells. Requires confirmation by conjunctival culture.	Vidarabine ointment 3% q3h or 1% iododeoxy-uridine or trifluridine 1%–2% solution, 1 drop q2h × 7–21 days (Kohl, 1992); for recurrent lesions, oral suppressive therapy with acyclovir 80 mg/kg/day divided q8h (AAP, 2003). Ophthalmologic consultation should be obtained for disease monitoring and determining length of therapy.

in preventing GC ophthalmia, but none of these agents reduced the incidence of chlamydial conjunctivitis in infants born to mothers with chlamydial infection. Other reports suggest that the incidence of chlamydial conjunctivitis may be decreased by using any of these agents for prophylaxis. However, many of these reports did not have adequate length of follow-up to document prevention of disease, and onset of symptoms may actually be delayed by prophylaxis (Laga et al., 1988; Schachter, 1989).

2. The major advantages of silver nitrate are low allergenic potential and prevention of emergence of resistant bacteria, which have caused nursery outbreaks of erythromycin-resistant staphylococcal conjunctivitis (Hedberg et al., 1990). It also is proven to be effective against penicillinase-producing *Neisseria gonorrhoeae*. The major disadvantages of silver nitrate are the frequent development of chemical conjunctivitis and decreased likelihood of eradicating already-established infection. Single-dose administration prevents evaporation and possible eye damage secondary to a more concentrated solution.

3. Another study indicates that 2.5% povidone-iodine ophthalmic solution is another effective prophylactic agent and is less toxic and more cost-effective than either silver nitrate or erythromycin (Isenberg et al., 1995).

SUPERFICIAL BACTERIAL INFECTIONS

A. **Scalp Infections:** Fetal monitoring sites and skin abrasions from delivery manipulations are predisposing sites for infection and abscesses. Etiologic agents include normal skin, vaginal and GI tract flora, as well as agents causing maternal infection. These include the following: *N. gonorrhoeae*, group B streptoccocus, *S. epidermidis*, *S. aureus*, *Haemophilus* spp., gram-negative bacteria, and herpes simplex virus. For scalp abscesses incision and drainage is usually sufficient therapy. However, exudate should be cultured and appropriate therapy administered for 5–7 days (or longer if cellulitis develops).

B. **Skin Infections** (Marcy and Klein, 1992)

1. Pustules: The most common skin infection is impetigo neonatorum, or pustular skin lesions caused by *S. aureus.* This can be diagnosed by Gram stain of pustular debris and is usually responsive to topical antibiotic therapy alone. However, systemic therapy may be needed if lesions are extensive or if systemic symptoms are present. Concomitant bacteremia may occasionally occur. These infections can be a source of nursery staphylococcal outbreaks. Syphilis and candidal infections may also present with pustular rashes.

2. Vesicles: These can be seen with herpes simplex virus, varicella, and a variety of bacterial agents. Vesicle fluid should be stained and cultured to rule out these infections.

3. Maculopapular rashes: These rashes occur frequently and are most commonly noninfectious in origin. Infectious etiologies include numerous viruses (especially enterovirus), *S. aureus,* and streptococcal species.

4. **Abscesses:** Abscesses usually occur in the scalp at fetal monitoring sites and are generally due to *S. aureus* but may be caused by streptococcal species or gram-negative organisms.

C. **Breast Infection** (Shinefield, 1990; Mustafa et al., 1992): Usually presents in week 2–3 after birth. Examination shows unilateral breast swelling with or without redness. Infants are not usually systemically ill unless subcutaneous infection spreads beyond the breast tissue. The most common pathogen isolated from needle aspiration or exudate is *S. aureus*, though coliform bacteria and group B streptococcus can be causative agents. Though mild cellulitis can be treated with appropriate parenteral antibiotic therapy alone, abscesses require surgical incision and drainage, as well as parenteral antibiotic therapy. Permanent breast tissue disfigurement can result from more extensive disease.

D. **Omphalitis** (Cushing, 1985; Mustafa et al., 1992): Periumbilical erythema in infants is seen with some frequency and is usually due to cutaneous irritation by the sharp edges of a dried umbilical cord. However, true infection of the umbilicus (omphalitis) can rapidly progress to diffuse cellulitis and even necrotizing fasciitis, a frequently lethal disease. Etiologic agents include group A or B streptococcus, *S. aureus*, *P. aeruginosa*, and gram-negative and anaerobic bacteria. Infection is frequently caused by mixed pathogens. Therefore, any infant with periumbilical erythema deserves close observation and, if it does not resolve, should have a WBC with differential, blood culture, culture of any drainage and of an aspirate of the cellulitic area, and broad-spectrum coverage pending culture results. Surgical debridement may be required for progressive infections (i.e., fasciitis). Lack of prompt resolution may suggest a deeper infection (e.g., urachal cyst remnant).

CHLAMYDIA

A. **Background and Epidemiology:** *Chlamydia trachomatis* is now the most common cause of venereal disease in the United States. Prevalence rates of the organism in pregnant women vary between 6% and 12%, and over 70% of these may be asymptomatic (Schachter et al., 1983). Prolonged rupture of membranes and preterm deliveries are increased in women with recent or active disease (Sweet et al., 1987).

B. **Neonatal Infections:** Acquisition of infection is generally thought to occur around the time of delivery via inoculation of the infant's eye or respiratory tract with infected maternal secretions. It appears that none of the agents recommended for prophylaxis effectively prevents chlamydial conjunctivitis (Hammerschlag et al., 1989). Because of the delayed onset of presentation of these infections (up to 6 or more weeks after delivery), infant disease may be missed unless close follow-up is carried out or symptoms become severe enough to warrant evaluation. In a prospective study of 131 infants born to mothers with incompletely treated chlamydial infections, 18% developed conjunctivitis and 16% pneumonia (Schachter et al., 1986).

1. Conjunctivitis: Acquisition of *C. trachomatis* occurs in approximately 50% of infants born vaginally to infected mothers and in some infants delivered

by cesarean section with intact membranes. The risk for conjunctivitis is 25% to 50% in infants who acquire *C. trachomatis*. Onset of symptoms is variable, from several days to 3-4 weeks, and presentation may be delayed by prophylactic therapy (Laga et al., 1988). The infant is usually otherwise clinically well, infection may be unilateral or bilateral, and discharge and edema range from minimal to severe. Ocular findings are usually present for at least 1–2 weeks. There may be an associated nasal discharge and/or vulvovaginitis in female infants. Outcome of untreated disease ranges from mild to scarring with impaired vision.

2. Pneumonia: The most serious chlamydial infection in neonates is pneumonia, which can be fatal if not treated, although this is rare. Of exposed infants, 3%–18% will develop pneumonia (Alexander and Harrison, 1983). Symptoms develop 3–11 weeks after birth (range, 2–19 weeks after birth). The infant is usually afebrile and has a recurrent staccato cough, tachypnea, rales, and occasional wheezing. Laboratory findings often include mild peripheral eosinophilia, eosinophils in the tracheal aspirate, CXR demonstrating hyperinflation, and bilateral diffuse infiltrates.

C. **Diagnosis:** In conjunctivitis, rapid diagnosis should be performed by Giemsa staining of scrapings of the lower palpebral conjunctiva. The presence of blue-stained intracytoplasmic inclusions within epithelial cells is diagnostic. Alternatively, and in many laboratories more commonly, the palpebral scrapings can be analyzed by fluorescent antibody test or enzyme immunoassay for the causative agent, although these are not as sensitive. These studies must be performed on conjunctival cells, not on exudate alone. Culture is also available. In pneumonia, diagnosis is often by clinical presentation, eosinophilia, and/or antigen detection or culture of a nasopharyngeal specimen. In children with pneumonia, an acute microimmuno-fluorescence serum titer of *C. trachomatis*–specific immunoglobulin (Ig) M of ≥1:32 is diagnostic. Serologic testing is not widely available.

D. **Prevention:** Because of the failure of ocular prophylaxis and the late onset of ocular and respiratory symptoms, the most effective strategy for preventing neonatal disease is screening and treatment of maternal infection during pregnancy. High-risk women should be screened early in pregnancy, and all women screened in the third trimester. Ocular prophylaxis is not reliably effective in preventing conjunctivitis or pneumonia.

E. **Therapy:** Treatment is with erythromycin estolate or ethylsuccinate orally for 14 days for conjunctivitis or pneumonia, the dose depending on the age and weight of the patient. Topical therapy for conjunctivitis is inefficient and unnecessary and does not eradicate nasopharyngeal colonization. Some experts recommend that infants born to mothers with active disease be treated with erythromycin. Mothers of neonates with chlamydial infection and their sexual partners should be treated for infection.

F. **Isolation:** Standard Precautions, including appropriate drainage and secretion precautions, are indicated for an infected mother and the neonate with conjunctivitis. Respiratory precautions are not necessary for the infant with pneumonia or respiratory symptoms.

GONORRHEA (GC)

A. **Background and Epidemiology:** During pregnancy, the incidence of infections due to *Neisseria gonorrhoeae* ranges from 1%–10% depending on the population, occurring more commonly in adolescents and those from lower socioeconomic classes (Gutman, 1992a). Disseminated disease is more common in teenagers (infected within one week of menstruation) and during pregnancy, but most infected women are asymptomatic. There is a high incidence of other concomitant venereal disease, particularly chlamydial infection.

B. **Fetal and Neonatal Effects and Disease:** Maternal infection increases the risk for spontaneous abortion, premature rupture of membranes, premature delivery, and chorioamnionitis and may result in perinatal distress, neonatal sepsis, arthritis, meningitis, scalp abscess, and ophthalmia (vaginitis, bacteremia, ectopic pregnancy) (Gutman, 1992a). Neonatal ophthalmia is the most common manifestation of gonococcal infection in neonates, occurring in 30%–40% of infants who do not receive ocular prophylaxis and who are born to infected women (Schachter, 1989). Diagnosis is made by identifying gram-negative diplococci on Gram stain of the conjunctival exudate and confirmed by positive culture of the exudate.

C. **Prophylaxis:** All pregnant women should have an endocervical culture for GC at the first prenatal visit with repeat testing during the third trimester for those at high risk for repeat infection. (Gram stains of material obtained from the endocervix of postpubertal females are less sensitive than culture for detection of infection, but they can be of help in the differential diagnosis of a patient with acute abdominal pain or when immediate therapy is indicated.) Prophylaxis against gonococcal conjunctivitis is achieved by administration of one of the recommended topical agents within an hour of birth (see "Neonatal Conjunctivitis" above).

D. **Therapy** (AAP, 2003c): Appropriate culture and sensitivity testing should be done for both *N. gonorrhoeae* and chlamydia. Syphilis and HIV should also be excluded. (All patients with presumed or proven gonorrhea should be evaluated for concurrent syphilis, hepatitis B virus, HIV, and *C. trachomatis* infections.) Mother and her partners need evaluation for gonococcal and chlamydial infection and appropriate therapy. Because of high incidence of penicillin-resistant GC strains, penicillin therapy is no longer considered adequate empiric therapy. Penicillin may be used once penicillin-susceptibility of the organism is established. All neonates with gonococcal infections, including conjunctivitis, require hospitalization for parenteral therapy.

   1. Local infections (conjunctivitis, scalp abscesses): Ceftriaxone 25–50 mg/kg/day (maximum 125 mg) IV or IM once; in neonates with jaundice, cefotaxime 100 mg/kg/day IV or IM once. With conjunctivitis, frequent saline eye irrigation should be performed until the discharge is resolved, and an ophthalmologic consultation is recommended.

   2. Systemic disease: 7 days of therapy with ceftriaxone 25–50 mg/kg/day IV or IM once daily; in neonates with jaundice, cefotaxime 50 mg/kg/day IV or IM divided bid for septicemia and arthritis. Meningitis should be treated for 10–14 days.

3. Infants born to mothers known to have gonorrhea should receive a single dose of ceftriaxone, 125 mg intravenously or intramuscularly; for premature and low-birth-weight infants, the dose is 25 to 50 mg/kg, to a maximum of 125 mg.

E. **Isolation:** Standard Precautions are recommended for infected mothers and neonates (including those with conjunctivitis).

SYPHILIS

A. **Background and Epidemiology:** The incidence of acquired and congenital syphilis increased dramatically in the United States during the late 1980s and early 1990s but has subsequently decreased. In one study, statistically significant independent predictors of congenital syphilis were the following: young maternal age, African-American, single marital status, absence of father's name on the birth certificate, previous pregnancy, substance abuse, and lack of prenatal care (Desenclos et al., 1992). Rates of infection remain disproportionately high in large urban areas and the rural South of the United States. Congenital syphilis usually results from transplacental passage of *Treponema pallidum,* and infection can occur throughout pregnancy. Rate of fetal transmission depends on stage of disease, being 70%–100% during primary disease, 90% with secondary syphilis, and slowly decreasing thereafter but averaging 30% during latent syphilis (Gutman, 1992b). Infection can be transmitted to the fetus at any stage of disease; the rate of transmission is 60% to 100% during secondary syphilis and slowly decreases with time. Much less commonly, an infant can be infected at birth by contact with an infectious maternal lesion. With untreated maternal disease, 45%–55% of pregnancies may result in abortion, stillbirth, or perinatal death (Ricci et al., 1989; Gutman, 1992b). Surviving infected infants may or may not have symptoms at birth.

B. **Clinical Manifestations and Laboratory Findings:** Spread hematogenously, syphilis can involve most organs. The incubation period for acquired primary syphilis typically is 3 weeks but ranges from 10 to 90 days. However, the infant may be asymptomatic. Infants may have hepatosplenomegaly, snuffles, lymphadenopathy, mucocutaneous lesions, osteochondritis and pseudoparalysis, edema, rash, hemolytic anemia, or thrombocytopenia at birth or within the first months of life. Characteristic clinical manifestations include the following:

1. Skeletal abnormalities: Useful diagnostically because they occur commonly (95% of symptomatic patients), are usually present at birth, and are not affected by maternal therapy (Mahboubi, 1981). These lesions are usually painful, but radiographic changes may occur in otherwise asymptomatic infants (Brion et al., 1991). Most changes occur in the metaphyses, ranging from radiolucent or radiopaque lines to metaphyseal destruction, osteitis, and periostitis, although there are no findings specific to congenital syphilis. These lesions gradually heal spontaneously, usually by 6 months of age.

2. Skin lesions: Copper-colored maculopapular rash, which is most severe on the hands and feet, may appear at 1–3 weeks with subsequent desquamation. Lesions present at birth may be bullous. Less commonly seen are mucous patches and fissures around the lips and anus. *Rhagades* refers to fissure scars radiating from the mouth.

3. Nasal discharge: Often referred to as "syphilitic snuffles," a bloody nasal discharge may occur, usually in the first week of life.

4. Late manifestations: Untreated congenital syphilis can cause a variety of findings, which present after 2 years of age, including bony and dental abnormalities, interstitial keratitis, and central nervous system disease (i.e., meningitis, paresis, tabes dorsalis, and hydrocephalus). Some consequences of intrauterine infection may not become apparent until many years after birth, such as interstitial keratitis (5–20 years of age), eighth cranial nerve deafness (10–40 years of age), Hutchinson teeth (peg-shaped, notched central incisors), anterior bowing of the shins, frontal bossing, "mulberry molars," "saddle nose," rhagades, and Clutton joints (symmetric, painless swelling of the knees).

C. **Laboratory Findings:** Frequently seen are the following: Coombs-negative hemolytic anemia and hyperbilirubinemia, abnormal liver function tests, nonhemolytic anemia, and thrombocytopenia. Elevated or decreased WBCs may be seen. No distinctive CSF findings occur, but there may be elevated WBCs and protein. Positive CSF VDRL is the only specific finding for CNS disease, but this may be negative in early neonatal disease and positive in an uninfected neonate with a high titer of transplacentally acquired VDRL antibody.

D. **Diagnostic Tests** (AAP, 2003d)

1. Definitive: Darkfield exam or direct fluorescent antibody of exudate or tissue. Many false negatives, so congenital syphilis cannot be ruled out with a negative test.

2. Presumptive: Must use both a nontreponemal and treponemal test together to make a diagnosis.

   a. Nontreponemal
      (1) Most frequently used test is the VDRL. Others include RPR (rapid plasma reagin test) and ART (automated reagin test). VDRL and RPR are equal in sensitivity and specificity.
      (2) Because nontreponemal tests are inexpensive and rapid, they are effective screening tests.
      (3) These tests are quantitative, so they can be used to follow efficacy of therapy.
      (4) Rising titer indicates active infection (new infection, reinfection, reactivation or treatment failure). A fourfold increase in titer after treatment suggests reinfection or relapse.
      (5) Titers fall with adequate therapy and become nonreactive within 1–2 years with primary, secondary, and congenital syphilis. A sustained fourfold decrease in titer of the nontreponemal test result after treatment demonstrates adequate therapy.

(6) Major disadvantages include false-negative results in early primary, latent acquired, and late congenital syphilis. Biologic false-positive results can be caused by certain viral infections (e.g., infectious mononucleosis, hepatitis, varicella, and measles), lymphoma, tuberculosis, malaria, endocarditis, connective tissue disease, pregnancy, abuse of injection drugs, laboratory or technical error, or Wharton jelly contamination when cord blood specimens are used.

(7) Only the VDRL nontreponemal test is used for cerebrospinal fluid testing.

b. Treponemal

(1) Treponemal tests currently in use are FTA-ABS and *T pallidum* particle agglutination (tP-PA) tests.

(2) Used to help establish a presumptive diagnosis when a nontreponemal test is positive.

(3) Disadvantages include expense and false-positive reactions, which occur with other spirochetal diseases.

(4) Remain positive for life, even with successful therapy.

(5) Antitreponemal IgM antibody testing is available in some reference laboratories but is not commercially available.

E. Screening for Disease

1. Maternal screening: All women should be screened with a nontreponemal test early in pregnancy and again at delivery. In high-risk patients, also screen at 28 weeks. If mother is treated during pregnancy, monthly titers are necessary throughout remainder of pregnancy to ensure adequate response (i.e., fourfold decrease in titer).

2. Neonatal screening: The serologic status of the mother needs to be determined before discharging each infant from the hospital. Many states also require cord blood serology. The burden of proof in deciding not to treat an infant for possible congenital syphilis rests with the physician caring for the infant.

F. When to Consider a Diagnosis of Congenital Syphilis: An infant should be evaluated for congenital syphilis when there is a positive maternal VDRL or RPR confirmed by a positive treponemal test and one or more of the following (AAP, 2003d):

1. Untreated, inadequately treated, or undocumented treatment of syphilis.

2. Syphilis during pregnancy treated with a drug other than penicillin.

3. Treatment less than 1 month before delivery (because this is too short an interim period to document adequate response to therapy).

4. Lack of documented maternal serologic response (fourfold decrease in nontreponemal antibody titer) to treatment.

5. Clinical evidence of neonatal syphilis.

G. Neonatal Evaluation for Suspected Congenital Syphilis

1. Physical examination.

2. Quantitative VDRL or RPR on baby. Serum is preferred over cord blood, which may give false-positive results. Note that a positive neonatal VDRL in an asymptomatic infant does not differentiate between occult disease and passive transfer of maternal antibodies. Likewise, false-negative tests can occur with maternal infection late in pregnancy or if very high levels of maternal antibody are present (prozone phenomenon).

3. Maternal FTA-ABS and quantitative VDRL or RPR.
4. CBC with differential, platelet count, blood smear.
5. Bilirubin and liver function tests.
6. Long-bone radiographs (unless the diagnosis has been established otherwise).
7. CSF cell count, glucose, protein, VDRL (RPR should not be used for CSF).
8. Ophthalmologic exam if symptomatic.
9. Specific test if indicated (i.e., CXR with respiratory symptoms).
10. Antitreponemal IgM on baby if available.

H. **Treatment for Newborns <4 Weeks of Age With Suspected or Proven Congenital Syphilis** (AAP, 2003d)

1. For neonates with proven or highly probable disease, definitive treatment should be given: aqueous crystalline penicillin G, 100,000–150,000 U/kg per day, administered as 50,000 U/kg per dose IV, every 12 hours during the first 7 days of life and every 8 hours thereafter for a total of 10 days OR penicillin G procaine, 50,000 U/kg per day IM, in a single dose for 10 days. Treatment should be given in the following cases:
   a. Physical or radiologic evidence of disease.
   b. Nontreponemal titer is >4 times higher than mother's titer.
   c. Nontreponemal titer is <4 times higher but still greater than mother's titer and serologic follow-up cannot be guaranteed.
   d. Reactive CSF VDRL or abnormal CSF analysis in an infant born to a mother with a history of syphilis.
   e. Maternal therapy that did not consist of documented, appropriate treatment or that failed to produce a fourfold or greater decrease in maternal nontreponemal antibody titer (especially if follow-up serology cannot be guaranteed).
   f. Any infant considered at risk for congenital syphilis and warranting evaluation, if full infant work-up cannot be performed.
   g. Positive placenta or umbilical cord test results for treponemes using DFA-TP staining or darkfield test.

2. An asymptomatic infant with a negative work-up whose mother has one of the following situations may be given aqueous crystalline penicillin G for 10–14 days (and if more than 1 day is missed, the entire course needs to be restarted) OR penicillin G procaine, 50,000 U/kg per day IM in a single dose for 10 days OR clinical follow-up at 1, 2, 3, 6, and 12 months and serologic follow-up at 2–3 months, 6 months, and 12 months to document declining nontreponemal antibody titers plus penicillin G benzathine 50,000 U/kg IM in a single dose:
   a. No history of penicillin therapy.
   b. Inadequate or no documentation of penicillin therapy.
   c. Treated with erythromycin or other nonpenicillin therapy.

      d. Treated less than 1 month before delivery with appropriate penicillin therapy.

      e. Serologic tests that fail to demonstrate a fourfold or greater decrease in antitreponemal antibody titer.

   3. An asymptomatic infant with a negative work-up whose mother has a history of appropriately treated syphilis with penicillin >1 month before delivery and one of the following situations may be treated by using clinical follow-up at 1, 2, 3, 6, and 12 months and serologic follow-up at 2–3 months, 6 months, and 12 months to document declining nontreponemal antibody titers plus penicillin G benzathine 50,000 U/kg IM in a single dose:

      a. Maternal titers that decreased fourfold for early syphilis and remained stable and low for late syphilis.

      b. Mother has no evidence of reinfection or relapse.

   4. Follow-up of infants treated for congenital syphilis: Clinical follow-up at 1, 2, 3, 6, and 12 months and serologic follow-up at 2–3 months, 6 months, and 12 months. If there is no decline in titers by 3 months, or if the titer does not become negative by 6 months, the infant should be retreated. CSF examinations should be performed on infants with initially abnormal CSF findings every 6 months until normal; retreatment should be done if CSF VDRL is positive at 6 months or if CSF abnormalities persist at 2 years.

   5. Untreated, asymptomatic infants whose mothers had a documented response to appropriate treatment for syphilis during pregnancy should have a monthly VDRL or RPR test performed until their nontreponemal test is negative.

 I. Isolation Procedures: For mother or infant being treated for syphilis, Standard Precautions are indicated. Additionally, gloves should be used when handling infected newborns until after 24 hours of therapy.

TUBERCULOSIS (TB)

 A. Congenital Infection: Congenital tuberculosis (TB) is rare. Women with isolated pulmonary TB generally do not pose a risk to infecting the infant until after delivery, when there is exposure to respiratory secretions. In utero infections involving multiple organs can occur by hematogenous spread with maternal miliary TB or very rarely in mothers with endometrial or cervical TB via infected amniotic fluid. Infection acquired at birth from infected secretions (women with tuberculous endometritis) may present with symptoms in the first month of life. Infants infected in utero may be asymptomatic or exhibit a variety of early or delayed symptoms, including prematurity, anorexia, irritability, fever, respiratory symptoms, and hepatosplenomegaly. Newborns suspected of having congenital TB should have a tuberculin skin test (TST), chest x-ray, lumbar puncture, cultures for *Mycobacterium tuberculosis,* and placental exam and culture. Treatment should be initiated if the physical exam or chest x-ray is abnormal.

B. Management of Asymptomatic Infants With Mothers or Household Contacts With Possible or Known TB (AAP, 2003e; Smith et al., 1992): Each case requires individual evaluation because of the complexity of treatment decisions. In most cases, an infectious disease specialist should be consulted. If mother or other household contacts have TB, management of the newborn is based on the category of maternal or household contact infection as follows:

1. Mother or household contact has a negative CXR: If the mother or household contact is asymptomatic, the mother or household contact may require treatment for TB infection, but the infant and infected person do not require separation, and the neonate does not require testing or therapy. All household members should have a TST and further evaluation. The mother usually is a candidate for treatment of latent tuberculosis infection (LTBI), a condition defined as occurring in patients who have no clinical or radiographic abnormalities suggesting TB but who have a positive tuberculin skin test. Treatment in LTBI involves daily isoniazid therapy for 9 months and provides significant protection against development of TB for at least 20 years.

2. Mother or household contact has an abnormal CXR: The neonate and the potentially infected person should be separated until the mother or household contact has been fully evaluated and, if active TB is found, started on therapy (see below). If the work-up for active TB is negative in the mother or household contact, the infant is at low risk for acquiring TB and separation of the neonate from the infected adult is not necessary. All household members should have a TST and further evaluation.

3. Mother or household contact has radiographic or clinical evidence of active and possibly contagious TB: This situation requires immediate reporting to the public health department so that the entire household can be evaluated quickly. The infant should be tested for HIV infection and managed as follows:

   a. Mother and infant should be separated if the mother is judged contagious (clinical or radiologic evidence of active disease). The infant should be evaluated for neonatal TB. If the mother (or household contact) has tuberculosis disease attributable to multidrug-resistant *M. tuberculosis* or has poor adherence to treatment and directly observed therapy (DOT, i.e., therapy in which patient is watched to make certain the dose is taken) is not possible, the infant should be separated from the ill mother or household member, and BCG immunization should be considered for the infant.

   b. Neonatal work-up for suspected congenital TB should include TST, CXR, and appropriate cultures (CSF and 3 consecutive days of first morning tracheal and/or gastric aspirates obtained via nasogastric tube). In addition to culture, smears for acid-fast bacilli should be done, cell analysis in CSF performed, and fluorescent detection methods used if available. A TST (5 TU of purified protein derivative [PPD] intradermally) should be placed, although results of this test are often not positive for the first 4–6 weeks and may remain negative even with active neonatal disease. Therefore, regardless of TST results, therapy should be initiated with isoniazid, rifampin, pyrazinamide, and streptomycin or kanamycin.

   c. If the neonatal work-up is negative, the infant should be given isoniazid until 3–4 months of age, when a TST is done. If the TST is negative and mother and household contacts with TB are adhering to treatments and are no longer infectious, isoniazid can be discontinued. Separation from the mother and/or household contact can be discontinued when the infant is receiving isoniazid. Isoniazid should be continued for 9 months if the repeat TST is positive but reassessment for disease is negative.

   d. If neonatal disease is suspected or diagnosed, the newborn should be treated with isoniazid, rifampin, pyrazinamide, and streptomycin or kanamycin, and consultation should be obtained from an infectious disease specialist. Mother and infant can resume contact after the mother is judged noncontagious and the mother and infant are receiving appropriate therapy.

   e. If therapy for maternal TB was initiated during pregnancy and maternal sputum is negative, separation of mother and infant is not necessary and the infant should be started on isoniazid prophylaxis (10 mg/kg/day). Prophylaxis can be discontinued at 3–4 months of age if a CXR and repeat TST are negative at that time. Prophylaxis should be continued for 9 months if the repeat TST is positive but reassessment for disease in the infant is negative.

  4. Breast-feeding is not contraindicated if the mother is receiving therapy. Breast-feeding mothers receiving isoniazid should also be treated with pyridoxine. Breast-fed infants do not require pyridoxine unless they are receiving isoniazid.

  C. **Management of Infants Born to Mothers with Treated TB** (Feigin, 1992): The highest maternal relapse rates occur in women immediately after delivery and if therapy occurred less than 5 years ago. Mother and infant need close follow-up, including maternal CXR after delivery and at 1, 3, and 6 months. Infant tuberculin testing should be done at 6 weeks and at 3, 6, 9, and 12 months.

  D. **Management of Infants Born to Mothers with Unclear TB Status:** At times when the maternal TB status is unclear (e.g., no prenatal care, language difficulties) and it is suspected the mother may be at risk for past or present TB infection, the infant should be managed as outlined above ("Management of Asymptomatic Infants With Mothers or Household Contacts With Possible or Known TB").

  E. **Isolation:** Most patients (mothers and newborns) who are receiving treatment require only Standard Precautions. Patients with the following require more than Standard Precautions: (1) cavitary pulmonary tuberculosis, (2) positive sputum AFB smears, (3) laryngeal involvement, (4) extensive pulmonary infection, or (5) suspected congenital tuberculosis. These patients should be placed in a negative-pressure hospital room. Caretakers and hospital personnel should wear personally fitted and sealed particulate respirators during patient contact. All family members and household contacts who visit should be managed with airborne precautions until they are documented not to have contagious TB. Other visitors should not be allowed to visit until it is documented that they do not have TB or are not contagious.

REFERENCES

Alexander ER, Harrison HR: Role of *Chlamydia trachomatis* in perinatal infection, *Rev Infect Dis* 5:713-719, 1983.

American Academy of Pediatrics. In Pickering LK, editor: *Red book: report of the committee on infectious diseases,* ed 26, Elk Grove Village, IL, 2003a, American Academy of Pediatrics.

American Academy of Pediatrics: Chlamydial infections. In Pickering, LK, editor: *Red book: report of the committee on infectious diseases,* ed 26, Elk Grove Village, IL, American Academy of Pediatrics, 2003b, pp 235-243.

American Academy of Pediatrics: Gonococcal infections. In Pickering, LK, editor: *Red book: report of the committee on infectious diseases,* ed 26, Elk Grove Village, IL, American Academy of Pediatrics, 2003c, pp 285-291.

American Academy of Pediatrics: Syphilis. In Pickering, LK, editor: *Red book: report of the committee on infectious diseases,* ed 26, Elk Grove Village, IL, American Academy of Pediatrics, 2003d, pp 596-607.

American Academy of Pediatrics: Tuberculosis. In Pickering, LK, editor: *Red book: report of the committee on infectious diseases,* ed 26, Elk Grove Village, IL, American Academy of Pediatrics, 2003e, pp 642-660.

Bomela HN, Ballott DE, Cory BJ, et al: Use of C-reactive protein to guide duration of empiric antibiotic therapy in suspected early neonatal sepsis, *Pediatr Infect Dis J* 19:531-535, 2000.

Brion LP, Manuli M, Rai B, et al: Long-bone radiographic abnormalities as a sign of active congenital syphilis in asymptomatic newborns, *Pediatrics* 88:1037-1040, 1991.

Bryan CS, John JF, Pai S, et al: Gentamicin vs cefotaxime therapy of neonatal sepsis, *Am J Dis Child* 139:1086-1089, 1985.

Centers for Disease Control and Prevention: Prevention of perinatal group B streptococcal disease: revised guidelines from CDC, *MMWR* 51(RR-11):1-22, 2002.

Cushing AH: Omphalitis: a review, *Pediatr Infect Dis* 4:282-285, 1985.

Desenclos J-C, A, Scaggs M, Wroten JE: Characteristics of mothers of live infants with congenital syphilis in Florida, 1987-1989, *Am J Epidemiol* 136:657-661, 1992.

Escobar GJ, De-kun L, Armstrong MA et al: Neonatal sepsis workups in infants ≥2000 grams at birth: a population-based study, *Pediatrics* 106:256-263, 2000.

Evans HE, Frenkel LD: Congenital syphilis. In Evans HE, editor: *Perinatal AIDS: clinics in perinatology,* Philadelphia, 1994, WB Saunders, pp 149-162.

Feigin RD, Adcock LM, Miller DJ: The immune system. In Fanaroff AA, Martin RJ, editors: *Neonatal-perinatal medicine,* ed 5, St Louis, 1992, Mosby-Year Book, pp 683-690.

Freedman RM, Ingram DC, Gross I, et al: A half century of neonatal sepsis at Yale, *Am J Dis Child* 135:140-144, 1981.

Garcia-Prats JA, Cooper TR, Schneider VF et al: Rapid detection of microorganisms in blood culture of newborn infants utilizing an automated blood culture system, *Pediatrics* 105:523-527, 2000.

Gerdes JS, Polin RA: Sepsis screen in neonates with evaluation of plasma fibronectin, *Pediatr Infect Dis J* 6:443-446, 1987.

Gerdes JS: Clinicopathologic approach to the diagnosis of neonatal sepsis, *Clin Perinatol* 18:361-381, 1991.

Gutman LT: Gonorrhea. In Feigin RD, Cherry JD, editors: *Textbook of pediatric infectious diseases*, ed 3, Philadelphia, 1992a, WB Saunders, pp. 540-552.

Gutman LT: Syphilis. In Feigin RD, Cherry JD, editors: *Textbook of pediatric infectious diseases*, ed 3, Philadelphia, 1992b, WB Saunders, pp 552-563.

Hammerschlag MR, Klein JO, Herschel M, et al: Patterns of use of antibiotics in two newborn nurseries, *N Engl J Med* 296:1268-1269, 1977.

Hammerschlag MR, Cummings C, Roblin PM, et al: Efficacy of neonatal ocular prophylaxis for the prevention of chlamydial and gonococcal conjunctivitis, *N Engl J Med* 320:769-772, 1989.

Harris MC, Deuber C, Polin RA, et al: Investigation of apparent false-positive urine latex particle agglutination tests for the detection of group B streptococcus antigen, *J Clin Microbiol* 27:2214-2217, 1989.

Hedberg K, Ristinen TL, Solar JT, et al: Outbreak of erythromycin-resistant staphylococcal conjunctivitis in a newborn nursery, *Pediatr Infect Dis J* 9: 268-273, 1990.

Isenberg SJ, Apt L, Wood M: A controlled trial of povidone-iodine as prophylaxis against ophthalmia neonatorum, *N Engl J Med* 332:562-566, 1995.

Kohl S: Postnatal herpes simplex virus infection. In Feigin RD, Cherry JD, editors: *Textbook of pediatric infectious diseases*, ed 3, Philadelphia, 1992, WB Saunders, pp 1558-1583.

Kushner I, Feldman G: Control of the acute phase response: demonstration of C-reactive protein synthesis and secretion by hepatocytes during acute inflammation in the rabbit, *J Exp Med* 148:466-477, 1978.

Laga M, Plummer FA, Piot P: Prophylaxis of gonococcal and chlamydial ophthalmia neonatorum, *N Engl J Med* 318:653-657, 1988.

Liu CH, Lehan C, Speer ME, et al: Degenerative changes in neutrophils: an indicator of bacterial infection, *Pediatrics* 74:823-827, 1984.

Luginbuhl LM, Rotbart HA, Facklam RR, et al: Neonatal enterococcal sepsis: case control study and description of an outbreak, *Pediatr Infect Dis J* 6:1022-1030, 1987.

Mahboubi S: Radiological findings in perinatal infections, *Clin Perinatol* 8:517-537, 1981.

Manroe BL, Weinberg AG, Rosenberg CR, et al: The neonatal blood count in health and disease. I. Reference values for neutrophilic cells, *J Pediatr* 95:89-98, 1979.

Marcy SM, Klein JO: Focal bacterial infections. In Remington JS, Klein JO, editors: *Infectious diseases of the fetus and newborn infant*, ed 3, Philadelphia, 1992, WB Saunders, pp 700-741.

Mathers NJ, Polhandt F: Diagnostic Audit of C-reactive protein in neonatal infection, *Eur J Pediatr* 146:147-151, 1987.

Mathieu PL: Comparison study: silver nitrate and oxytetracycline in newborn eyes: a comparison of the incidence of conjunctivitis following the instillation of silver nitrate or oxytetracycline into the eyes of newborn infants, *Am J Dis Child* 95:609-611, 1958.

Matorras R et al: Chemoprophylaxis of early-onset intrapartum group B streptococcal disease, *Eur J Obst Gynecol* 40:57-62, 1991.

Mustafa MM, McCracken GH Jr: Perinatal bacterial diseases. In Feigin RD, Cherry JD, editors: *Textbook of pediatric infectious diseases*, ed 3, Philadelphia, 1992, WB Saunders, pp 891-924.

Nelson JD: Antibiotic therapy for newborns. In Nelson JD. editor: *Pocketbook of pediatric antimicrobial therapy*, ed 9, Baltimore, 1993, Williams & Wilkins, pp 8-17.

Philip AGS: *Neonatal sepsis and meningitis*, Boston, 1985, GK Hall & Co, pp 76, 92.

Philip AGS, Hewitt JR: Early diagnosis of neonatal sepsis, *Pediatrics* 65:1036-1041, 1980.

Placzek MM, Whitelaw A: Early and late neonatal septicemia, *Arch Dis Child* 58:728-731, 1983.

Pyati SP, Pildes RS, Ramamurthy RS, et al: Decreasing mortality in neonates with early-onset group B streptococcal infection: reality or artifact, *J Pediatr* 98:625-627, 1981.

Rabalais GP, Bronfin DR, Daum RS: Evaluation of commercially available latex agglutination test for rapid diagnosis of group B streptococcal infection, *Pediatr Infect Dis J* 6:177-181, 1987.

Ricci JM, Fojaco RM, O'Sullivan MJ: Congenital syphilis: The University of Miami/Jackson Memorial Medical Center experience, 1986-1988, *Obstet Gynecol* 74:687-693, 1989.

Rodwell RL, Leslie AL, Tudehope DI: Early diagnosis of neonatal sepsis using a hematologic scoring system, *J Pediatr* 112:761-767, 1988.

Rodwell RL, Taylor K, Tudehope DI, et al: Hematologic scoring system in early diagnosis of sepsis in neutropenic newborns, *Pediatr Infect Dis J* 12:372-376, 1993.

Saltz GR, Linnemann CC, Brookman RR, et al: *Chlamydia trachomatis* cervical infection in female adolescents, *J Pediatr* 98:981-985, 1981.

Sanchy PJ, Siegel JD, Cushion NB, et al: Significance of a positive urine group B streptococcal latex agglutination test in neonates, *J Pediatr* 116:601-606, 1990.

Schachter J: Why we need a program for the control of *Chlamydia trachomatis*, *N Engl J Med* 320:802-804, 1989.

Schachter J, Grossman M, Sweet RL, et al: Prospective study of perinatal transmission of *Chlamydia trachomatis*, *J Am Med Assoc* 255:3374-3377, 1986.

Schachter J, Stoner E, Moncada J: Screening for chlamydial infections in women attending family planning clinics: evaluations of presumptive indicators for therapy, *West J Med* 138:375-379, 1983.

Schrag SJ, Zell ER, Lynfield R: A population-based comparison of strategies to prevent early-onset group B streptococcal disease in neonates, *N Engl J Med* 347:233-239, 2002.

Schwersenski J, McIntyre L, Bauer CR: Lumbar puncture frequency and cerebral spinal fluid analysis in the neonate, *AJDC* 145:54-58, 1991.

Sherman MP, Goetzman BW, Ahlfors CE, et al: Tracheal aspiration and its clinical correlates in the diagnosis of congenital pneumonia, *Pediatrics* 65:258-263, 1980.

Shinefield HR: Staphyloccal infections. In Remington JS, Klein JO, editors: *Infectious diseases of the fetus and newborn infant*, ed 3, Philadelphia, 1990, WB Saunders, pp 866-900.

Smith MHD, Starke JR, Marquis JR: Tuberculosis and opportunistic mycobacterial infections. In Feigin RD, Cherry JD, editors: *Textbook of pediatric infectious diseases*, ed 3, Philadelphia, 1992, WB Saunders, pp 1321-1362.

Sweet RL, Landers DV, Walker C, et al: *Chlamydia trachomatis* infection and pregnancy outcome, *Am J Obstetr Gynecol* 156:824-831, 1987.

Velaphi S, Siegel JD, Wendel GD, et al: Early-onset group B streptococcal infection after a combined maternal and neonatal group B streptococcal chemoprophylaxis strategy, *Pediatrics* 111:541-547, 2003.

Visser VE, Hall RT: Urine culture in the evaluation of suspected neonatal sepsis, *J Pediatr* 94:635-638, 1979.

Weiss MG, Ionides SP, Anderson CL: Meningitis in premature infants with respiratory distress: role of admission lumbar puncture, *J Pediatr* 119:973-975,1991.

Wiswell TE, Hachey WE: Multiple site blood cultures in the initial evaluation of neonatal sepsis in the first week of life, *Pediatr Infect Dis J* 10:365-369, 1991.

20 Viral Infections

Jan Paisley, MD ▪ *Patti J. Thureen,* MD ▪ *Mark J. Abzug,* MD

Neonatal viral infections account for a large proportion of the infections that comprise the *TORCH* acronym, which includes *t*oxoplasmosis, *o*ther infections (syphilis, human immunodeficiency virus [HIV], enteroviruses, and varicella), *r*ubella, *c*ytomegalovirus (CMV), and *h*erpes simplex virus (HSV). Rubella, CMV, and some other less commonly occurring viruses such as lymphocytic choriomeningitis virus (LCM) are transferred transplacentally. These infections should be suspected when an infant is born with intrauterine growth retardation (especially if growth restriction is symmetrical with microcephaly), hepatospenomegaly, thrombocytopenia (petechiae or ecchymoses), or cerebral calcifications. Other viruses (e.g., HSV and enteroviruses) are commonly transferred at or around the time of delivery, and especially if maternal antibodies have not had time to pass to the infant prior to delivery, the infant can present with a fulminant sepsis-like syndrome including fever, disseminated intravascular coagulopathy (DIC), liver failure, respiratory distress/failure, shock, myocarditis/cardiomyopathy, or meningitis. Many of these infections can also be transferred horizontally postnatally.

HEPATITIS B VIRUS (HBV)

A. **Background and Epidemiology** (Robinson, 2000; AAP, Red Book, 2003): There are approximately 300,000 primary HBV infections per year and approximately 1.25 million HBV carriers in the United States. Approximately 5%–8% of the total U.S. population has been infected and 0.2%–0.9% of the total population are chronically infected. In highly endemic areas, including China, Southeast Asia, Eastern Europe, Middle East, Africa, the Amazon Basin, and some Caribbean and Pacific Islands, 70%–90% of the adult population has been infected and 8%–15% have chronic infection. HBV carriers have an approximate 25% risk for death due to HBV-related liver disease (cirrhosis, chronic active hepatitis, or chronic persistent hepatitis) or due to primary hepatocellular carcinoma. In the United States, the highest prevalence rates are in Asian immigrants, IV drug users, Alaskan Indians, Pacific Islanders, homosexual men, and household contacts of chronic HBV carriers. Overall about 1–2 per 1000 pregnancies are complicated by acute hepatitis B infection and 5–15 per 1000 pregnancies are complicated by chronic infection in the United States.

Although only 6%–10% of older children and adults who are infected will develop chronic HBV infection, 25%–50% of children 1-5 years and >90% of infants who are perinatally infected will develop chronic HBV infection. Neonatal infections usually occur in the perinatal period from exposure to infected maternal secretions or blood; in utero infection occurs rarely. Of infants born to mothers who are hepatitis B surface antigen (HbsAg)–positive, 30%–40% will become infected if they are not given hepatitis B immunoglobulin (HBIG) and hepatitis B vaccine (HepB vaccine) after birth (Armstrong, 2001). The highest risk for perinatal transmission (70%–90%) has been found to be with HBsAg-positive, HBeAg-positive, and HBeAb-negative mothers whose infants are not given HBIG and hepatitis B vaccine after birth. If the mother is HBsAg-positive but HbeAg-negative, the risk for perinatal infection is 5%–20%. Overall, the risk for infection in infants born to HBsAg-positive mothers is decreased by ~95% to ~1%–3% when HBIG and hepatitis B vaccine are given within 12 hours of birth. Some studies have shown that HepB vaccine alone (without HBIG), when started at birth, is ~85% effective in preventing hepatitis B infection even in HBeAg-positive mothers (Lolekha, 2002). However, at this time it is recommended to give both HepB vaccine and HBIG at birth to infants born to HBsAg-positive mothers. Breast-feeding has not been shown to increase the transmission rate of hepatitis B.

B. **Laboratory Tests and Their Interpretation in HBV Infections** (AAP Red Book, 2003; Edwards, 1988; Robinson, 2000): Figure 20-1 illustrates the time course appearance of the various tests described below.

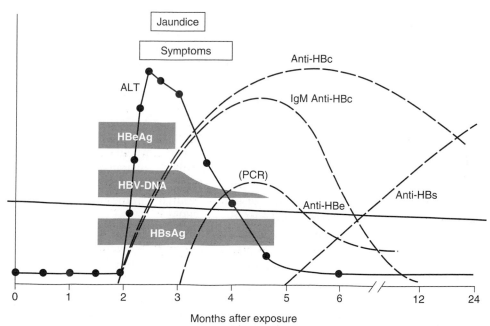

FIGURE 20-1 ● The clinical, virologic, and serologic courses of a typical case of acute hepatitis B. *Anti-HBc,* antibody to hepatitis B core antigen. *Anti-HBs,* antibody to hepatitis B surface antigen. *Anti-HBe,* antibody to hepatitis B e antigen. *HBeAg,* hepatitis B e antigen. *HBV-DNA,* hepatitis B DNA. *HBsAg,* hepatitis B surface antigen. *ALT,* alanine aminotransferase. *PCR,* polymerase chain reaction. (With permission from Mandell GL, Douglas DL, Bennett JE: *Principles and practice of infectious diseases,* ed 5, 2000, Churchill-Livingstone.)

1. Hepatitis B surface antigen (HBsAg): Positive in both acute and chronic infection. However, HBsAg may become negative in acute infection as clinical condition improves but before anti-HBs appears. Persistent HBsAg positivity after acute infection (especially past 6 months) denotes a chronic carrier state.

2. Antibody against hepatitis B surface antigen (anti-HBsAg): Indicates past HBV infection but can also be used to determine immune status after vaccination (it is the only antibody that develops with effective vaccination).

3. Total antibody against hepatitis B core antigen (anti-HBc): Indicates acute or past HBV infection. It does not become positive with hepatitis B vaccination, whereas the presence of both anti-HBsAg and anti-HBc indicates resolved infection. Chronic HBV carriers generally have HBsAg and anti-HBc.

4. IgM antibody against hepatitis B core antigen (IgM anti-HBc): Present during acute but not chronic infection. Will be positive in acute cases when HBsAg has disappeared but anti-HBsAg not yet present. Usually not present in perinatal HBV infection.

5. Hepatitis B e antigen (HBeAg): Marker of viral replication. Indicates highly infectious status.

6. Antibody against hepatitis B e antigen (anti-HBe): Indicates lower probability for transmitting infection.

7. Cord blood specimens cannot be used to diagnose neonatal infection because of possible contamination with maternal blood or secretions and because of possible transient transplacental passage of maternal antigens.

C. **Clinical and Laboratory Manifestations in the Infant:** The incubation period for acute infection is 45–160 days with an average of 90 days. Most infants infected in utero or perinatally are asymptomatic at birth. Jaundice occurs <3% of the time, with direct hyperbilirubinemia occurring later than indirect hyperbilirubinemia. Fulminant fatal hepatitis B is very rare. Other possible symptoms include prematurity, poor feeding, vomiting, and poor weight gain. In infants infected at delivery or after birth, antigen is not present for at least 2–5 months, after which infected infants are usually HBsAg-positive. Infants who become chronically infected are at risk for development of chronic hepatitis, cirrhosis, and/or hepatocellular carcinoma.

D. **Treatment/Prophylaxis** (AAP Red Book, 2003; AAP/ACOG, 2002; also see Chapter 12 for full hepatitis B immunization schedule). The AAP Committee on Infectious Diseases has recommended that routine serologic screening of all pregnant women be performed and priority be given to universal immunization of all infants and children. Ideally, maternal screening for HBsAg is done early in pregnancy, with repeated testing late in pregnancy for HBsAg-negative women who are at high risk for acquiring the infection.

The appropriate HBV prophylaxis for the neonate should be determined according to the mother's status (AAP Red Book, 2003, AAP/ACOG, 2002) (Table 20-1). The two available monovalent or single antigen hepatitis B vaccines that have been approved to use at birth are Recombivax HB (5 μg/0.5 mL) pediatric formulation (Merck & Co.) or Energix-B (10 μg/0.5 mL) [GlaxoSmithKline]. For neonates, the dose is 0.5 mL of either vaccine IM in

● TABLE 20-1
Neonatal Schedule for Hepatitis B Vaccine and HBIG Administration for Prevention of Perinatal Transmission of Hepatitis B*

Maternal Status	Dosing Schedule	Age
Neonates of HBsAg-positive mothers	HepB vaccine #1 (0.5 ml IM)	At birth (within 12 hours)
	HBIG (0.5 ml IM)	At birth (within 12 hours)
	HepB vaccine #2 (0.5 ml IM)	1–2 months
	HepB vaccine #3 (0.5 ml IM)	6 months
	Check HBsAg and anti-HBs 1–3 months after HepB vaccine series finished, and if infant is HbsAg and HbsAb (anti-HBs) negative, reimmunize with 3 doses at 2-month intervals and retest	7–9 months
	Infants with birth-weight <2 kg will need first dose repeated at 1 month or when weight >2 kg, second dose at 2–3 months, and third dose at 6–7 months	
Neonates of HBsAg-negative mothers	HepB vaccine #1 (0.5 ml IM)	At birth (preferably before hospital discharge) to 2 months
	HepB vaccine #2 (0.5 ml IM)	1–2 months after first dose
	HepB vaccine #3 (0.5 ml IM)	6–18 months
	Infants with birth-weight <2 kg should have initial immunization delayed until weight >2 kg	
Neonates of mothers with unknown HbsAg status (HbsAg should be drawn on mother at birth)	HepB vaccine #1 (0.5 ml IM)	At birth (within 12 hours)
	HBIG (0.5 ml IM) Further management dependent on mother's HbsAg result	At birth (within 12 hours if birth-weight <2 kg) If birth-weight ≥2 kg, HBIG should be given if HbsAg is positive within 7 days of birth

HepB, hepatitis B; *HBIG*, hepatitis B immune globulin; *IM*, intramuscularly; *HBsAg*, hepatitis B surface antigen.
*Adapted from Pickering LK, editor: *Red book: report of the committee on infectious diseases,* ed 26, Elk Grove Village, IL, 2003, American Academy of Pediatrics; American Academy of Pediatrics and American College of Obstetricians and Gynecologists: Perinatal infections. In *Guidelines for perinatal care,* ed 5, Elk Grove Village, IL, 2002, American Academy of Pediatrics and American College of Obstetricians and Gynecologists.

the anterolateral thigh. Both vaccines have been shown to produce protective antibody with a complete series in >95% of recipients, with minimal side effects including pain at the injection site (3%–29%) and fever ≥37.7° C (1%–6%). Anaphylaxis has occurred in 1/600,000; no deaths have been attributed to the vaccines (MMWR, 2003).

1. Infants born to HBsAg-positive mothers: These infants need to have their first hepatitis B vaccine (0.5 mL IM) along with hepatitis B immune globulin (HBIG) (0.5 mL IM) administered at a different site from the vaccine, and both vaccines should be given within 12 hours of life. As noted above, only a single-antigen hepatitis B vaccine should be given, not the combination vaccines that are given later in the immunization series to infants. The skin at the injection sites should be well cleansed before the injection to avoid inoculation of the virus contaminating the skin. The local or state health department needs to be notified that the infant has been born and the dates that the HBIG and HepB vaccine were given. The mother needs to be educated and given written materials regarding the importance of her baby completing the HepB vaccination schedule on time including the second vaccine at 1–2 months of age and the third vaccine at 6 months. For premature infants weighing <2 kg at birth the vaccine and HBIG should be given within the first 12 hours of birth; however, the first immunization will not count as part of the series and will need to be repeated when the infant is >2 kg or 1–2 months of age, the second 1–2 months later, and the third 6 months later. Serologic testing including HBsAg and quantitative anti-HBs (HbsAb) should be performed 1–3 months after the third vaccine. Infants who are HBsAg-positive are chronically infected and will need long-term medical management. Infants who are HBsAg negative are at ongoing risk for horizontal infection from their mother and must be documented to have an immune status defined as an anti-HBs concentration of >10 mIU/ml. If the titer is <10 mIU/ml, the infant should receive either another 3-dose schedule starting immediately (1 month and 6 months later followed by repeat serology testing for anti-Hbs) or, alternatively, 1–3 additional doses with anti-HBs titers 1 month after each until documented >10 mIU/ml. Note that these recommendations are for infants >2 kg in weight at birth. Guidelines for preterm infants <2 kg in weight at birth can be found in the AAP Red Book, 2003 edition.

2. Infants born to HBsAg-negative mothers: First dose of hepatitis B vaccine should be administered at birth (preferably before hospital discharge) to 2 months at the latest. The second dose should be given 1–2 months later and the third dose at 6–18 months. If the neonate weighs <2 kg at birth, the first dose should be delayed until the infant is >2 kg, or the dose should be repeated after 2 kg since immunogenicity cannot be guaranteed in this group. The Immunization Action Coalition (IAC) is now recommending that all infants born to HBsAg-negative mothers receive their first HepB vaccine before discharge from the nursery. Since the new combination vaccines cannot be given prior to 6 weeks of age, this requires a separate monovalent vaccination. The reasons for the IAC recommendation

include the following possibilities: the mother converted from a negative to positive status after her screening was done; she was improperly screened with the wrong test panel (i.e., HBsAb instead of HBsAg); the results were misinterpreted or mistranscribed; or she was positive and the results were not forwarded to the hospital. State and local hepatitis coordinators have reported more than 500 medical errors regarding perinatal hepatitis B prevention over a 3-year period, causing many children to unnecessarily become chronically infected with hepatitis B and at least one infant to die. Numerous lawsuits are pending against both the practitioners and hospitals involved with these cases *(www.immunize.org)*.

3. Infants born to mothers with unknown HBsAg status: Maternal HBsAg should be drawn as soon as possible. The infant should be given HBV vaccine within the first 12 hours of life, and, if the maternal HbsAg comes back positive, the infant should be given HBIG as soon as possible, at least within the first 7 days of life. If the baby is born with a birth-weight of <2 kg and the mother's HBsAg is unknown, it is recommended that the infant be given HBV vaccine within 12 hours of birth and, if the maternal HbsAg status cannot be determined within the first 12 hours of life, HBIG 0.5 mL IM given within 12 hours of birth, since immunogenicity of the vaccine alone cannot be guaranteed. The remaining vaccination schedule should be followed as outlined above depending on whether the mother is HBsAg-positive or -negative.

E. **Isolation Procedures:** Infants born to HBsAg-positive mothers should be cared for with Standard Precautions since a small percentage of these infants are also infected. No special isolation is required. Immediately after birth, the infant should be handled with gloves until all maternal blood is removed (note that this procedure is now recommended in all births).

F. **Breast-Feeding:** Although hepatitis B virus is secreted in breast milk, breast-feeding does not increase the risk for an infant acquiring hepatitis B infection and therefore is not contraindicated if above immunoprophylaxis recommendations have been followed. However, it is recommended that special precautions be taken when storing breast milk of an HBsAg-positive mother in the nursery and that, ideally, it not be stored in the same location as the breast milk for other neonates in order to protect those who have not received appropriate immunoprophylaxis (AAP/ACOG, 2002).

OTHER HEPATITIS VIRUSES

A. **Hepatitis A Virus** (HAV) (AAP Red Book, 2003; AAP/ACOG, 2002): HAV rarely is transmitted perinatally, and there is no evidence that the virus is a teratogen. The rare occurrence of vertical transmission of the virus from an infected mother to the infant appears to result in mild neonatal disease. Vertical transmission has resulted in spread of infection in nurseries by fecal-oral contamination. Both mother and infant should have Contact Precautions, with particular care in handling urine and stool. Breast-feeding is not contraindicated. Immunoglobulin administration to the infant (0.02 mL/kg) has been recommended by some if the mother is symptomatic 2 weeks before delivery to 1 week after delivery, but the efficacy of this therapy has not been determined. HAV vaccine is now available, but universal immunization is not recommended at the present time. Although safety of hepatitis A vaccine in pregnancy has not been established, the risk to the fetus should be very low.

B. **Hepatitis C Virus** (HCV) (Red Book, 2003; AAP/ACOG, 2002): Seroprevalence among pregnant women in the United States is low (1%–2%). Among HCV-positive pregnant women, maternal-infant vertical transmission occurs in about 5%, but this occurs only in women who are positive for HCV RNA at delivery. However, coinfection of pregnant women with HIV increases the risk for vertical HCV transmission. Persistent infection occurs in 75%–85% of people infected with HCV, with chronic hepatitis developing in 60%–70% and cirrhosis in 10%–20% of these people. Infection is spread primarily by parenteral exposure to blood and blood products with 60%–90% of IV drug users and hemophiliacs receiving clotting factors prior to 1987 being infected. Sexual transmission among monogamous couples is uncommon; infection is present in only 1.5% of spouses without other risk factors. At this time universal screening is not recommended during pregnancy because of low incidence of disease, frequent false-positive results with screening tests, and no proven interventions to interrupt vertical transmission. Immune globulin manufactured in the United States does not contain antibodies to HCV and is unlikely to prevent infection following exposure. Neither immunoglobulin nor antiviral agents are recommended for postexposure prophylaxis of neonates born to women with HCV. Infants born to mothers with known prior HCV infection should have their skin well cleansed before their vitamin K injection to prevent inoculation at the time. They should then be tested for anti-HCV after 1 year of age (to avoid detection of passively acquired maternal antibody). If earlier diagnosis is desired, PCR for HCV RNA may be performed at 1–2 months of age. Although HCV is secreted in breast milk, HCV transmission via breastfeeding has not been documented, and the infection rate among breast-fed infants is similar to that in formula-fed infants. According to current guidelines of the U.S. Public Health Service, maternal HCV infection is not a contraindication to breast-feeding. The decision to do so should be based on an informed discussion between the woman and her health care provider (AAP/ACOG, 2002). Abstaining from breast-feeding is suggested if nipples are cracked or bleeding.

C. **Hepatitis D Virus** (HDV): HDV can be transmitted by blood or blood products, injection drug use, or sexual contact, as long as HBV also is present in the patient. Maternal infection of the fetus has been described but is rare. Infant testing is not recommended. No specific therapy is warranted, but Standard Precautions are recommended. Effective prophylaxis against hepatitis B virus transmission will prevent HDV transmission.

HERPES SIMPLEX VIRUS (HSV)

A. **Background and Epidemiology** (AAP Red Book, 2003; AAP/ACOG, 2002): The prevalence of HSV infections has increased 30% in the past few decades

(AAP/ACOG, 2002). Approximately 20%–30% of childbearing women have serologic evidence of prior HSV-2 infection. However, most do not have a history of genital ulcers. Neonatal HSV infection can be devastating, resulting in serious morbidity and mortality. Incidence estimates range from 1 in 3000 to 1 in 20,000 births, with about 25% of these infections due to HSV-1 and 75% by HSV-2. Most neonatal HSV infections are acquired during passage through the infected vaginal canal during birth or by ascending infection, sometimes even through intact membranes. Rarely, postnatal HSV infection can occur from parents, hospital personnel, or other infected neonates via contact with infected mouth, hands, or breasts. Most newborns infected with HSV are delivered to women who have asymptomatic or unrecognized infections. A neonate born vaginally to a mother with asymptomatic or symptomatic primary HSV has a 33%–50% risk for acquiring HSV infection. With recurrent disease, the risk for transmission during a vaginal delivery is <5%.

B. Clinical Findings
  1. Congenital or intrauterine infection: Approximately 5% of neonatal HSV infections occur as a result of intrauterine transmission. Less than 50 cases have previously been described. HSV often has a severe presentation, with frequent chorioretinitis, microcephaly, micro-ophthalmia, small-for-gestational-age status, skin lesions and scarring, hydranencephaly, and possible cataracts present at birth or within the first 24–48 hours (Bale, 2002).
  2. Neonatal infection (AAP Red Book, 2003; Volpe, 2000): Neonatal HSV infection is rarely, if ever, asymptomatic and is often very severe with high mortality and morbidity rates. Initial symptoms can occur anytime between birth and 4–6 weeks of age and can range from a few vesicles on the skin to dissemination to every major organ. HSV infections acquired at the time of delivery or in the neonatal period are usually categorized into one of three presentations as described below. Maternal history and physical examination are usually not helpful in making the diagnosis (unless active herpetic vesicles are present at delivery) since most mothers are asymptomatic at the time of transmission.
     a. Local: Localized infection generally involves the skin (vesicles or bullae), eye (conjunctivitis, keratitis, or retinitis), or mouth (ulcers). Presents most frequently during first or second week of life and accounts for approximately 40% of all HSV infections. The initial lesions will often present at areas of trauma such as fetal scalp electrodes.
     b. CNS: Most overt symptoms are seizures and encephalitis. Occurs most commonly during second to fourth weeks of life and accounts for approximately 35% of all HSV infections.
     c. Disseminated: Presents with general symptoms suggestive of bacterial sepsis plus hepatitis, encephalitis, pneumonitis, and frequently DIC. Involves liver, adrenals, skin (75% with rash, usually vesicular; may not be present at time of initial presentation of symptoms), lungs, CNS (60%, including seizures, irritability, coma, abnormal tone), and eyes (chorioretinitis and conjunctivitis). Usually presents during the first 2 weeks of life and accounts for ~25% of all HSV infection.

C. Diagnosis

1. Culture: HSV is relatively easy to culture, and special transport media can be used if immediate tissue culture is not possible. A cotton swab for culture should be obtained from the eyes, nasopharynx or oropharynx, rectum, and skin vesicles (if present) in all symptomatic infants (a single mucosal swab can be sent for culture with the eyes, nasopharynx/ oropharynx, and rectum swabbed in that order), as well as from suspicious maternal perineal lesions. Infant CSF, urine, and blood should also be cultured. The yield of CSF culture in neonates with CNS disease is <50%. Polymerase chain reaction (PCR) has a much higher yield in CSF and should be performed on CSF if this test is available. Cutaneous and mucosal cultures are preferably obtained 24–48 hours after delivery to differentiate transient colonization from true infection but should be done immediately in symptomatic infants or infants with typical lesions. Viral identification in culture typically requires 1–3 days.

2. Other rapid identification tests: These include direct fluorescent antibody staining of vesicle scrapings and enzyme immunoassay antigen detection in vesicle or body fluids. These tests are as specific as cultures but less sensitive. Polymerase chain reaction (PCR) is very sensitive for detecting HSV DNA in CSF or other fluids but has the limitation of possible false-positive results. Also, PCR is currently available only in research or specialized laboratories.

D. Treatment of Documented or Suspected Infection: Parenteral acyclovir is the treatment of choice for neonatal HSV. The dosage of acyclovir is 20 mg/mg/dose IV every 8 hours for 14 days for localized disease limited to the skin, eye, and mouth and for 21 days for disseminated or CNS infection. Relapse of skin, eyes, and mouth and CNS disease can occur, and the value of long-term suppressive or intermittent acyclovir for neonates with skin, eye, and mouth relapse and/or disease is being evaluated. Infants with ocular involvement should be treated with a topical medication (1%–2% trifluridine, 1% iododeoxyuridine, or 3% vidarabine) in addition to parenteral therapy, and an ophthalmology consultation should be obtained (Kimberlin, 2001; AAP Red Book, 2003).

E. Prognosis: Approximately half of all infants with untreated infection die, with high morbidity in survivors. Morbidity and mortality are highest in those infants with CNS or disseminated disease. Early initiation of antiviral therapy has been proven to favorably affect the outcome of neonatal HSV disease. In a total of 186 neonatal patients with HSV infection from 1981–1997, improvement of outcome was shown with the higher dose of acyclovir at 20 mg/kg/dose compared with historical controls receiving 10 mg/kg/dose for CNS and disseminated disease. With the higher dose acyclovir, the survival rate for disseminated disease increased from ~40%–70% and for CNS disease from ~80% to ~95%. The survival rate for both treatment groups for localized (skin, eye, and mouth) disease was 100%. Of disseminated HSV disease patients in the higher dose treatment group, 83% were developing normally at 12 months of age, compared with 60% in the lower dose treatment group.

Patients with CNS disease had similar development at 12 months, with 31% of the higher dose treatment group being normal compared with 29% in the lower dose treatment group. Of infants with localized (skin, eye, and mouth) disease, 100% in the higher dose treatment group were normal, compared with 98% in the lower dose treatment group at 12 months (Kimberlin, 2001).

F. **Prevention**

1. Primary infection: For neonates born vaginally to women with suspected or documented active primary HSV infection at the time of delivery (where neonatal infection rates may be as high as 50%), empiric acyclovir 20 mg/kg/dose IV every 8 hours after birth pending neonatal culture results should be considered. (Other experts suggest obtaining cultures at 24–48 hours and initiating treatment only if cultures become positive.) Recommendations for acyclovir use after cesarean section are less clear, but acyclovir administration should be considered, particularly with rupture of membranes >4–6 hours.

2. Reactivation: For known exposure to active recurrent infection at vaginal delivery (where transmission rate is <5%) or cesarean section delivery, cultures from the newborn should be obtained 24–48 hours after birth, but most experts feel therapy does not need to be initiated unless the infant is symptomatic, premature, has acquired open wounds during delivery, or has other factors that put the infant at higher risk for acquiring infection. If cultures become positive, or if symptoms develop, acyclovir therapy should be initiated. Similarly, neonatal surface cultures can be considered for newborns born to mothers with a history of recurrent genital herpes and no lesions present at delivery, although they are not routinely recommended.

3. All persons with herpes labialis (cold sores) should follow strict handwashing guidelines, avoid lesion contact with the infant, and wear a surgical mask when holding the infants until the lesion is crusted and dry. Breast-feeding is acceptable with maternal disease if the lesions are not on the breast and provided the mother uses good handwashing technique and covers active lesions.

4. Infants who are at risk for HSV, even if culture-negative, need to be carefully followed for a minimum of 6 weeks. Education of parents and caregivers about the signs of neonatal HSV is crucial, since some of these babies may be discharged home before the culture results becoming available.

G. **Isolation Procedures:** Women with HSV-1 or HSV-2 lesions should be managed with Contact Precautions throughout their hospitalization. They should be taught about their infection and about hygienic measures to prevent postpartum transmission to the neonate. They should be instructed to wash hands carefully and use a clean barrier to ensure that the neonate does not come into contact with lesions or infectious material. Breast-feeding is permitted if there are no lesions in the breast area and all other lesions are covered. People with cold sores (herpes labialis) or herpes stomatitis should not kiss or nuzzle the neonate until lesions have cleared. Careful handwashing and wearing a disposable surgical mask are helpful in protecting the neonate. Neonates born vaginally (or by cesarean delivery if membranes have ruptured) to mothers with active lesions should be physically separated from other neonates and managed with Contact Precautions. Infants born to mothers with a past history of infection but without active lesions at delivery do not require isolation, although good handwashing technique needs to be reinforced. Infants with HSV infection should be isolated throughout the illness and managed with Contact Precautions (AAP/ACOG, 2002).

VARICELLA-ZOSTER VIRUS (VZV)

A. **Background and Epidemiology:** Varicella is one of the most highly communicable human diseases, with 90% of susceptible household contacts becoming infected with exposure. It is now preventable with the use of a live attenuated vaccine. First exposure with this virus causes chickenpox (varicella), and reactivation of the latent virus causes zoster (shingles). Chickenpox develops in approximately 0.05% of pregnant women. If chickenpox develops before 20 weeks gestation, the fetus has approximately a 2% risk for developing fetal varicella syndrome (Bale, 2002). The incubation period for chickenpox ranges from 10–21 days but is generally 14–16 days. Viremia occurs 1–2 days before the onset of the rash, and contagiousness begins with viremia and can last as long as 5 days after the rash onset or until the last pox lesion has scabbed over.

B. **Neonatal Clinical Manifestations:** Maternal infection during pregnancy can produce three different syndromes.
  1. Congenital varicella syndrome: Approximately 2% of women who contract chickenpox during the first or early second trimester have infants with abnormalities that may include cutaneous scarring (cicatrix); eye abnormalities, including chorioretinitis, microphthalmia, cataracts, and Horner syndrome; prematurity; limb hypoplasia; and mental retardation, microcephaly, hydrocephalus, seizures, extremity paralysis, and other neurologic abnormalities (Bale, 2002).
  2. Perinatal chickenpox: Occurs within the first 10 days of life. The most severe cases occur with onset of maternal rash close to delivery (5 days before to 2 days after delivery). In these instances virus passes transplacentally to the infant, but a sufficient maternal antibody response has not developed to protect the infant. Fetal infection rate is 24%–50%. Disease is usually disseminated with a mortality rate of 20%–30%; death is usually secondary to pneumonia. Less severe neonatal infections similar to the disease seen in older children generally occur when maternal rash onset is more than 5 days before delivery, there has been adequate time for maternal antibody to develop and pass across the placenta to protect the infant, and the infant is not extremely premature (Baley, 2002).
  3. Neonatal zoster: Very rare; presumably occurs following mild and undetected fetal varicella infection (occurring as a result of maternal varicella during gestation), with reactivation of VZV at birth (Baley, 2002). Zoster following in utero infection may also occur later in infancy or early childhood.

C. **Diagnosis:** Diagnosis is generally by history and clinical presentation in the mother and infant. Immunofluorescent stain or PCR for VZV DNA can differentiate varicella lesions from herpes simplex lesions. Viral cultures from vesicular fluid are also definitive, but it is difficult to obtain rapid results from these cultures.

D. **Prophylaxis:** Varicella-zoster immune globulin (VZIG) 125 U IM is recommended for infants born to a mother who develops chickenpox within 5 days before to 2 days after delivery, for premature infants with known postnatal exposure who are <28 weeks or weigh ≤1000 g regardless of maternal status, and for exposed premature (>28 weeks) infants whose mothers have not had varicella. VZIG is not recommended for healthy term infants exposed postnatally or for an infant whose mother develops a rash more than 48 hours after delivery, although it may be considered for an exposed newborn with severe skin disease (AAP Red Book, 2003). VZIG prevents development of varicella in about half of exposed infants and prevents most severe neonatal varicella disease (Bakshi, 1986). It should be given as soon as possible but may be effective if administered up to 4 days after delivery or exposure. Maternal VZIG during pregnancy may not protect the fetus from varicella infection (Stiehm, 1992) but is indicated to protect a seronegative, varicella-exposed mother from severe infection. Although varicella vaccine is now available, data on its use in the newborn period are not available and it is recommended for infants >12 months of age.

E. **Treatment:** Neonates who develop varicella with severe clinical disease should be treated with intravenous acyclovir.

F. **Infection Control** (AAP Red Book, 2003; AAP/ACOG, 2002): "Exposure" to an infected varicella case includes hospitalization in the same room containing either 2–4 beds, being in an adjacent bed in a ward, face-to-face contact, or physical contact. All susceptible patients and hospital workers exposed to an infected infant or mother must be identified and the following procedures implemented:
   1. VZIG should be given to susceptible immunocompromised individuals, susceptible pregnant women, premature infants >28 weeks gestation if mother is susceptible, and all infants <28 weeks gestation.
   2. Discharge all exposed patients before 8 days after rash onset in index case. If not possible, use strict isolation (see below) days 8–21 after rash onset in index case (to day 28 if VZIG was given).
   3. Exposed staff should not have patient contact days 8–21 after rash onset in index case (28 days after receiving VZIG).

G. **Isolation Procedures** (AAP Red Book, 2003; AAP/ACOG, 2002): In addition to Standard Precautions, both Airborne and Contact Precautions (i.e., strict isolation, if possible in a negative pressure room) are recommended for most exposures, including:
   1. Infected mothers and neonates: for at least 5 days after rash onset and for duration of vesicular eruption.
   2. Hospitalized nonimmune pregnant women who have been exposed to varicella: from days 8–21 after rash onset in the index patient and thereafter if the pregnant woman develops varicella.
   3. Neonates born to mothers with varicella: while hospitalized or until day 21 if there is a prolonged hospital stay.

4. If either mother or infant received VZIG while hospitalized: until day 28 after exposure.

HUMAN IMMUNODEFICIENCY VIRUS (HIV)

A. **Background and Epidemiology** (AAP Red Book, 2003; AAP/ACOG, 2002; Fowler, 2000, Workowski, 2002): Worldwide an estimated 12 million women and 1.1 million children have been infected with HIV. In the United States, approximately 6000 HIV-infected women give birth each year. In the absence of any intervention, the risk for infection for a neonate born to an HIV-seropositive mother is approximately 25% (range 13%–39%). Infants who are breast-fed have an additional 12%–14% risk for becoming infected. The risk for HIV transmission can be reduced to <2% by following antiretroviral regimens, practicing obstetrical interventions, and avoiding breast-feeding.

B. **Clinical Manifestations and Prognosis of Neonates Infected with HIV** (Baley, 2002; Krist, 2002): Almost all infected infants are asymptomatic at birth. Most untreated infected infants begin to demonstrate symptoms within the first 1–2 years of life. However, a small percentage of infants, usually following intrauterine infection, will have rapidly progressive disease with onset within the first month or two after delivery. In general, most opportunistic infections do not occur until later in the course of an infant's disease with the exception of *Pneumocystis carinii*, which may occur in the first months of life. Common symptoms of untreated HIV in the infant include recurrent bacterial infections (otitis media, sinusitis, bacteremia, pneumonia, meningitis), persistent or recurrent candidiasis, hepatosplenomegaly, lymphadenopathy, chronic diarrhea, failure to thrive, and developmental delay.

C. **Diagnosis** (AAP Red Book, 2000; AAP/ACOG, 2002): Transplacental transfer of antibody complicates the diagnosis of infant infection, making early diagnosis dependent on detection of virus (viral culture), virus RNA (HIV RNA PCR), or virus DNA (HIV DNA PCR). Infants born to HIV-infected women should be tested by HIV DNA PCR during the first 48 hours, between 2 weeks and 2 months of age, and at 3–6 months of age. Umbilical cord samples should not be used for the initial test after birth because of possible contamination with maternal blood. Any time an infant tests positive, testing should be repeated as soon as possible to confirm the diagnosis. An infant is considered infected if two separate HIV DNA PCRs are positive. Infection of the neonate is reasonably excluded if two HIV DNA PCRs at or beyond 1 month of age are negative, with at least one done at ≥4 months of age, or if two HIV antibody tests (e.g., ELISA, Western blot, or immunofluorescence antibody test) done >1 month apart at >6 months of age are negative. Approximately 93% of infected infants have a positive HIV DNA PCR by 2 weeks of age and almost all do by 1 month. A single HIV DNA PCR assay has a 95% sensitivity and 97% specificity at or after 1 month of age. Virus culture for HIV is available in only a few laboratories and requires up to 28 days for positive results, so generally it has been replaced by the more sensitive DNA PCR. HIV ICD (immune complex dissociated) p24 Ag assays are less sensitive than DNA PCR, with false-positive results in the first month, so these are not recommended. HIV RNA PCR may be used to diagnose HIV infection if the result is positive but cannot rule out infection if the result is negative. Consultation with a pediatric infectious disease specialist is indicated for any neonate suspected of having HIV infection.

D. **Prevention of Perinatal HIV Transmission** (AAP Red Book, 2003; AAP/ACOG, 2002; Krist, 2002; Fowler, 2000).

1. Obstetric HIV transmission factors (Box 20-1): Early diagnosis and treatment of the pregnant woman can dramatically decrease the risk for perinatal transmission of HIV. Through early treatment with antiretroviral medications to decrease the mother's viral load (especially with combination antiretroviral therapy) and appropriate obstetrical management, the transmission rate of HIV can be decreased from ~25%–30% to < 2%. Current guidelines suggest that treatment with antiretroviral medications be prescribed for pregnant women in the same manner as for nonpregnant adults.

2. Postnatal neonatal care of the HIV-exposed infant: After birth, the infant's skin should be cleansed well with a disinfectant with antiviral properties such as chlorhexadine before any invasive procedures of the skin (such as vitamin K injection, hepatitis B vaccine injection, AccuCheck, blood draws, or IV starts) to prevent inoculation of HIV virus from the skin. Other invasive procedures around the time of delivery such as DeLee suctioning,

---

● BOX 20-1
OBSTETRIC FACTORS FOR HIV TRANSMISSION FROM MOTHER TO FETUS/NEWBORN

Increasing HIV Transmission Risk
- Maternal viral load >1000 copies/mL (especially if >50,000 copies/mL)
- Low CD4+ lymphocyte count (~<500 cells/mL)
- Primary HIV infection during pregnancy
- Other sexually transmitted diseases
- Chorioamnionitis
- Artificial rupture of membranes (ROM)
- ROM >4 hours before delivery
- Invasive monitoring (e.g., fetal scalp electrodes)
- Instrumented deliveries (forceps, vacuum)
- Vaginal delivery (especially if maternal viral load >1000 copies/mL)
- Premature delivery at <37 weeks

Decreasing HIV Transmission Risk
- Prenatal and intrapartum antiretroviral drugs
- Elective cesarean section before onset of labor and rupture of membranes (especially if maternal viral load >1000 copies/mL)
- Vaginal disinfectant if prolonged ROM and vaginal delivery
- Avoidance of any invasive procedures in neonate during delivery and after birth (e.g., fetal scalp electrode, DeLee suctioning, intubation, unless necessary for meconium)

fetal scalp monitoring, and intubation should be limited whenever possible. Measures should be taken to make sure the infant is not at risk for other vertically transmitted, sexually transmitted diseases, such as congenital syphilis, HSV, chlamydia, hepatitis B, and hepatitis C, by checking the mother's prenatal labs and closely evaluating the infant. Currently it is recommended that the exposed neonate be treated with zidovudine 2 mg/kg per dose every 6 hours for 6 weeks, beginning by 8–12 hours after delivery, following maternal prophylaxis (usually with a treatment regimen that includes PO zidovudine prior to delivery, then IV zidovudine during delivery; zidovudine plus lamivudine and nevirapine have also been shown to be effective prophylaxis during the peripartum period). Combination treatment of the exposed neonate can be considered in high-risk situations. These recommendations evolve rapidly, and it is recommended that consultation with a pediatric infectious disease specialist, HIV clinic, the CDC *(www.cdc.gov)*, or the HIV/AIDS Treatment Information Service *(www.hivatis.org)* be obtained for current treatment recommendations. Serial testing should be initiated within 48 hours of birth as outlined under "Diagnosis" above. *Pneumocystic carinii* pneumonia (PCP) prophylaxis with trimethoprim-sulfamethoxasole is recommended beginning at 4–6 weeks of age and continuing until 1 year of age or until HIV infection is definitely excluded. Continuation beyond 1 year in HIV-infected infants is based on CD4 lymphocyte counts. Breast-feeding is contraindicated unless there is no availability of infant formulas. Oral poliovirus vaccine should not be administered to HIV-exposed infants.

E. **Isolation Procedures:** Standard Precautions should be strictly followed by all persons caring for HIV-positive women and their offspring. Gloves should be worn when handling the infant until blood and amniotic fluid have been removed from the neonate's skin and for contact with blood or blood-containing fluids and for procedures that entail exposure to blood. Other special isolation precautions are not necessary unless the infant has another coexisting infection such as HSV, which may require isolation. Note that some institutions do not identify infants born to HIV-positive women, reinforcing the need for Standard Precautions in the care of all patients.

CYTOMEGALOVIRUS (CMV)

A. **Background and Epidemiology:** CMV is currently the most common intrauterine infection, with ~1% of all newborns infected in utero and excreting CMV at birth. Fortunately, 90% of these infants are asymptomatic and only ~5% have severe involvement. Among pregnant women in the United States, 50%–60% of middle-class women are seropositive as compared with 90% of women of lower socioeconomic status. Vertical transmission from mother to infant occurs with both maternal primary infection and reactivation; sequelae are much more likely following primary infection. Approximately 2% of women will have a primary CMV infection during pregnancy. Transplacental infection of the fetus occurs in 30%–40% of these pregnancies, resulting in symptomatic neonatal disease in 5%–10% and long-term sequelae (e.g., deafness, mental retardation) in 10%–20% overall. The risk for transplacental infection with recurrent maternal infection is only 1%. Nearly all of these infected infants are asymptomatic at birth. Infection can also occur during delivery by exposure in the maternal genital tract or postpartum from infected maternal secretions or from breast milk. These infections are usually asymptomatic except in premature infants who have a higher risk for symptoms due to lack of maternal antibody transfer and underdeveloped immune systems.

B. **Clinical Manifestations** (Baley, 2002; Fowler, 1997; Noyola, 2001; Pass, 2002; Rivera, 2002; Stagno, 2001; Volpe, 2000)

1. Maternal: Most women are asymptomatic during either primary infection or reactivation. Up to 10% develop a mononucleosis-like illness and, less commonly, hepatitis, thrombocytopenia, anemia, myocarditis, or aseptic meningitis with primary infection.

2. Congenital infection

   a. Symptomatic at birth: Severe congenital infection usually occurs when the infant is infected early in a pregnancy of a woman with primary infection. Symptoms can include growth retardation (20%–50%), prematurity (20%–50%), hepatosplenomegaly (75%–100%), microcephaly (20%–50%), jaundice (50%–75%), petechiae or ecchymoses (usually related to thrombocytopenia; 75%–100%), pneumonia (0%–20%), chorioretinitis (0%–20%), inguinal hernias (20%–50%), sensorineural hearing loss (50%–60%; frequently progressive or occurring later after birth), periventricular intracranial calcification (50%), and seizures (10%–25%). These infants have a poor prognosis, with up to a 20%–30% mortality and ~90% of patients with intracranial calcifications having severe neurologic sequelae, compared with ~30% of patients with normal CT scans.

   b. Asymptomatic at birth: Among the ~90% of congenitally infected infants who are asymptomatic at birth, 5%–15% may have long-term sequelae. The most common sequela is sensorineural hearing loss, occurring in 7%–8%, followed by decreased IQ (<70 in 3%–4%); microcephaly, seizures, or paresis (2%–3%); chorioretinitis or visual difficulties (2%–3%); and school problems. Important to note is that the hearing loss has been shown to be delayed in 18% of the infants with eventual hearing loss. The median age of detection is 27 months (range, 25–62 months). It also has been shown to be progressive in 50%, with the median age of first progression at 18 months (range, 2–70 months). Therefore, serial follow-up hearing screens through school age are recommended for all children diagnosed with symptomatic or asymptomatic congenital CMV. (See "treatment" below.)

3. Perinatal or postpartum infection: Transmission can occur via passage through the birth canal, via breast milk, or from blood transfusion. The majority of these infections are, and remain, asymptomatic. Rarely, CMV pneumonitis has been reported after the 4- to 12-week incubation period. There do not appear to be any long-term sequelae. Severe disease has occurred in premature infants infected with CMV via blood transfusion.

Symptomatic CMV has also occurred in premature infants fed maternal breast milk. Pasteurization of milk appears to inactivate CMV and freezing milk at −20°C (−4°F) will decrease viral titers but does not reliably eliminate CMV and may decrease the nutritional value of the milk.

C. **Diagnosis** (AAP Red Book, 2003; AAP/ACOG, 2002; Baley, 2000; Pass, 2002): Diagnosis of CMV infections is problematic because most maternal and non-congenital disease is asymptomatic, prolonged viral shedding often follows infection, and disease reactivation is common. Congenital CMV is diagnosed by viral isolation from the infant's urine in the first 2–3 weeks of life. This can be accomplished by traditional viral cultures, which require up to 2 weeks to yield results, rapid culture methods (shell vial assay), which can give results in 24 hours, or polymerase chain reaction (PCR), which can detect very small amounts of CMV DNA. It is uncertain whether the use of PCR offers additional benefit since newborns with congenital CMV infection shed large amounts of virus from urine and saliva for extended periods of time (years). The detection of anti-CMV IgM may also be used to diagnose infection. However, this offers no advantage over urine viral cultures or PCR, requires invasive blood drawing as opposed to noninvasive urine collection, is less sensitive, and is subject to false-positive results. Identification of CMV in the urine beyond 3 weeks of age does not distinguish among congenital, perinatal, or postnatal infection.

D. **Treatment** (AAP Red Book, 2003; Baley, 2002; Pass, 2002)
   1. Antiviral treatment: Ganciclovir, foscarnet, and cidofovir have been shown to be beneficial for treatment of adults with CMV retinitis, especially in HIV-infected patients. However, no antiviral agents are currently approved for treatment of congenital CMV. A phase III randomized trial in neonates with central nervous system disease due to congenital CMV infection that compared 6 weeks of intravenous ganciclovir treatment with no treatment showed significant benefit in the treatment group, particularly lack of progressive hearing loss. The treatment group did have a higher rate of neutropenia than the placebo group (63% versus 20%), and questions remain whether the benefit of treatment will be sustained over time; thus the implications of these results for clinical practice are still unclear. Nevertheless, treatment can be considered for newborns with evidence of central nervous system disease (including ocular or auditory involvement) or other severe end-organ disease. There is currently no proven therapy for CMV exposure.
   2. Management of congenital CMV: Children with congenital CMV are at risk for developmental delay, neurologic abnormalities, mental retardation, impaired vision, and hearing loss as previously discussed. Early detection of hearing loss is particularly important because of its importance to speech development. Because of the risk for delayed or progressive hearing loss, serial hearing tests are recommended in the newborn period and at 3, 6, 12, 18, 24, 30, and 36 months of age and then annually to school age. Retinal disease associated with CMV has also been reported to develop several weeks after birth; therefore follow-up eye exams after birth are rec-

ommended in the newborn period, at 12 months, at 3 years, and at ~5 years unless otherwise recommended by the ophthalmologist. Neurologic exams and developmental assessments should be done by the primary care physician at each well-child examination (Pass, 2002).

E. **Prevention** (AAP/ACOG, 2002; Baley, 2002; Pass, 2002): Pregnant women, particularly any known to be CMV seronegative, should be advised to use good handwashing technique. No other strategies to prevent congenital infection have been developed. Blood products given to neonates, especially premature infants, should be treated to reduce the potential for CMV transmission (filtration, freezing in glycerol) or should be obtained from CMV-seronegative donors. Likewise, donated breast milk can be pasteurized or frozen or be acquired from seronegative donors to reduce CMV transmission.

F. **Isolation Procedures** (AAP/ACOG, 2002; Baley, 2002; Pass, 2002): Because of the frequency of in utero infection, approximately 1% of all neonates excrete CMV in their urine. Neither symptomatic or diagnosed asymptomatic infants with CMV require isolation, but Standard Precautions, particularly for pregnant caretakers, should be enforced. Proper handwashing after exposure to secretions is especially important for these pregnant personnel.

RUBELLA

A. **Background and Epidemiology** (AAP Red Book, 2003; Baley, 2002; MMWR, 2001; Zimmerman; 2001): Since licensure of the rubella vaccine in the United States in 1969, the number of total rubella cases has dramatically decreased from 57,600 in 1969 to 267 in 1999. The number of congenital rubella cases has also dramatically declined by 99% during this time period, with only 6 cases reported in 1999. Rubella infections in the United States now predominantly occur in foreign-born residents from countries that have no rubella vaccination programs. In particular, Hispanics accounted for >70% of cases and 81% of congenital rubella cases from 1997–1999. Rubella is usually a mild and often asymptomatic infection in children and adults. Up to two thirds of pregnant women who are infected with rubella are asymptomatic. However, infection during pregnancy can cause a wide range of fetal and neonatal outcomes depending on the gestational age at the time of maternal infection.

B. **Congenital Infection** (AAP Red Book, 2003; Bale, 2002; Baley, 2002; MMWR, 2001; Volpe, 2000): Both the incidence of transmission to the fetus and the effects of infection on the fetus are dependent on the timing of maternal infection during pregnancy. Maternal rubella infection prior to 11 weeks has been reported to cause a 90% fetal infection rate, with 90%–100% of infected newborns having congenital defects. Maternal infection at 11–20 weeks is associated with a 50% fetal infection rate and 30% congenital defect rate. Maternal infection at 20–35 weeks causes ~30% to 50% fetal infection rate and at >35 weeks causes ~100% fetal infection rate. Newborns who were infected at >20 weeks are generally asymptomatic at birth, without evidence of congenital anomalies. As with CMV infection, infants born with asymptomatic rubella infection can develop consequences later; the most common is progressive hearing loss, followed by risk for learning disabilities, eye damage, endocrinopathies, vascular disease, panencephalitis, and developmental delay. Many of the symptoms of congenital rubella syndrome are similar to those seen in congenital CMV and toxoplasmosis, including petechiae or ecchymoses (35%), microcephaly (25%), intrauterine growth retardation (60%), hepatosplenomegaly (35%), sensorineural hearing loss (60%), cataracts (30%; often bilateral) and chorioretinitis (10%; often with a "salt and pepper" appearance). A unique feature of congenital rubella is congenital heart disease, which occurs in up to 70% of those infected in the first 8 weeks of gestation; the most common lesion is patent ductus arteriosus, followed by or in combination with pulmonary artery or pulmonary valvular stenosis. Other features particularly suggestive of congenital rubella include bony radiolucencies (~20%–50%) and dermal erythropoiesis ("blueberry muffin" rash; ~20%).

C. **Diagnosis:** Diagnosis of congenital rubella infection in an infant with suggestive abnormal findings can be made by detection of virus from nasal secretions, throat swab, urine, blood, or CSF. Specific cell lines are required for cultivation of rubella virus. It is most consistently isolated from nasal specimens, with a sensitivity of approximately 50%–80%. The sensitivity is increased with the use of PCR. Rubella-specific IgM detection in the infant's blood or demonstration of stable or rising rubella IgG titers in serial sera obtained over several months can also be used to make a presumptive diagnosis. Virologic diagnosis of congenital rubella infection after 1 year of age is difficult.

D. **Management and Therapy:** Susceptible pregnant women or pregnant women with unknown immune status who develop symptoms compatible with rubella or who are exposed to rubella infection should undergo serologic testing to determine whether they are previously rubella-immune or whether they have recently acquired infection. Postexposure prophylaxis with immune globulin may be considered but does not always prevent fetal infection. There is no specific antiviral therapy for congenital rubella or for amelioration of progressive disease after birth.

E. **Prevention:** All pregnant women should be screened for rubella immunity whether or not they have received prior rubella immunization (even though vaccine failures are rare). If possible, susceptible pregnant women should avoid exposure to infected persons. Pregnant women should not be given the vaccine (a live virus vaccine) because of the small risk for transplacental transmission of vaccine virus (1.2%–1.8%). However, seronegative women should be vaccinated with measles-mumps-rubella vaccine postpartum before discharge from the hospital. Although vaccine virus is excreted in breast milk and can be transmitted to neonates, it has not led to symptomatic disease, and breast-feeding is not a contraindication to vaccination.

F. **Isolation Procedures:** Respiratory and urinary secretion of virus may occur for several months or more after birth, and Contact Precautions should be used with all infants suspected of having congenital rubella for the duration of the hospitalization. Infants with congenital rubella are considered contagious until 1 year of age unless they are shown to be repeatedly culture-negative before this time.

NONPOLIOVIRUS ENTEROVIRUSES (EV)

A. **Background and Epidemiology** (AAP Red Book, 2003; AAP/ACOG, 2002; Abzug, 1993; Abzug, 2001; Baley, 2002): Neonatal enterovirus (EV) infections are common, especially during the summer and fall in temperate climates. Most neonatal enteroviral disease presents as a mild nonspecific febrile illness (viral meningitis) or, more rarely, as an overwhelming sepsis-like syndrome (myocarditis and/or meningoencephalitis).

  1. Mild disease: Most newborns with mild illness have acquired infection postnatally or horizontally after birth, usually from a family member. Findings often include fever, irritability, poor feeding, vomiting and/or diarrhea, rash, respiratory distress, and aseptic meningitis. The course is almost always self-limiting with an expected full recovery even with evidence of meningitis.

  2. Severe sepsis-like syndrome: This generally is a consequence of vertical transmission before or around the time of birth following recent maternal infection, often in the absence of transplacental antibodies for the infecting virus. Onset of illness typically occurs within 2–5 days of birth, and findings often include fever or hypothermia, shock, disseminated intravascular coagulopathy (DIC), hepatitis and liver failure, myocarditis/cardiomyopathy, respiratory distress/failure, and meningitis and/or encephalitis. The presentation can mimic disseminated HSV or bacterial sepsis. Isolated meningoencephalitis or myocarditis also occurs. Mortality in severe disease approaches 50%, but if the infant survives, a full recovery often ensues.

B. **Diagnosis:** Cultures for viral isolation should be obtained from throat, rectum, serum, urine, and involved clinical sites (e.g., CSF). Polymerase chain reaction (PCR) may add to the diagnostic yield, particularly for CSF and serum.

C. **Management and Therapy:** There is no specific antiviral therapy available for enterovirus infections. Pleconaril is an experimental medication undergoing clinical evaluation for treatment of severe neonatal enteroviral infection. Intravenous immune globulin can be used for life-threatening neonatal disease, but proof of efficacy is lacking. Pediatric infectious disease consultation is recommended in cases of suspected severe neonatal enteroviral infections to discuss current recommended treatment.

D. **Prevention:** Nursery outbreaks of enteroviral infections occasionally occur. Methods used to interrupt transmission include infection control strategies with contact isolation. Prophylactic immune globulin has also been used.

E. **Isolation Procedures:** Contact Precautions are indicated for infants with proven infection and those suspected to have disease based on maternal history.

HUMAN PAPILLOMAVIRUS (HPV)

A. **Background and Epidemiology** (AAP Red Book, 2003; AAP/ACOG, 2002): Genital warts caused by human papillomavirus (HPV) are common. Fortunately, the risk for a neonate born to a mother with genital warts of developing subsequent laryngeal papillomatosis, which typically presents at

2–3 years of age, is very small. The protective value of cesarean section delivery is unknown and therefore is not recommended to protect the neonate from HPV infection.

B. **Treatment:** Treatment of laryngeal papillomatosis consists of repeated surgical excision; interferon treatment is under investigation.

C. **Prevention:** Mothers with HPV and their neonates do not require any special isolation precautions other than Standard Precautions.

HUMAN PARVOVIRUS

A. **Background and Epidemiology** (AAP Red Book, 2003; AAP/ACOG, 2002; Baley, 2002): Parvovirus B19 is the cause of erythema infectiosum, commonly presenting with a "slapped cheek" appearance and lacey-appearing rash about 7–10 days after onset of constitutional symptoms such as fever, malaise, myalgias, and headaches. The risk for transplacental transmission to the fetus during pregnancy is 20%–33%. Most infected fetuses have no complications. Risk for fetal hydrops/death (~2%–6%) is maximal with maternal infection in the first half of pregnancy.

B. **Diagnosis:** Serology and antigen or DNA detection are the mainstays of diagnosis.

C. **Therapy:** Intrauterine blood transfusion has been used successfully.

LYMPHOCYTIC CHORIOMENINGITIS (LCM)

A. **Background and Epidemiology** (AAP Red Book, 2003; Bale, 2002; Baley, 2002): Infected mice and hamsters can infect humans via direct contact, ingestion of material contaminated by excreta, and inhalation of infected aerosols. Approximately 5% of the population is seropositive.

B. **Clinical Manifestation:** Infection symptoms often include a biphasic fever lasting as long as 1–3 weeks, malaise, myalgia, retro-orbital headache, photophobia, anorexia, and nausea. Intrauterine infection can mimic congenital CMV and toxoplasmosis, producing chorioretinopathy, macrocephaly or microcephaly, hydrocephalus, or intracranial calcifications, as well as intrauterine death.

C. **Diagnosis:** Diagnosis is made by serologic testing or viral isolation.

D. **Treatment:** There is no current treatment available.

E. **Prevention:** Pregnant women should be advised to avoid any contact with hamsters and mice and their excreta.

REFERENCES

Abzug MJ: Prognosis for neonates with enterovirus hepatitis and coagulopathy, *Pediatr Infect Dis J* 20(8):758-763, 2001.

Abzug MJ, Levin MJ, Rotbart HA: Profile of enterovirus disease in the first two weeks of life, *Pediatr Infect Dis J* 12: 820-824, 1993.

American Academy of Pediatrics: Cytomegalovirus infection. In Pickering LK, editor: *Red book: report of the committee on infectious diseases,* ed 26, Elk Grove Village, IL, 2003, American Academy of Pediatrics, pp 259-262.

American Academy of Pediatrics: Enterovirus (nonpolio) infections. In Pickering LK, editor: *Red book: report of the committee on infectious diseases,* ed 26, Elk Grove Village, IL, 2003, American Academy of Pediatrics, pp 269-270.

American Academy of Pediatrics: Hepatitis A. In Pickering LK, editor: *Red book: report of the committee on infectious diseases,* ed 26, Elk Grove Village, IL, 2003, American Academy of Pediatrics, pp 309-318.

American Academy of Pediatrics: Hepatitis B. In Pickering LK, editor: *Red book: report of the committee on infectious diseases,* ed 26, Elk Grove Village, IL, 2003, American Academy of Pediatrics, pp 318-336.

American Academy of Pediatrics: Hepatitis C. In Pickering LK, editor: *Red book: report of the committee on infectious diseases,* ed 26, Elk Grove Village, IL, 2003, American Academy of Pediatrics, pp 336-340.

American Academy of Pediatrics: Hepatitis D. In Pickering LK, editor: *Red book: report of the committee on infectious diseases,* ed 26, Elk Grove Village, IL, 2003, American Academy of Pediatrics, pp 340-341.

American Academy of Pediatrics: Herpes simplex. In Pickering LK, editor: *Red book: report of the committee on infectious diseases,* ed 26, Elk Grove Village, IL, 2003, American Academy of Pediatrics, pp 344-353.

American Academy of Pediatrics: Human immunodeficiency virus infection. In Pickering LK, editor: *Red book: report of the committee on infectious diseases,* ed 26, Elk Grove Village, IL, 2003, American Academy of Pediatrics, pp 360-382.

American Academy of Pediatrics: Human papillomaviruses. In Pickering LK, editor: *Red book: report of the committee on infectious diseases,* ed 26, Elk Grove Village, IL, 2003, American Academy of Pediatrics, pp 448-451.

American Academy of Pediatrics: Lymphocytic choriomeningitis. In Pickering LK, editor: *Red book: report of the committee on infectious diseases,* ed 26, Elk Grove Village, IL, 2003, American Academy of Pediatrics, pp 413-414.

American Academy of Pediatrics: Parvovirus B19. In Pickering LK, editor: *Red book: report of the committee on infectious diseases,* ed 26, Elk Grove Village, IL, 2003, American Academy of Pediatrics, pp 469-461.

American Academy of Pediatrics: Rubella. In Pickering LK, editor: *Red book: report of the committee on infectious diseases,* ed 26, Elk Grove Village, IL, 2003, American Academy of Pediatrics, pp 536-541.

American Academy of Pediatrics: Varicella-zoster infections. In Pickering LK, editor: *Red book: report of the committee on infectious diseases,* ed 26, Elk Grove Village, IL, 2003, American Academy of Pediatrics, pp 672-686.

American Academy of Pediatrics and American College of Obstetricians and Gynecologists (AAP/ACOG): Perinatal infections. In *Guidelines for perinatal care,* ed 5, Elk Grove Village, IL, 2002, American Academy of Pediatrics and American College of Obstetricians and Gynecologists.

Armstrong GL: Childhood hepatitis B virus infections in the United States before hepatitis B immunization, *Pediatrics* 108(5):1123-1128, 2001.

Bakshi SS, Miller TC, Kaplan M et al: Failure of varicella-zoster immunoglobulin in modification of severe congenital varicella, *Pediatr Infect Dis* 5:699-702, 1986.

Bale JF: Congenital infections, *Neurol Clin* 20(4):1039-1060, 2002.

Baley JE, Toltzis P: Viral infections. In Fanaroff AA, Martin RJ: *Neonatal-perinatal medicine: diseases of the fetus and infant,* ed 7, St Louis, 2002, Mosby, pp 764-767.

Edwards MS: Hepatitis B serology—help in interpretation, *Pediatr Clin North Am* 35(3):503-515, 1988.

Fowler KB et al: Progressive and fluctuating sensorineural hearing loss in children with asymptomatic congenital cytomegalovirus infection, *J Pediatr* 130:624-630, 1997.

Fowler MG, Simonds RJ, Roongpisuthipong A: HIV/AIDS in infants, children, and adolescents—update on perinatal HIV transmission, *Pediatr Clin North Am* 47(1):21-38, 2000.

Kimberlin DW et al: Safety and efficacy of high-dose intravenous acyclovir in the management of neonatal herpes simplex virus infections, *Pediatrics* 108(2): 230-238, 2001.

Krist AH: Practical therapeutics—management of newborns exposed to maternal HIV infection, *Am Fam Phys* 65(10): 2049-2061, 2002.

Lolekha S et al: Protective efficacy of hepatitis B vaccine without HBIG in infants of HBeAg-positive carrier mothers in Thailand, *Vaccine* 20(31-32):3739-3743, 2002.

Morbidity and Mortality Weekly Report: Control and prevention of rubella: evaluation and management of suspected outbreaks, rubella in pregnant women, and surveillance for congenital rubella syndrome, *MMWR/CDC* 50(RR-12), 2001.

Morbidity and Mortality Weekly Report: Hepatitis A and B vaccines (Appendix), *MMWR/CDC* 52(RRo1):34-36, 2003.

Noyola DE et al: Early predictors of neurodevelopmental outcome in symptomatic congenital cytomegalovirus infection, *J Pediatr* 138:325-331, 2001.

Pass RF: Cytomegalovirus infection, *Pediatr Rev* 23(5):163-170, 2002.

Rivera LB et al: Predictors of hearing loss in children with symptomatic congenital cytomegalovirus infection, *Pediatrics* 110(4): 462-467, 2002.

Robinson WS: Hepatitis B virus and hepatitis D virus. In Mandell GL, Douglas DL, Bennett JE: *Principles and practice of infectious diseases*, ed 5, 2000, Churchill Livingstone, pp 1652-1678.

Shapiro CN: Epidemiology of hepatitis B, *Pediatr Infect Dis J* 12(5):433-437, 1993.

Stagno S: Cytomegalovirus. In Remington JS et al, editors: *Infectious diseases of the fetus and newborn infant*, ed 5, Philadelphia, 2001, WB Saunders.

Stiehm ER: Passive immunization. In Feigin RD, Cherry JD, editors: *Textbook of pediatric infectious diseases*, ed 3, Philadelphia, 1992, WB Saunders, pp 2261-2288.

Volpe JJ: Viral, protozoan, and related intracranial infections. In Volpe JJ: *Neurology of the newborn*, ed 4, Philadelphia, 2000, WB Saunders, pp 737-747.

Volpe JJ: Viral, protozoan, and related intracranial infections—TORCH infections. In Volpe JJ: *Neurology of the newborn*, ed 4, Philadelphia, 2000, WB Saunders, pp. 718-726.

Workowski KA, Levine WC: Sexually transmitted diseases treatment guidelines—2002, *MMWR* 51(RR-6), May 10, 2002.

Zimmerman L, Reef SE: Incidence of congenital rubella syndrome at a hospital serving a predominantly Hispanic population, El Paso, Texas, *Pediatrics* 107(3):E40, 2001.

Isolation Procedures

Patti J. Thureen, MD

A. **Categories of Isolation:** In 1996 the Hospital Infection Control Practices Advisory Committee of the Centers for Disease Control and Prevention (CDC) issued new guidelines for isolation practices for hospitalized patients (Garner, 1996). This committee designated two major categories of infection control practices: *Standard Precautions,* which is an expanded set of the previously designated "Universal Precautions," and *Transmission-Based Precautions,* which provide guidelines for the care of patients with specific pathogens or syndromes in which the pathogenic organism may be spread by airborne, droplet, or contact routes. These guidelines are simpler than the prior 1988 recommendations (Centers for Disease Control and Prevention, 1988), but they are intended to be supplemented by guidelines developed by each hospital for its own specific patient population. The Standard and Transmission-Based Precaution guidelines are discussed in more detail below, and specific disease isolation is indicated under each disease section (Garner, 1996; American Academy of Pediatrics, 2003). Comprehensive infection control guidelines can also be found at the Centers for Disease Control and Prevention (CDC) website *(www.cdc.gov/ncidod/hip/guide/guide.htm).*

B. **Standard Precautions:** These guidelines, intended for the care of *all* patients, were developed to protect patients and health care workers from blood-borne and other body fluid–borne infections. They are designed to prevent cutaneous (particularly nonintact skin) and mucous membrane exposure to blood and body fluids, including feces, nasal secretions, sputum, sweat, tears, urine, and emeses. These precautions apply *even if there is no visible blood* in the body fluids. The guidelines for prevention of exposure to blood-borne pathogens are now mandated in hospitals by the Occupational Safety and Health Administration (OSHA) and are to apply to all patients (OSHA, 1991). The most recent Standard Precaution guidelines include the following:

1. Hand cleansing: *Hand hygiene before* and *after* **every patient contact is the single most important method to prevent and control infections in the health care setting.** Immediate handwashing or washing of other body surfaces is necessary if contaminated with blood and body fluids. This applies even if gloves are used, and hands should be washed immediately after glove removal. Hands should be thoroughly washed after all patient contact regardless of whether or not there was obvious contact with body fluids. Hands should be cleaned with either a waterless antiseptic agent or with soap and water. Recent CDC guidelines note that

the order of efficacy for reducing bacteria are (1) alcohol-based hand rubs, (2) antiseptic soaps and detergents, and (3) non-antimicrobial soaps. These guidelines recommend alcohol-based hand rubs as the routine method of hand hygiene, with soap and water for visibly soiled hands (Boyce and Pitter, 2002).

2. Barrier precautions to prevent cutaneous and mucous membrane exposure to blood, body fluids, secretions, and excretions and contact with any items that might be contaminated with these fluids. Barriers include:
   a. *Gloves* (clean, nonsterile) should be worn when contacting blood and body fluids, mucous membranes, open skin, or items soiled by blood and body fluids. Hand hygiene should be performed immediately after glove removal. New gloves should be used with new patient contact and before touching noncontaminated items or surfaces.
   b. *Masks, face shields, and protective eyewear* should be used when patient contact or procedures may potentially generate splashes, sprays, or droplets of blood, body fluids, secretions, or excretions that might come in contact with the mucous membranes of the eyes, nose, and mouth.
   c. *Nonsterile gowns or aprons* should be used during patient contact or procedures likely to generate splashes, sprays, or droplets of blood, body fluids, and secretions that may contaminate caregiver skin or clothing. Contaminated gowns should be promptly removed.

3. Patient care equipment that might be contaminated should be handled and cleaned in a manner that prevents skin and mucous membrane exposure and clothing contamination.

4. Soiled linen should be handled, transported, and cleaned in a manner that prevents skin and mucous membrane exposure and clothing contamination.

5. "Sharps Program" needs to be in place to prevent blood-borne pathogen exposure by needlestick and other sharp object injuries during cleaning, using, or disposing of these items.

6. Mouth-to-mouth resuscitation should be avoided and be replaced by use of readily available resuscitation and ventilation equipment.

C. **Transmission-Based Precautions** (Table 21-1): These guidelines are for patients with suspected or proven infection that requires measures **in addition to Standard Precautions** in order to prevent spread of infection. They are based on preventing transmission by one of three routes:

1. *Airborne transmission*: Occurs when the infectious agent is disseminated either by microorganisms in dust particles or in evaporated droplets, which can remain airborne for prolonged periods. The organisms can by spread widely by air currents and then inhaled or deposited on a susceptible person. Therefore special air handling and ventilation are required to prevent transmission.

2. *Droplet transmission*: This occurs when infectious droplets are generated during coughing, sneezing, talking, or procedures such as suctioning and bronchoscopy. These droplets travel short distances and may contact a susceptible individual's eyes, nose, or mouth. Because these droplets do not remain suspended, special air handling and ventilation measures are not required.

● TABLE 21-1
Centers for Disease Control Recommendations for Transmission-Based Precautions*

	Airborne Transmission	Droplet Transmission	Contact Transmission
Private room	Yes, with negative air pressure ventilation	Preferred but not required; cohorting of infants with same infection acceptable	Preferred but not required; cohorting of infants with same infection acceptable
Masks	Yes, with respiratory protective device indicated if infectious pulmonary tuberculosis suspected	Yes, for close patient contact (≤3 feet)	No
Gowns	No	No	Yes
Gloves	No	No	Yes
Examples	Measles, tuberculosis, varicella, or disseminated zoster	Rubella, pertussis, influenza, adenovirus, mumps, parvovirus B19, invasive meningococcal or *H. influenzae* infection, *M. pneumoniae* infection	Multidrug-resistant bacteria, herpes simplex, cutaneous infections, impetigo, disseminated herpes zoster, viral conjunctivitis, lice, scabies, diarrheal infection in incontinent or diapered patients (*C. difficile*, *E. coli* 0157: H7, *Shigella*, rotavirus, hepatitis A), uncontained abscesses or cellulitis; young children with RSV, parainfluenzae or enteroviral infections

*Note that Transmission-Based Precautions are to be done in addition to Standard Precautions.
Data derived from Garner JS: Guidelines for isolation precautions in hospitals, *Infect Control Hosp Epidemiol* 17:53-80, 1996; American Academy of Pediatrics: Infection control for hospitalized children. In Pickering LK, editor: *Red book: report of the committee on infectious diseases*, ed 26, Elk Grove Village, IL, 2003, American Academy of Pediatrics, pp 146-154; American Academy of Pediatrics and American College of Obstetricians and Gynecologists (AAP/ACOG): Perinatal infections. In *Guidelines for perinatal care,* ed 5, Elk Grove Village, IL, 2002, American Academy of Pediatrics and American College of Obstetricians and Gynecologists.

3. *Contact transmission*: This is the most common route for transmission of hospital-acquired infections. There are two types of contact transmission:
   a. Direct contact: This involves direct person-to-person transmission of a microorganism from an infected or colonized person to a susceptible host. This type of transmission frequently occurs during patient care.

  b. Indirect contact: This type of transmission occurs when a susceptible host comes in contact with a contaminated object such as gloves, dirty dressings, dirty linen or instruments, or when contaminated hands transmit infection from one patient to another because of failure to thoroughly wash hands between patients.

D. Nursery Infection Control Measures (AAP/ACOG, 2002).

 1. *Routine, thorough handwashing between examining patients is the single most important means to control hospital-acquired infection.*

 2. Initial handwashing: On entering the nursery, the following should be performed:

  a. Uncover arms to above the elbow. Remove rings, watches, and bracelets.

  b. Use one of the following types of scrub procedures:

   (1) If providing care for infants who are very susceptible to infection, before performing invasive procedures, or after caring for an infected infant, use an antiseptic (antimicrobial) preparation. Chlorhexidine gluconate (4%) or iodophor antiseptics are preferred, although the latter is more drying to the skin. For nursery outbreaks of *S. aureus* infections, hexachlorophene-based antiseptics are useful.

   (2) For routine handwashing in the nursery, batericidal soap and water may be sufficient.

   (3) Note that liquid soap dispensers may become contaminated.

   (4) Foams and gels when applied to *clean hands* appear to be the best method for decreasing the bacterial count on the hands (see above).

  c. At the start of a work shift, thoroughly scrub all areas to a point above the elbows for 3 minutes. Then rinse and dry thoroughly with paper towels.

  d. Clean fingernails with nail cleaning stick. Fingernails should be trimmed short, and no false fingernails or opaque nail polish should be permitted.

  e. Handwashing is required even if gloves have been worn. Wash immediately after removal of the gloves.

 3. Handwashing between patient contact and after touching contaminated objects:

  a. Perform a 10-second wash.

  b. Use soap and vigorous rubbing, without a brush.

 4. Attire

  a. Short-sleeved hospital attire ("scrub" clothes) should be hospital-laundered and worn by all nursery personnel. Cover gowns are not required as long as strict handwashing is enforced.

  b. Those who examine neonates should be certain that clothing or unscrubbed skin do not touch the infant or equipment.

  c. When an infant is held by nursing staff, other personnel or parents, a long-sleeved gown should be worn over the clothing. This gown can be discarded after use, or it may be maintained for use exclusively for that infant. If the latter is done, the exclusive-use gown should be changed regularly.

      d. For infants with known or suspected infection, cover gowns should be discarded before handling another patient. A dedicated cover gown may be used for up to 8 hours for that infant.

      e. Sterile, long-sleeved gowns, caps, beard masks, and masks should be used for surgical procedures.

      f. Hand jewelry should not be worn in the nursery while caring for infants.

      g. Sterile gloves should be used during deliveries and all invasive procedures. Disposable, nonsterile gloves may be used for care of patients in isolation or to protect the caregiver from contamination during procedures.

      h. All personnel should realize that handling dirty diapers with bare hands can produce heavy contamination and transient colonization of the hands that cannot be easily eliminated with handwashing. These microorganisms can be readily transmitted between infants.

   5. All visitors should be screened for highly contagious infections before being admitted to the nursery.

E. Neonatal Linen and Trash Disposal (AAP/ACOG, 2002).

   1. Linen provided to the nursery does not need to be sterile but should be clean and transported to the nursery in covered carts.

   2. Either cloth or disposable diapers are acceptable.

   3. Soiled linen should be placed in impervious plastic bags in hampers that are easy to clean and disinfect. Soiled cloth diapers should never be rinsed in the nursery.

   4. Linen and all diapers (either cloth or disposable) should be sealed in plastic bags and removed from the nursery at least every 8 hours. Bags of linen should be taken to the laundry at least twice a day.

   5. Nursery linens and cloth diapers should be laundered separately from other hospital linen and with products designed to retain softness.

F. Intravascular Flush Solutions (AAP/ACOG, 2002).

   1. Sterile, unpreserved flush solution should be provided by the pharmacy. Solutions containing benzyl alcohol preservative are no longer used in neonates because their use has been associated with metabolic acidosis and death.

   2. If the flush solution contains heparin, the heparin should be added in the pharmacy if possible.

   3. Flush solutions should be timed and dated when they are opened. They should be kept at room temperature no longer than 8 hours before being discarded.

REFERENCES

American Academy of Pediatrics: Infection control for hospitalized children. In Pickering LK, editor: *Red book: report of the committee on infectious diseases,* ed 26, Elk Grove Village, IL, 2003, American Academy of Pediatrics, pp 146-154.

American Academy of Pediatrics and American College of Obstetricians and

Gynecologists (AAP/ACOG): Perinatal infections. In *Guidelines for perinatal care*, ed 5, Elk Grove Village, IL, 2002, American Academy of Pediatrics and American College of Obstetricians and Gynecologists.

Boyce JM, Pitter D: Guidelines for hand hygiene in health-care settings, *MMWR* 51(RR-16). October 25, 2002.

Centers for Disease Control and Prevention: Update: Universal Precautions for prevention of transmission of human immunodeficiency virus, hepatitis B virus, and other bloodborne pathogens in health care settings, *MMWR* 37:377-382, 387-388, 1988.

Department of Labor, Occupational Safety and Health Administration: Occupational exposure to bloodborne pathogens: final rule, *Fed Reg* 56:64175-64182, 1991.

Garner JS: Hospital Infection Control Practices Advisory Committee. Guidelines for isolation precautions in hospitals, *Infect Control Hosp Epidemiol* 17:53-80, 1996.

Discharge Planning and Follow-Up Care

Preparation for the care of a healthy newborn should be a continuous process that begins when a woman first becomes aware of her pregnancy. Childbirth education classes provide information about the care and development of a newborn, the impact on the family, and preparation for bringing the baby home. After the birth of the baby, education can be individualized for each newborn and its family. Care providers must assess the family's educational background, and current need for infant care instruction in order to provide appropriate information necessary for a smooth transition to the home.

The care provider must also assess the infant's course in the hospital to determine when the infant is medically ready for discharge. Discharge criteria must be carefully evaluated to ensure that an infant is healthy at the time of discharge.

Discharge Planning and Follow-Up Care

22 Parental Preparation

Jane Deacon, RNC, MS, NNP

ASSESS PARENT READINESS FOR DISCHARGE TEACHING

A. Physical conditions that may limit comprehension of discharge teaching, include medications, pain, exhaustion, and substance abuse.

B. Psychosocial conditions that may affect the ability to understand discharge teaching instructions, include age, cultural background, language barriers, knowledge base, previous experience, socioeconomic status, developmental level, and emotional disorders.

TEACHING TECHNIQUES

A. **Small Group:** Parents are gathered in a quiet setting and taught using a lecture format with demonstrations. Information includes physical care and feeding of the infant, safety, infant behavior and development, and signs of illness. Parents have the opportunity to ask questions and participate in demonstrations.

B. **Individualized:** Information is taught and demonstrated to mother and/or father in a one-on-one setting. Information can thereby be individualized.

C. **Audiovisual Materials:** Films, videos, and hospital television programs may be available to supplement individual or group teaching.

D. **Printed Material/Booklets:** Supplement to individual or group teaching activities. Parent education materials in the form of booklets, pamphlets, baby magazines, and handouts are also freely distributed by various baby product companies and are usually available in nurseries.

E. **Internet Sites:** May be helpful to obtain information on child care. Suggest those sites that have accurate, current information and those that are sponsored by well known, reliable organizations. Warn families that information on the Internet may not be accurate or reflect accepted medical practice. Information obtained from Internet sites should be discussed with their primary care provider.

EDUCATION CONTENT FOR DISCHARGE TEACHING

A. **Bathing**
   1. Gather all supplies and equipment before beginning the bath. Supplies include the following: sink or tub, clean washcloth, towel, mild soap, baby shampoo, soft hair brush/comb, alcohol on cotton-tipped swabs for umbilical cord care, cotton balls, and clean clothes.

2. Caution against leaving baby unattended on an unprotected surface or in the bath tub. Demonstrate by keeping one hand on the baby at all times to prevent falls or slipping in the tub. Caution against devices that keep baby propped up in the tub, because these can allow an infant to slip down into the water and drown.
3. A washcloth placed in the bottom of the tub will help prevent the baby from slipping.
4. A bath every 2 to 3 days is sufficient if the face and diaper area is kept clean; bath may be given at any time during the day.
5. The room should be warm and free of drafts. The water should be warm to touch, not hot.
6. Sponge-bathe until the umbilical cord has fallen off and, if circumcised, until the circumcision site is healed.
7. Bathe from "clean to dirty" beginning with the face.
   a. Do not use soap on the face.
   b. Wipe each eye from the inner canthus to the outer canthus with wet cotton balls.
   c. Clean ears with a washcloth, not cotton-tipped swabs. Wash behind the ears because regurgitated milk may accumulate there.
   d. Wash neck. If the infant is reclining, lift the shoulders slightly with hand placed under the shoulders; if infant is held sitting up, lift chin to wash neck. Infants have naturally short necks, which can make it difficult to clean neck folds.
   e. Bathe the rest of the body, cleaning the diaper area last.
   f. Shampoo the hair either before the bath begins or after the baby has been washed and dried.
      (1) Shampoo the head while holding the baby in a football position with one hand, thus freeing the other hand to wash the head.
      (2) The soft spot will not be injured by washing over it.
      (3) Use baby shampoo and a soft brush.
      (4) Rinse well and towel dry the hair.

B. **Umbilical Cord Care**
   1. Clean with each diaper change and at bath time. Dip cotton-tipped swabs in alcohol and clean at the base where the cord meets the skin. (The base of the cord may be below skin level.)
   2. Demonstrate folding diapers and clothing away from the cord to keep the area dry.
   3. Cord will fall off in 1 to 2 weeks. A drop or two of blood may be visible when the cord drops off.
   4. Encourage the family to notify the health care provider if bleeding or oozing continues or if there is circumferential erythema around the umbilical site, a foul odor, or drainage.

C. **Skin Care/Rashes/Jaundice:** Lotions or creams applied to the skin are not necessary and may cause irritation. If a lotion is used, an unscented, non–alcohol-based product should be selected. The skin of most babies is dry and peels for the first 2–3 weeks, after which it will be soft and smooth.

1. A number of marks or rashes are normal.
    a. Erythema toxicum is a benign rash with a white center surrounded by an area that is flat and red (Color Plate 3). This may come and go on various sites of the face, trunk, and limbs. It can occur up to 3 months of age. Lotions and creams may exacerbate the condition.
    b. Milia is another normal finding that manifests as multiple yellow or pearly white papules about 1 mm in size occurring on the brow, cheeks, and nose. No treatment is necessary. It resolves spontaneously during the first few weeks after birth.
    c. Epstein's pearls are the oral counterpart of facial milia. These are white pearly papules on the midline palate that resolve spontaneously and require no treatment.
2. Jaundice of the face and chest may be noticeable in the first week of life. It may be visible into the second week in some breast-fed infants.
    a. Caution parents about jaundice that extends to cover the entire body and lower extremities.
    b. Advise them to notify the health care provider if jaundice extends to the lower extremities.

D. **Voiding and Stooling Patterns**
1. Expect two to six wet diapers a day for the first 1–2 days and six to eight thereafter. Wet diapers indicate adequate oral intake. Advise parents to notify the health care provider if there is no urine output for over 12 hours. With disposable diapers it may be difficult to tell if the baby voided. Advise to tear apart the diaper liner and examine the diaper padding or use a cloth diaper.
2. Expect stooling each day but remind parents that the infant will establish an individual pattern. Stools change from dark meconium to seedy yellow or yellow/green in the first few days of life.
    a. Bowel movements vary according to the type of feeding. Formula-fed infants have one to several soft, formed, light yellow to green/brown stools per day. Breast-fed infants usually stool more frequently and have liquid yellow stools.
    b. Infants may turn red in the face during bowel movements. Regardless of such "straining," if the stools are soft, constipation is not a problem. A constipated stool is small, firm to hard, and generally consists of several pieces/balls. If constipation is a problem, notify the health care provider.
    c. An increased number of stools, an abnormal or unexpected change in the color or consistency of stools, blood or mucus with stools or a water ring may indicate diarrhea or other serious problem. Instruct parents to notify the health care provider if diarrhea is suspected. Caution parents on how rapidly an infant can become dehydrated.

E. Diaper Area
1. Clean the diaper area with mild soap and water with each diaper change.
    a. Diaper rash is caused by irritation from urine and stool being held against the skin. Emphasize that prompt cleaning after wetting or stooling will prevent most diaper rashes.
    b. If redness occurs in the diaper area, change more frequently. If an ointment is needed, a barrier type such as petrolatum jelly, Desitin®, or A&D-ointment® may be helpful. Exposing the area to air may also be helpful in treating a diaper rash. Use of a powder or lotion may exacerbate a diaper rash. Notify the health care provider if the rash resembles pinpoint red raised areas (monilial rash) or if the rash persists.
2. Clean females by separating the labia and cleaning away stool from front to back. A white vaginal discharge in the first few days of life is normal.
3. Clean males by wiping away all stool from under and around the scrotal area.
    a. If infant is uncircumcised, explain that the foreskin should not be forcibly retracted. The foreskin will loosen naturally later in life (age 2–5) and does not require extensive care.
    b. If infant is circumcised, a small amount of bleeding may occur during the first few hours after the procedure. If a Gomco device or Mogen clamp is used, petrolatum gauze dressing should be applied around the penis to prevent adherence of the diaper. No dressing is used with the Plastibell®; petrolatum should be avoided since this could loosen the string
    c. Avoid wipes containing alcohol; advise to cleanse with clear water for the first few days until healing is evident.
    d. Instruct parents to observe and report unusual edema, erythema, bleeding, and drainage. Describe the appearance of normal granulation tissue during the healing process. Reinforce the need for sponge baths until the circumcision is healed.

F. Fingernail Care:
Keep nails short to prevent scratching the face. Fingernails may be filed with an emery board. Scissors or clippers may be used to trim the nails. Caution against accidentally clipping the skin or tips of the fingers.

G. Bulb Syringe:
Instruct to position the infant's head to one side. Before inserting into baby's mouth, compress the bulb firmly so that air and any secretions are expressed. Insert the bulb in one side of the mouth and slowly release, drawing in secretions. Remove from the mouth and empty the bulb by compressing it several times. Demonstrate cleaning the bulb syringe by washing in hot, soapy water. Demonstrate squirting water in and out of the syringe, rinsing with clean water, and allowing it to dry. Caution parents against excessive nasal suctioning unless drainage is interfering with infant's ability to breathe or eat comfortably. Excessive suctioning will cause more secretions and may damage mucosal membranes.

FEEDING (see also Chapter 8)

    A. **Breast-Feeding:** Encourage 8–12 feeds per 24 hours.

        1. Offer both breasts at each feeding. Alternate starting breast to ensure adequate stimulation and emptying.

        2. Duration of feed should not be limited; rather, infant should nurse until satisfied. By day 3–5 infant should be suckling 5–10 minutes per breast.

        3. Feeding interval should be 1 1/2 to 3 hours with one 4- to 5-hour interval at night.

        4. Position infant comfortably either in the cradled, football hold, or side-lying position.

    B. **Formula Feeding**

        1. Most newborns will take 1 to 2 ounce of formula per feeding every 2–4 hours in the first 24–48 hours of life; thereafter, volume of feedings in the first month will increase to 12–24 ounces/day; the interval between feedings will increase to every 3–4 hours with a longer interval at night.

        2. Advise that formula must be stored in the refrigerator and should not be allowed to sit out longer than 1 hour. Warm formula by placing in a pan of hot water. Test on the inside of the wrist. Caution that microwaving causes uneven heating and is not recommended.

        3. Position the bottle so that the nipple is filled with milk. Rub the palate with the nipple to stimulate sucking.

        4. Encourage burping after every 1 to 2 ounces and at the end of the feeding to help remove swallowed air, which could cause distension and discomfort. Demonstrate common burping positions.

        5. Encourage family to read and follow mixing instructions of the formula packaging. Instruct to mix no more than a 24-hour supply at one time, pour into small, clean bottles, and refrigerate. Demonstrate mixing of formula.

        6. Discourage saving the remainder of a feed since bacteria can grow in the formula. Bottles, nipples, and plastic rings should be cleaned in hot, soapy water or in a dishwasher. There is no need for sterilization unless family lives in an area with an unclean water supply.

INFANT BEHAVIOR

    A. **Crying**

        1. Assure parents that they will soon learn to distinguish hunger and pain cries from fussy behavior. All infants cry in the early weeks of life for many reasons including hunger, discomfort, fatigue, boredom, and overstimulation. Sometimes no specific cause is determined.

        2. Infants cry approximately 60–90 minutes a day during the first 3 weeks of life. By 2–3 weeks of age, babies begin a different type of crying that is fussy in nature. It may occur at the same time every day. Usual comfort measures may not stop crying.

        3. Normal, well-cared-for babies cry. Parents should be taught that if obvious needs have been met, crying behavior is a part of infant behavior and does not necessarily mean the parent is doing anything wrong.

4. Once causes for crying have been eliminated and comfort measures tried, the infant may need to "cry it out" and can be placed in a crib in a quiet room.
   a. Although this is stressful for parents, reinforce that leaving the infant in a safe environment for 15 minutes may be enough time to allow the infant to fall asleep.
   b. Parents should check on the infant after 15 minutes; if the infant is still crying, they should retry comfort measures and put infant back to bed if necessary.
   c. Several 15-minute sessions may be required before the infant is asleep.
5. Crying may increase to 2–4 hours per day by 6 weeks and gradually decrease by 3 months of age.

B. **Comfort Measures:** The following measures may be helpful for a crying baby:
   1. Feed/burp.
   2. Change diaper.
   3. Check clothing for comfort/warmth.
   4. Swaddle or wrap securely in soft blankets.
   5. Hold until baby falls asleep.
   6. Rock baby.
   7. Decrease environmental stimulation by turning down the lights, decreasing noise, limiting activity in room.
   8. Offer pacifier.
   9. Walk or rock while holding.
   10. Place in baby swing.
   11. Give baby a bath.
   12. Play soothing music.
   13. Gently massage baby's body.
   14. Take a stroller ride.
   15. Take a car ride.
   16. Carry in soft front carrier.

C. **Colic**
   1. Characterized by irritable crying for no obvious reason, for more than 3 hours a day. It usually takes place during the late afternoon or early evening on at least 3 days a week (Murray et al, 2002). It occurs in 10% to 20% of all infants beginning in the first 2 to 3 weeks of life (Grover, 2002).
   2. Colic may continue for 4–6 months.
   3. The cause is unknown. Allergies, parental stress, immaturity of the GI system, or CNS have been investigated.
   4. Infants cry as though in pain, draw their knees to their abdomen, and may pass gas. Crying is intense, causes parental stress, and can be a factor in poor parent-infant bonding and child abuse. Parents need to discuss colic behavior with their care provider.
   5. Pharmacologic agents such as antispasmodics, antiflatulents, or sedatives may be required in severe cases.

D. **Awake/Asleep Behavior**
   1. Expect the infant to sleep 15–20 hours per day in the first month, progressing to longer sleep periods at night and shorter periods during the day.

2. By 12 weeks of age, most babies sleep 5 hours at night and will progressively increase sleep time at night to coincide with awake time during the day.
3. Established patterns may be interrupted during illness, teething, and growth spurts.
4. Infants should be positioned on the back for sleep. Prone positioning has been associated with sudden infant death syndrome (SIDS). Soft objects such as pillows or stuffed toys should not be placed in the crib, because these can cause suffocation (AAP, 2000).

E. **Developmental Milestones:** Emphasize to parents that there is a range of normal for developmental tasks. Every baby is an individual, and differences between babies should be expected.
1. The infant will grow rapidly during the first year of life. In the first 6 months, the infant will gain an average of 1.5 lb and grow 1 inch per month.
2. Newborns can see objects 6–8 inches from their eyes and prefer designs in black and white or human faces. Babies will stare at objects that interest them and learn to follow them by turning in their direction.
3. Babies can locate the general direction of sounds.
4. Head control is achieved by the end of the third month.
5. Smiling begins by 3–5 weeks and cooing and babbling by 2–3 months. Babies enjoy being talked to and will respond with a flurry of activity from their arms and legs.

MEDICAL CARE

A. **When to Call the Health Care Provider**
1. Breathing difficulties.
2. Seizures, loss of consciousness.
3. Lethargy, irritability.
4. Decreased feeding for 24 hours.
5. Vomiting more than 1–2 entire feeds in 1 day or projectile vomiting.
6. No urine output for more than 12 hours.
7. Bowel movements that are black, watery, loose, or of increased frequency.
8. Reddened umbilical site.
9. Redness, drainage, swelling, foul odor around circumcision site.
10. Jaundice covering abdomen/extremities.
11. Pustules/rashes other than normal newborn rashes.
12. White patches in the mouth that remain after the mouth is gently wiped with a wet cloth or cannot be removed with gentle scraping.
13. Temperature under 97.7° F (36.4° C) or over 100° F (37.8° C) axillary. Demonstrate temperature taking and reading a thermometer.
14. "Ill looking"

B. **Weight**
1. Expect weight loss in the first week of life.
2. Caution about signs of dehydration (lack of voiding, tenting skin, dry mouth, excessive irritability, or sleepiness).

C. **Fontanel:** Is palpable until closure at approximately 12 to 18 months of life. It is not extremely fragile but should be protected from trauma.

D. **Smoking**
  1. Respiratory infections are frequent in infants who are exposed to smoke from cigarettes.
  2. Smoking is one factor in sudden infant death syndrome (Murray et al, 2002).
  3. Parents who smoke should be encouraged to quit. If they continue to smoke, they should smoke only outside the home, because smoke is absorbed by infants even when smoking occurs in another room in the house. Also advise not to smoke in the car.

E. **Cardiopulmonary Resuscitation**
  1. Generally not a part of discharge teaching due to time constraints.
  2. Encourage parents to take a class in CPR through their health care provider, the American Red Cross, or the hospital.

F. **Follow-Up Medical Care**
  1. Stress the importance of regular medical check-ups. These visits include developmental milestone assessment, physical examination, immunizations, and emotional support and guidance for parents.
  2. The first visit should be within 48 hours of discharge for infants discharged before 48 hours of age (AAP/ACOG, 2002).

G. **Phone Numbers:** Provide numbers for the hospital nursery, health care provider, and emergency rescue (911) on a card and encourage parents to place near the phone for easy access.

SAFETY

A. Protect infant from infection by limiting exposure to crowds, sick individuals, or toddlers the first month of life.

B. Avoid excessive sun exposure (>15 minutes).

C. Stress importance of car seat restraint. Information about specific state laws on child restraints should be reviewed. Inform parents that properly installed child safety seats may reduce the chance of fatal injury to infants in case of a collision (AAP, 1999; Lang and Stewart, 1999).

D. Reinforce that seats must be used properly. Directions from the manufacturer must be followed for safe and effective use. Car seats must be approved for use in cars. Caution against using infant seats designed for home use, because these are not adequate to protect a child in a car. Infant car seats should be positioned to face the rear of the car until the baby is 1 year old or weighs 20 lb. This is generally considered the time it takes before the bone structure is adequately mineralized and able to withstand a forward impact in a five-point harness restraint (Stevens, 1997). Children should not be placed in a seat in which an air bag could deploy during a collision.

E. Encourage parents to examine toys for small, loose parts that could obstruct airways, as well as rattles containing small objects that could choke the baby if the rattle breaks.

F. If a pacifier is needed, encourage a one-piece pacifier that cannot come apart and cause choking.

G. Advise to remove from baby's reach any items that could be harmful and to put all medication and toxic substances out of children's reach.

H. Check crib to be sure crib slats are no greater than 2 3/8 inches apart. The mattress should be firm, and pillows should be avoided. This reduces the risk for suffocation. All paint used on the crib or in the infant's environment should be lead-free. Avoid soft stuffed animals or other objects placed in the crib that could suffocate the baby.

I. Keep crib away from windows with curtains, blinds, or shade cords that could accidentally wrap around the neck and strangle the baby.

J. Do not hang any toys with strings over the crib. They could accidentally strangle the baby if they fall or get pulled into the crib by an active baby.

K. Encourage parents to keep the number of the Poison Control center near the telephone.

L. Do not leave an infant alone with a pet.

PARENT EDUCATION DOCUMENTATION

Document teaching activities on a hospital-approved form and place in the permanent record. (See Appendix E for Patient Education Sheet.)

REFERENCES

American Academy of Pediatrics (AAP): Safe transportation of newborns at hospital discharge, *Pediatrics* 104(4):986-987, 1999.

American Academy of Pediatrics (AAP), Task Force on Infant Sleep Position and Sudden Infant Death Syndrome: Changing concepts of sudden infant death syndrome: implications for infant sleeping environment and sleep position, *Pediatrics* 105(3):650-656, 2000.

American Academy of Pediatrics (AAP) and American College of Obstetricians and Gynecologists (ACOG): *Guidelines for perinatal care,* ed 5, Elk Grove, IL, 2002, American Academy of Pediatrics.

Grover G: Crying and colic. In Berkowitz CD, editor: *Pediatrics: a primary care approach,* ed 2, Philadelphia, 2002, WB Saunders, pp 111-114.

Lang NJ, Stewart DD: Safe travel in the car: what parents need to know, *Mother Baby J* 4(4):13-18, 1999.

Lowdermilk D, Perry SE, Piotrowski KA: *Maternity nursing,* ed 6, St Louis, 2003, Mosby, p 770.

Moran BA: Substance abuse in pregnancy. In Mattson S, Smith JE, editors: *Core curriculum for maternal newborn nursing,* ed 2, Philadelphia, 2000, WB Saunders, pp 545-563.

Murray SS, McKinney ES, Gorrie TM: *Foundations of maternal newborn nursing,* ed 3, Philadelphia, 2002, WB Saunders.

Stevens K: Nursing care of newborns. In Nichols FG, Zwelling E, editors: *Maternal-newborn nursing: theory and practice,* Philadelphia, 1997, WB Saunders, p 1162.

23 Discharge Assessment

Jane Deacon, RNC, MS, NNP

PHYSICAL EXAMINATION

A. When to Perform: A physical examination should be performed and documented in anticipation of discharge (Figure 23-1 is a sample of the newborn documentation record). Performing the exam with parents present can assure them of the infant's physical condition. Questions can be answered and the need for continued follow-up care can be reinforced.

B. Components of the Physical Examination

1. General evaluation: Review any concerns the nurse may have. Observe color, tone, and behavioral state.

2. Morphology: Evaluate congenital abnormalities and the need for follow-up before or after discharge.

3. Head: Palpate anterior and posterior fontanel. Check sutures for mobility. Palpate for caput succedaneum, which should begin resolving by the second day of life. Differentiate caput (crosses sutures) from cephalohematoma (confined to single bone). Observe for molding. Note abrasions, lacerations, or forceps marks (especially over/near eyes) for healing or signs of infection.

4. Eyes: Visualize red reflexes. Observe for chemical conjunctivitis (rare with erythromycin) or subconjunctival hemorrhages. Observe for normal spacing of eyes or downward slant (seen in Down syndrome).

5. Ears: Assess for set and position. Note preauricular tags or pits. Ask about any history of renal disease if tags and/or pits are detected. Observe for patent canals.

6. Nose: Assess patency of nares. Observe for septal dislocation or deviation.

7. Mouth: Observe for natal teeth, mucoid cysts, and Epstein's pearls. Inspect hard and soft palate for clefts. Note size and position of tongue.

8. Neck: Palpate for masses such as cystic hygromas, cysts, and goiter. Observe for webbing or redundant skin.

9. Chest: Auscultate for breath sounds. Observe for symmetry of chest, respiratory rate and effort, grunting, flaring, and retractions.

10. Heart: Auscultate for cardiac rate and rhythm. Note murmurs. Evaluate need for cardiac consultation (murmur >grade 1, cyanosis, decreased pulses, and perfusion). Assess capillary refill. Palpate brachial and femoral pulses.

11. Abdomen: Palpate for kidneys, liver, and spleen. Observe for distension. Assess umbilical cord for redness, foul odor, and discharge.

NEWBORN RECORD

PRENATAL
Mother's Name_____
Age____ G____ P___LC___TAB___SAB____
Blood type_____ Antibody Screen_____
HbsAG___STS___Rubella___GBS___Other_____
Past OB/Medical Hx/ Family Hx_____
_____
_____
LMP_____EDC_____
Prenatal Care Provider_____
Medications_____
_____
US findings_____
Complications_____
_____

LABOR
Spont_____Induced_____ Augmented_____
Reason_____
ROM (hrs)_____ Maternal abx_____
Labor Complications_____

DELIVERY
Date_____Time_____ Presentation _____
SVD_____C/S _____ Reason _____
Nuchal cord_____3 Vessel Cord ☐Yes ☐No
Anesthesia_____

APGARS

SIGN	1	5
HR		
RR		
Tone		
Reflex		
Color		
Total		

RESUSCITATION
O2 BB__CPAP__ BM vent__ETT__CPR__Meds__
_____
_____
_____

GROWTH PARAMETERS
Birth Wt._____ gms _____ %
Length:_____ cms _____ %
OFC: _____ cms _____ %

PHYSICAL EXAMINATION

Date	Age(hrs)	Sex	T	HR	RR	Gestational age:		Wks		Exam	
			Nl	Abnl	Admission		Nl	Abnl	Discharge		
Skin (Color, perfusion, rash, bruising)											
Head (Trauma, molding, caput/ceph, fontanelles, sutures)											
Eyes (Vessels, red relflex, conjunctiva, cornea)											
Ears/Nose/Mouth/Palate (Position, pits, tags, ext canal/patent nares/clefts, teeth)											
Neck (Masses, trachea)											
Chest/Lungs (Symetry, retractions, breath sounds)											
Heart/Pulses (PMI, rhythm, murmurs)											
Abdomen (Liver, spleen, kidneys, masses, umbil)											
Skeletal (Back, extremities, hips, clavicles)											
Genitalia/Anus (Female: clitoromegaly, patent hymen Male: testes, penis; anus patent)											
Neurologic (Tone, head lag, activ, behavior, reflex)											
Other											

Admission Assessment/Plan_____
_____
_____

Discharge Assessment/Plan_____
_____
_____
_____
_____

DISCHARGE
Discharge Wt. _____ Bl type_____
Hep B Vaccine_____Hearing Screen ☐ Pass ☐ Fail
Medications_____
Referrals_____
Feeding method_____
Followup Provider_____Date/Time_____
SIGNATURE_____

FIGURE 23-1 ● Newborn record. (From University Hospital, Denver, Colorado.)

12. Skeletal: Palpate clavicles for fractures. Check hips for subluxation or dislocation. Inspect extremities for polydactyly, syndactyly, supernumerary digits, and positional or structural foot abnormalities.
13. Genitals: Inspect female infant for patent vagina, presence of vaginal tags, discharge, or pseudomenses. Observe male infant for descended testicles, hydroceles, and hypospadias. If circumcised, observe for healing, bleeding, or signs of infection.
14. Skin: Observe for rashes, Mongolian spots, nevi, cafe au lait spot, and presence of jaundice.
15. Neurologic: Assess for tone, suck, Moro reflex, grasp, rooting, behavioral state, and cry. Observe for palsies of upper extremities or face secondary to birth injuries.

PHYSIOLOGIC FUNCTIONS

A. **Abnormal Events During Hospitalization:** Evaluate that abnormal transition events or subsequent problems such as those listed below have resolved before discharge.
   1. Cardiovascular: Central cyanosis, significant or persistent murmur, weak pulses, poor perfusion.
   2. Respiratory: Tachypnea, grunting, flaring, stridor, retractions persisting for more than 1 hour after birth, or oxygen requirement of greater than 30% for >4 hours.
   3. Gastrointestinal: No stool by 24 hours of life, poor feeding, vomiting, abdominal distension.
   4. Genitourinary: No urine output by 24 hours of life, distended bladder, poor urinary stream.
   5. Thermoregulation: Hypothermia or hyperthermia.
   6. Hypoglycemia.
   7. Behavior: Excessive irritability or crying, poor tone, decreased activity, poor suck, jitteriness.
B. **Vital Signs**
   1. Normal body temperature (36.5° C–37° C) documented while normally clothed and swaddled.
   2. Documented waking heart rate between 120–160 (range may vary from 80 during sleep to 180 when active and crying).
   3. Normal respiratory rate between 30–60 without signs of respiratory distress (grunting, flaring, retracting, cyanosis, apnea, stridor, rales).
   4. Systolic blood pressure between 50 mm Hg and 80 mm Hg. Four extremity blood pressures should be taken if a murmur is audible. A 20-mm Hg difference between arm and leg should be investigated for the possibility of congenital heart disease.
C. **Feeding**
   1. The mother must demonstrate the ability to feed her infant either by breast or bottle.

2. Breast-feeding infants should demonstrate successful latching onto the breast, with rhythmic, continuous sucking movement for 10–15 minutes per breast every 1½–3 hours.
3. The infant should awaken for feeds or be easily roused.
4. Formula-feeding infants should take 1–2 ounces every 3–4 hours with a minimum of encouragement. Infants who do not demonstrate appropriate feeding ability are at high risk for dehydration. These infants should be carefully monitored until successful feeding behavior is established.

D. **Elimination Pattern**
   1. A minimum of one void and one stool should be documented in the first 24 hours of life.
   2. Delay circumcision until a void is documented. Counsel parents to report first void after circumcision, especially if discharge occurs soon after the circumcision.
   3. Advise parents to notify the health care provider if there has been no urine for 12 hours or no stool for 2 days.

E. **Weight Loss**
   1. The average weight loss is 5%–7% over 3–4 days.
   2. A weight loss of >10% may indicate inadequate intake. Evaluate feeding history or any evidence of excessive losses.
   3. Reweigh the baby if scale error may be a possibility. Close follow-up of an infant is necessary if weight loss is >7% at discharge. Infants who have >10% weight loss should be closely evaluated for feeding problems and should remain in the hospital until weight loss has stabilized.

F. **Jaundice**
   1. Evaluate jaundice evident in the first 24 hours of life.
   2. Consider evaluating jaundiced infants who:
      a. Have a blood group incompatibility or "set-up."
      b. Have a risk for excessive jaundice such as bruising.
      c. Have an inexperienced mother who may not be able to recognize progressive jaundice.
      d. Are SGA, of low birth weight, and/or slightly preterm infants.
      e. Are not aggressively feeding at the time of discharge.
   3. Minimal evaluation should include blood type of mother and baby, Coombs test, total bilirubin level, and hematocrit (see Chapter 14 for treatment).

G. **Congenital Abnormalities** (see also Chapter 7): Review plan for treatment of congenital anomalies with parents.

H. **Perinatal Infection:** Evaluate infants for risk of perinatal infection (see Chapters 19 and 20).

I. **Laboratory Evaluation**
   1. Prenatal labs: Review prenatal labs for maternal blood type, antibody screen, hepatitis B screen, and syphilis status.
   2. Glucose screen (if indicated) should be 45 mg/dL or greater. If initial screen was <45 mg/dL, a subsequent normal blood glucose should be documented.

3. Newborn genetic screen should be obtained before discharge.
4. Hematocrit should be 45%–65%. Risk factors for anemia include blood loss before or after delivery, increased destruction (hemolysis) of red blood cells, and impaired red blood cell production. Those at risk for polycythemia include infants with intrauterine hypoxia, infants of diabetic mothers, small-for-gestational-age infants, and twins (one may be donor and the other a recipient in twin-to-twin transfusion syndrome). Other risk factors include maternal fetal transfusion, delayed cord clamping, or chromosomal abnormalities.
5. Total bilirubin if significant jaundice is present.

J. **Hepatitis B Immunization** (AAP/ACOG, 2002)
   1. Recommended by the AAP at birth, 1 month, and 6 months.
   2. Hepatitis B immune globulin (HBIG) is recommended if mother's HBsAg status is positive (see also Chapter 20).

K. **Vitamin K and Eye Prophylaxis:** Administration of each should be documented.

L. **Hearing Screen:** Recommended in the newborn period (National Institute of Health, 1993).

EARLY DISCHARGE (< 48 HOURS) CONSIDERATIONS

A. Infants born by uncomplicated vaginal delivery who have a normal newborn course are generally eligible for discharge at 48 hours of age. The benefits of early discharge and the adverse effects of increased readmission rates continue to be evaluated. The Newborns' and Mothers' Health Protection Act of 1996 provides for stays of 48 hours after vaginal birth and 96 hours after cesarean delivery. The following criteria for early discharge and postdischarge follow-up have been established by the American Academy of Pediatrics (AAP, 1995):
   1. Uncomplicated antepartum, intrapartum, and postpartum courses for both mother and baby.
   2. Vaginal delivery.
   3. Knowledgeable family member or other support person including health care providers are available to assist mother at home in the first few days after discharge.
   4. No unresolved family, environmental, or social risk factors. These risk factors include, but are not limited to, untreated parental substance abuse/positive urine toxicology results in the mother or newborn; history of child abuse or neglect; mental illness in a parent who is in the home; lack of social support, particularly for single, first time mothers; no fixed home; history of untreated domestic violence; teen mother, particularly if other conditions above apply. When these or other risk factors are present, the discharge should be delayed until the issues are resolved or a plan to safeguard the infant is in place.
   5. Designated physician-directed source of continuing medical care for mother and baby is identified.

6. Definitive plan is established for follow-up within 48 hours after discharge. The follow-up visit can take place in a home or clinical setting. Personnel must be skilled in newborn assessment and care. The results of the visit should be reported to the infant's physician on the day of the visit.

7. Term infant (38–42 weeks gestation), single birth, with birth weight appropriate for gestational age.

8. Vital signs are documented as normal and stable for 12 hours preceding discharge: respiratory rate below 60 per minute, heart rate of 100 to 160 beats per minute, and axillary temperature of 36.1° to 37° C in open crib with appropriate clothing.

9. Infant has urinated and passed at least one stool.

10. Infant has completed at least two successful feedings and demonstrates the ability to coordinate sucking, swallowing, and breathing while feeding.

11. Physical examination reveals no abnormalities that require continued hospitalization.

12. No evidence of excessive bleeding at circumcision site for at least 2 hours after circumcision.

13. No evidence of significant jaundice in first 24 hours after birth.

14. The following laboratory data are available and reviewed as clinically indicated: maternal syphilis, hepatitis B surface antigen, cord or infant blood type, and direct Coombs test.

15. Plan for performing screening tests in accordance with state regulations is identified. A system for repeating the test must be ensured during the follow-up visit.

16. Initial hepatitis B vaccine is administered or a scheduled appointment for its administration has been made within the first week of life.

17. Mother has the knowledge, ability, and confidence to provide adequate care for her baby and has received education regarding breast-feeding or bottle-feeding (the breast-feeding mother-infant dyad should be assessed by trained staff regarding nursing position, latching on, adequacy of swallowing, and mother's knowledge of urine-stool frequency); cord, skin, and infant genital care; ability to recognize signs of illness and common infant problems, particularly jaundice; and infant safety.

PSYCHOSOCIAL EVALUATION

A. **Social Evaluation:** Such an evaluation should be completed to identify conditions that may place the infant at risk for safety and well-being. A social service consult should be requested if concerns exist or any of the following conditions are present:

1. Adolescent mother.
2. Lack of prenatal care.
3. Unwanted/unplanned pregnancy.
4. Relinquishment.
5. Inadequate support system.
6. Recent/current family stressors.

7. History of emotional disorders in mother/father.
8. Severe physical limitations of a parent that may interfere with adequate parenting.
9. Physical illness of mother necessitating prolonged hospitalization.
10. Mental retardation of mother that may interfere with adequate parenting.
11. Substance abuse in the home.
12. Positive toxicology screen on mother/infant.
13. History of Child Protective Service contact, child abuse/neglect, or children removed from parental care.
14. Negative interaction between mother and father.
15. Domestic violence.
16. Inadequate food or other essentials.
17. Inadequate housing/living arrangements/homelessness.
18. Incarceration of mother/father.

B. **Further Evaluation:** If the social worker recommends further evaluation, the infant should be maintained in the hospital until cleared for discharge by social services. The infant may be placed on a court or police hold if circumstances warrant keeping a child beyond usual discharge time (see also Chapter 13).

OTHER CONSIDERATIONS

A. **Adoption** (see also Chapter 13).
B. **Individuals with Disabilities Education Act (IDEA):** Governmental act passed in 1993 to identify individuals at risk for developmental delays. Part H of this act seeks to define those newborns who are at risk so that they may be evaluated and referred to proper agencies for developmental follow-up. Infants who are determined to be at risk should be referred to the identified agency responsible for the act (may be administered by different agencies as determined by the state; eligibility may vary by state). Eligible infants include those with conditions associated with significant developmental delays:
1. Chromosomal syndromes such as Down syndrome.
2. Congenital syndromes or conditions such as central nervous system (CNS) malformations, brain abnormalities, or fetal alcohol syndrome.
3. Sensory impairments such as hearing or vision impairment.
4. Metabolic disorders such as hypothyroidism, lipidoses, maple syrup urine disease, galactosemia, phenylketonuria (PKU).
5. Pre- and perinatal conditions such as TORCH (toxoplasmosis, other infections, rubella, cytomegalovirus, and herpes simplex) infections, intraventricular hemorrhage, teratogens, seizures, cerebral palsy, intrauterine exposure to illegal drugs, positive human immunodeficiency virus (HIV) status, meningitis.

DOCUMENTATION

A. A copy of the newborn record should be given to the family and a copy sent to the identified follow-up care provider. The record should include information about prenatal lab results, pregnancy, labor and delivery, resuscitation record, growth parameters, gestational age assessment, physical examination, discharge weight, results of any laboratory analysis, and hepatitis B (HBV) administration (see Figure 23-1).

B. Individualized discharge instructions should be given to parents to use as a reference for specific care guidelines (Figure 23-2).

C. A medical evaluation for discharge checklist may help the care provider identify problems or issues that may need follow-up after discharge (Figure 23-3).

Nursery Discharge Instructions

FEED YOUR BABY
☐ At the breast for 10–15 minutes per breast every 2 to 3 hours on demand.
☐ _____ formula at least 1–2 ounces every 2–4 hours on demand. Your baby will start taking more formula in a few days.

MEDICAL CARE FOR YOUR BABY
Some families will have a visit from a nurse after discharge.
You ☐ will ☐ will not have a visit from a nurse 1–2 days after your baby is discharged from the hospital.
You have chosen _____ for your baby's medical care.
The phone number is _____
The address is_____
Your baby should be seen by your doctor or at your clinic:
    ☐ 2–3 days after discharge.
    ☐ One week after discharge
    ☐ Other_____
Call for an appointment as soon as possible.

CIRCUMCISION CARE
If your baby was circumcised, the care for the circumcised penis is:
    ☐ **Plastibell method:** Clean with clear water only. Do not use alcohol or Vaseline on the circumcision site. The plastic ring will come out as the skin heals (about 7–10 days). Do not pull on the ring at any time as this could cause bleeding. Do not put the baby in a bathtub until after the plastic ring has fallen off. A white, yellow, sticky substance around the tip of the penis is normal. Watch for signs of infection such as swelling, pus, redness, or bad smell. Call your baby's doctor or clinic if you notice any of these signs.
    ☐ **Gomco or Mogen method:** Clean with clear water only. Place Vaseline on the tip of the penis for several days to prevent the penis from sticking to the diaper. Do not use alcohol on the penis. Do not put the baby in a bathtub until the circumcision site is completely healed (about 7–10 days). A white, yellow, sticky substance around the tip of the penis is normal. Watch for signs of infection such as swelling, pus, redness, or bad smell. Call your baby's doctor or clinic if you notice any of these signs.

MEDICATIONS
☐ Your baby has no medications.
☐ Your baby is taking: _____
Instructions:_____

SPECIAL MEDICAL CARE
☐ Your baby does not need medical care from a specialist.
☐ Your baby needs special medical care for:
Dr. _____
Appointment date and time: _____
Location: _____

Parent Signature_____ **Nurse Signature**_____ **Date**_____

FIGURE 23-2 ● Nursery discharge instructions.

Pt. Name:
Medical Record #:

Date of Birth:
Date of Discharge:

MEDICAL EVALUATION FOR DISCHARGE CHECKLIST

	YES	NO	N/A	LAB	ISSUE	FOLLOWUP/PLAN
PHYSICAL EXAM						
Exam WNL or does not require further hospitalization						
PHYSIOLOGIC FUNCTIONS						
Abnl events during hosp stay resolved						
Vital signs normal						
Feeding well						
Voiding						
Stooling						
Weight loss <5–7%						
Jaundice absent						
Anomaly present. Treatment plan made and discussed with family						
Low infection risk						
Normal hearing screen						
LABORATORY RESULTS						
Prenatal labs (Bl type, Hep B, syphilis)						
Normal glucose screen						
Newborn genetic screen drawn						
Hematocrit WNL						
Bilirubin WNL						
MEDICATIONS						
Hepatitis B						
Vitamin K						
Eye prophylaxis						
EARLY DISCHARGE (<48°)						
Early DC considerations evaluated						
PSYCHOSOCIAL						
Social issues resolved						
Adoption issues resolved						
I.D.E.A. Part H eligibility criteria absent						

*If any response is NO, identify issue and FU/PLAN

FIGURE 23-3 ● Medical evaluation for discharge checklist.

REFERENCES

American Academy of Pediatrics, Committee on Fetus and Newborn: Hospital stay for healthy term newborns, *Pediatrics* 96(4):788-790, 1995.

American Academy of Pediatrics (AAP) and American College of Obstetricians and Gynecologists (ACOG): *Guidelines for perinatal care*, ed 5, Elk Grove Village, IL, 2002, American Academy of Pediatrics.

National Institutes of Health: *NIH consensus statement: early identification of hearing impairment in infants and young children.* Rockville, MD, 1993, NIH.

24 Postdischarge Care

Jane Deacon, RNS, MS, NNP

POSTDISCHARGE SUPPORT

A. **Nursery Support:** Many nurseries encourage parents to call if they have questions about their infant. Some nurseries call parents 2–3 days after discharge. All calls should be documented on an identified form. Information discussed should include feedings, voiding and stooling pattern, breast-feeding issues, circumcision healing, jaundice, parental concerns, and whether a follow-up medical appointment has been made. If significant concerns are identified, parent should be encouraged to contact the follow-up care provider.

B. **Breast-Feeding Support:** Lactation follow-up for breast-feeding parents should be available, because most problems after discharge are feeding-related. Many hospitals have a lactation specialist whom parents can call with breast-feeding issues.

C. **Physician-Directed Nursing Follow-Up Clinics:** Provided as a service for infants discharged at 24 hours or less. Infants return to the hospital nursery 1 day after discharge, and assessments are made regarding feeding, jaundice, weight, circumcision site, umbilical site, and general health by qualified staff (i.e., nurse practitioner, physician, RN). Nursing clinics can be an alternative to the first primary care provider visit or for families who have not yet selected a follow-up care provider or those families who have special concerns. The primary care provider is notified with the results of the follow-up visit. (See Appendix E for Early Newborn Follow-Up Visit data sheet.)

D. **Visiting Nurse Service:** Home visits made after early discharge may be provided by a visiting nurse service.

FIRST FOLLOW-UP VISIT

A. **Timing:** AAP recommends (Gilstrap and Oh, 2002) that for newborns discharged before 48 hours after delivery an appointment be made for the neonate to be examined within 48 hours of discharge.

B. **Location:** The first visit can be provided by a hospital-based early follow up clinic, visiting nurse service, or primary care provider.

EVALUATION OF THE INFANT AT THE FIRST VISIT

See Appendix E for Health Maintenance Visit record.

A. **Discussion of Parental Concerns/Problems**

    B. **Review of Mother's History/Nursery Course**
    C. **Present Status**
       1. Weight.
       2. Feeding behavior.
       3. Elimination pattern.
       4. Waking/sleeping patterns.
       5. Development.
       6. Behavior.
       7. Family interaction.
       8. Family support system.
    D. **Vital Signs**
    E. **Measurements/Growth Parameters**
    F. **Physical Examination**
    G. **Anticipatory Guidance Information**
       1. Nutrition.
       2. Integration of infant into family.
       3. Safety.
       4. Development.
       5. Health promotion.
       6. Immunization plan.
       7. Appointment set for next follow-up visit.

REFERENCES

Gilstrap LC, Oh W, editors: *Guidelines for perinatal care*, ed 5, Elk Grove Village, IL, 2002, American Academy of Pediatrics and The American College of Obstetricians and Gynecologists, p 214.

Parental Advice Guidelines for Newborn Care

PHYSICAL CARE

Bathing Your Baby

General Information

It is not necessary to bathe your baby every day. Baths may be given every 2–3 days if the face and diaper area are kept clean. Baths may be given at any time during the day. The room in which the bath is given should be warm and free from drafts. The temperature of the water should be warm, not hot, to the touch. Gather all the supplies needed before you start the bath. Never leave the baby unattended on an unprotected surface. Keep one hand on the baby at all times to prevent falls. Never leave your baby unattended in the water; an infant can drown in 1 inch of water. Sponge-bathe the baby until the umbilical cord has fallen off and the circumcision site is healed. Submerging the cord may cause infection and can delay its drying out and falling off.

Supplies

1. Sink or tub
2. Washcloth and towel
3. Mild soap
4. Baby shampoo
5. Soft hair brush/comb
6. Alcohol and cotton-tipped swabs for umbilical cord care
7. Clean clothes

Bath/Shampoo Instructions

Begin with washing the face. Do not use soap on the face. Soap can be used from the neck down. First wipe each eye, then the rest of the face. Use clean water and a clean cloth. Dry gently. Clean ears with a wet washcloth, not cotton swabs. Wash behind the ears since regurgitated milk may accumulate there. Wash the neck by lifting the shoulders slightly with the hand placed under the shoulders. Lift the chin slightly to wash between skin folds. Continue to wash the rest of the body with mild soap, rinsing well. Wash the diaper area last. Lift baby from tub or sink and place on a clean dry towel. Dry well. If hair is to be shampooed, wrap baby in towel and hold in a "football" position with one hand, freeing the other hand to wash the head. The soft spot will not be injured by washing over it. Use baby shampoo and a soft brush. Rinse well and towel-dry the hair. Do not use a blow dryer to dry the baby's hair—the temperature is too hot for a baby's skin. Comb hair if necessary. Diaper and dress the baby in clean dry clothes.

Skin Care, Umbilical Cord Care, Fingernails/Toenails

Skin Care

Your baby has sensitive skin that requires special care. Between baths skin should be cleaned with water alone; soap can dry the skin and should be used with baths only. Dry well to prevent chafing. Newborn skin does not require any ointments, creams, or powders. These products can block pores and irritate skin, causing rashes. If skin is dry or cracked and a lotion is desired, choose an unscented, non–alcohol-based product. The skin may normally be dry and peel for the first 2–3 weeks, after which it will be soft and smooth. If your baby's skin is particularly sensitive, you may want to wash his or her clothes separately, using a mild laundry soap such as Ivory Snow® or Dreft®. Rinse twice with water.

Keep your baby out of direct sunlight. Babies' skin will sunburn in as little as 15 minutes. Discuss sunscreens with your heath care provider. If your baby gets sunburned, notify your health care provider as soon as possible.

Babies may have rashes that are normal. Some of these are listed below. If your baby has a rash that does not seem to be one listed here, call your health care provider.

1. Milia: Tiny white or yellow raised spots found on the cheeks nose, eyelids, chin, or forehead. These spots disappear on their own without treatment.
2. Neonatal acne: These resemble pimples and appear at 2–4 weeks of age. They disappear by 6–8 months without treatment.
3. Cradle cap: Oily, crusty scales on the top of the head. To remove, apply mineral oil and gently scrub with a very soft brush as you shampoo.
4. Heat rash: Red areas that occur around the creases or folds when baby sweats. Decrease sweating by dressing the baby in the same layers of clothing that keep you comfortable.

Umbilical Cord Care

It is important to keep the umbilical cord clean and dry. Clean the cord with each diaper change until it has fallen off. Dip cotton-tipped swabs in rubbing alcohol and clean at the base where the cord meets the skin. The base may be below skin level. Fold diapers and clothing away from the cord to keep the area dry. The cord should fall off in 1–2 weeks. There may be a drop or two of blood visible when the cord drops off. This is normal. Notify your health care provider if bleeding or oozing continues or if there is redness around the umbilical site, foul odor, or drainage from the umbilical cord site.

Fingernails/Toenails

Fingernails and toenails should be kept short so that babies will not scratch themselves. The nails are very soft, and care should be taken to keep from clipping the skin. Use baby scissors or clippers to trim the nails. An emery board may be used to file the nails. Trim the nails straight across and round out the corners to prevent unintentional scratches to your baby and others. Do not tear or bite the infant's nails—this can lead to infection. The best time to trim the nails is when your baby is in a deep sleep.

Elimination Patterns

Expect two to six wet diapers a day for the first 1–2 days and six to eight thereafter. Wet diapers indicate adequate oral intake. Notify your health care provider if the baby has not had a wet diaper in over 12 hours.

Expect stooling each day; however, remember that each infant will establish an individual pattern. Stool color will change from a dark green-black tarry substance to seedy yellow or yellow-green in the first few days of life. Bowel movements vary according to the type of feeding. Breast-fed infants stool more frequently than formula-fed infants, often with each feeding, and the stools tend to be loose and yellow in color. Formula-fed infants usually have one to two soft, formed stools per day.

Infants may turn red in the face during bowel movements. If the stools are soft, constipation is not a problem. A constipated stool is small, firm to hard, and generally consists of several pieces. If constipation is a problem, notify your health care provider.

An increased number of stools, a change in the color or consistency of stools, blood or mucus with stools, or a water ring may indicate diarrhea or other serious problems. Notify your health care provider if any of these symptoms occur.

Diaper Area Care, Preventing Diaper Rash

Diaper Area Care

Change baby's diaper as frequently as the baby wets or stools. After removing the diaper, rinse baby's bottom with a wet washcloth. Be sure all urine and stool have been removed. After the buttocks area is cleaned, wash the genital area. In males, carefully clean the scrotum and the area around and under the scrotum. In females, separate and clean between the folds of the genitals from front to back. A white or clear vaginal mucous discharge is normal for the first few days of life.

Preventing Diaper Rash

Most diaper rash is caused by irritation from urine and stool held against the skin by diapers. Keeping the area as clean and dry as possible will prevent most diaper rash. Occasionally, prepared wipes may irritate baby's skin and cause diaper rash. If a rash does occur, continue to keep the baby clean and dry, using only water for diaper changes. After the skin is dry, apply an ointment such as Desitin®, Vaselin®, or A&D ointment® with each diaper change. Allowing the area to be exposed to air will help the area dry and heal quickly. Do not use powder or lotion on the rash since this may aggravate it. Some diaper rashes are caused by infections, so if the rash does not improve after 2–3 days of treatment or worsens at any time, call your health care provider.

Diapers and Diaper Care

Diapers

Disposable diapers are convenient but tend to be more expensive than cloth diapers. Diaper services may be a less expensive option than disposable diapers and may be more convenient than laundering cloth diapers at home. Buying and laundering cloth diapers is the least expensive option. Many cloth diapers are made with Velcro fasteners, which are more convenient than diaper pins. Some also have a plastic cover on the outside, making them more convenient than plain cloth diapers. Many families prefer a combination of cloth for routine use and disposable for travel and day care. Either disposable or cloth diapers are suitable choices. Infants wearing cloth diapers will need to be changed more frequently, because urine and stood are held against the skin, which will lead to diaper rash. Disposable diapers have a lining that pulls moisture away from baby's skin, keeping it drier than cloth diapers.

Diaper Care

To launder cloth diapers, rinse out any stool in the toilet bowl immediately and soak them in a diaper pail filled with plain water, detergent/water, or a bleach solution. There is no need to prerinse diapers with urine only. When there is enough for a load, launder them in a washing machine with hot water, a mild detergent, and bleach. Double-rinse all diapers. Diapers can be softened and freshened by adding either one half cup vinegar or a commercial fabric softener to the rinse cycle. Drying in a clothes dryer will also soften diapers.

Foreskin Care and Circumcision Care

Foreskin Care

The uncircumcised penis should be cleaned with water at the time of diaper changes and bathing. Do not attempt to force the foreskin back over the penis. This could damage the penis, causing pain, bleeding, and possible scarring. The foreskin will begin to retract normally over time. This may take from 3–5 years.

Circumcision Care

A small amount of bleeding may occur after circumcision. Vaseline should be placed over the end of the penis to prevent the head of the penis from sticking to the diaper. If a plastic ring (Plastibell) was used for the circumcision, Vaseline should not be used because it may cause the string to slip off. The Plastibell ring will come out as the site heals (approximately 7–10 days). It should not be pulled out. Clean the head of the penis with clear water only. During healing, a light, sticky, yellow drainage will form over the head of the penis. This is part of the normal healing process and should not be cleaned off or removed. Your health care provider should be notified if any other drainage, redness, swelling, or foul odor is observed.

Feeding

Breast-Feeding

Feed the baby as often as he or she seems interested. Babies will develop their own schedule. Nursing baby every 2–3 hours the first several days will stimulate the milk supply and may minimize breast engorgement. Feed from both breasts at each feeding, beginning on the last side finished at the previous feed. Feed from 10–20 minutes per breast. Position the infant so that you and the infant are comfortable, with the baby cradled across your body or at your side in the "football" hold or lying beside you. If the baby seems sleepy, unwrap the clothing, change the diaper, talk to the baby, stroke the cheek. Guide the baby's mouth to the breast. To obtain a good latch, the baby's mouth should be open wide and should pull one fourth to one half of the areola into the mouth. Don't allow the baby to go more than 4 hours between feeds in the first few weeks. Once the baby is nursing well (every 2–4 hours, 10–15 minutes per breast), you can allow the baby to sleep as long as he or she wants at night. Generally, by this time, the baby will actively demand feeds.

Signs that indicate breast-feeding is successful include the following:

1. Breast milk comes in 2–4 days after delivery.
2. Breasts feel full before a feed and soften after a feed.
3. Nipples become less tender.
4. Let-down occurs. This is a tingly sensation with milk dripping from the breast when a feeding is due.
5. Baby is nursing 8–10 times a day.
6. Baby nurses for 10-20 minutes per breast.
7. Baby demands feeds and is satisfied after a breast-feed.
8. Baby has six to eight wet diapers per day.
9. Baby stools several times per day. Stool color changes in the first few days of life from green to yellow and is loose in consistency.
10. Mother and baby are happy with the experience.

Formula Feeding

Formula-fed infants generally take 1–2 oz of formula every 2–4 hours. When it is time for a feed, position the baby so that both you and the baby are comfortable. Hold the baby in your arms positioned on your lap with the head elevated several inches above the lower body. Tilt the bottle to allow milk to enter the nipple. Stimulate the lips or palate with the nipple to introduce it to the baby. The baby should start sucking. Burp the baby ever 1–2 oz by sitting the baby upright with the back straight and rub or gently pat the back. You may also hold the baby on your chest with baby's head above your shoulders and gently pat his or her back. Be sure to keep one hand on the back of the head, because infants do not have head control yet. Some infants spit up a little formula after a feed or with a burp. This is generally not a problem. If the infant spits up most of the feed for several consecutive feedings, notify your health care provider.

The infant may take 12–24 oz of formula per day. This will increase as the baby grows. Formula must be stored in the refrigerator and should not be allowed to sit out longer than 1 hour. Warm the formula by setting the bottle of formula in a pan of hot water. Test the temperature of the formula before feeding baby by sprinkling some on the inside of the wrist. It should not feel hot. If it does, allow it to cool before offering it to the baby. Microwaving formula is not recommended because it causes uneven heating.

Read and follow mixing instructions of the formula can. Do not add extra ingredients. Use the exact amount of water specified. Mix no more than a 24-hour supply at one time, put into small, clean bottles, and refrigerate. Do not save the remainder of a bottle for another feed, since bacteria can grow in the formula and make the baby ill. Clean baby bottles, nipples, and plastic rings in hot, soapy water and scrub with a bottle brush. A dishwasher will also provide adequate cleaning.

INFANT BEHAVIOR
Crying

All babies cry! Infants cry approximately 60–90 minutes a day during the first 3 weeks of life. By 2–3 weeks of age babies begin a different type of crying that is fussy in nature. It may occur at the same time every day, and usual comfort measures may not stop the crying. If obvious needs have been met, crying behavior is considered a part of normal infant behavior. You will soon learn to distinguish hunger and pain cries from fussy behavior. Infants cry in the early weeks of life for many reasons, including hunger, discomfort, fatigue, boredom, and overstimulation. Sometimes, no specific cause is determined.

Once causes for crying have been eliminated and comfort measures tried, the infant may be placed in a crib in a quiet room, even if crying continues. Although this can be stressful for parents, leaving the infant in a safe environment for 15 minutes may be enough time for the infant to fall asleep. You should check on the infant after 15 minutes and if the infant is still crying, retry comfort measures and put back to bed if necessary. Several 15-minute sessions may be required before the infant is asleep. Crying may increase to 2–4 hours/day by 6 weeks of age and gradually decrease by 3 months of age.

Comfort measures include the following.
1. Feed/burp.
2. Change diaper (observe for signs of diaper rash).
3. Check clothing for comfort/warmth (observe for tags that may be scratching or irritating the skin).
4. Swaddle or wrap securely in soft blankets.
5. Hold until baby falls asleep.
6. Rock baby in a rocking chair.
7. Decrease environmental stimulation by turning down the lights, decreasing noise, and limiting activity in room.
8. Offer a pacifier.
9. Walk or rock baby while holding.
10. Place in baby swing.
11. Bathe the baby.
12. Play soothing music/sing to baby.
13. Gently massage baby's body.
14. Take baby for a stroller or car ride.
15. Carry in a soft front carrier.

Colic

Colic affects approximately 10%–15% of infants. Characteristically, colic is intense, inconsolable crying in an otherwise healthy, well-fed child. The bouts of crying usually last 1–2 hours or longer. Colic usually begins during the second to third week of life and is usually over by 3 months of age. This fussy crying is harmless for your baby. The cause of colic is unknown. Colic is not usually caused by abdominal pain or excessive gas. Methods of consoling a baby who is "colicky" include motion, warmth, holding securely, infant swing, car ride, stroller ride, pacifier, massage, warm bath, or riding in a soft front pack. If the baby has been fed and changed and consoling methods have been tried, place baby in the crib and allow to cry for 15 minutes. If crying persists after 15 minutes, pick up the baby and try consoling methods again. It may take several 15 minute sessions before the baby falls asleep. Notify your health care provider if the cry seems to become a more painful one; if the crying lasts for more than 3 hours; if the colic begins after 1 month of age; if diarrhea, vomiting, or constipation occurs; if the baby is inconsolable; or if the caretaker is exhausted and frustrated.

Waking/Sleeping Behavior

You can expect the baby to sleep 15–20 hours/day in the first month, progressing to longer sleep periods at night and shorter periods during the day. By 2 weeks of age most babies sleep 5 hours a night and will progressively increase sleep time at night to coincide with awake time during the day. Established patterns may be interrupted during illness, teething, and growth spurts.

Development

Newborns can see objects 6–8 inches from their eyes. Studies show that they prefer designs in black and white. Babies can hear and locate the general direction of sounds. Head control is achieved by the end of the third month. Smiling begins by 3–5 weeks and cooing and babbling by 2–3 months. Babies enjoy being talked to and will respond with a flurry of activity from their arms and legs.

RECOGNIZING ILLNESS

Keep your health care provider's name and telephone number handy, as well as emergency phone numbers (e.g., 911). Notify your health care provider if you observe any of the following:
1. Breathing difficulties.
2. Convulsions, loss of consciousness (rhythmic movements such as jerking extremities, blinking, sucking/lip smacking, and bicycling movements of legs are all signs of convulsions).
3. Lethargy (excessive drowsiness), more irritability than usual.
4. Decreased feeding for 24 hours.
5. Vomiting more than one or two entire feeds in 1 day or projectile vomiting.
6. Bowel movements that are black, watery, loose, or of increased frequency.
7. Reddened umbilical site.
8. Redness, drainage, swelling, foul odor around circumcision site.
9. Jaundice covering abdomen/extremities.
10. Pustules/rashes/blisters other than normal newborn rashes.
11. White patches in the mouth that remain after the mouth is gently wiped with a wet cloth or fail to be removed with gentle scraping.
12. Temperature <97.7° F (36.4° C) or >100° F (37.8° C).
13. Baby that is "ill looking."
Behaviors that may concern parents but are neither abnormal nor indicate illness include:
1. Quivering of chin or lower lip when preparing to cry.
2. Hiccups: Small harmless spasms of the diaphragm muscle.
3. Sneezing: Helps the baby clean the nose of mucus, dust, lint, milk curds.

4. Wet burps after feeding: Small amount of milk that comes up with a burp.
5. Straining/red face with bowel movements.
6. Startle reflex: A response to noise or movement; the extremities extend outward and move to center, after which baby may cry.
7. Trembling/jitteriness of extremities in nonrhythmic fashion, usually while crying.
8. Yawning.
9. Cross-eyes: This is due to immature muscle control and will improve as muscle strength improves.
10. Passing gas.
11. Coughing: Removes secretions from the airway.
12. Irregular breathing/noisy breathing: May occur in an otherwise content and comfortable looking infant who does not appear to be in distress.

Taking a Temperature

If you are concerned that your baby may have a fever, take a temperature and have this information available when you call your health care provider. Place the bulb of the thermometer under the baby's armpit and hold the baby's arms down by the side. Hold the thermometer securely in place for 3 minutes. This is an *axillary* temperature. Rectal temperatures are not safe for a baby and not recommended. Axillary temperatures are as accurate as rectal temperatures.

A normal temperature is between 97.7° F (36.5° C) and 98.6° F (37.0° C). The following is a centigrade to Fahrenheit conversion scale:

36.5° C = 97.7° F
37.0° C = 98.6° F
37.8° C = 100.0° F
38.3° C = 101.0° F
38.9° C = 102.0° F
39.4° C = 103.0° F
40.0° C = 104.0° F

Using a Bulb Syringe

A bulb syringe can be helpful in clearing the baby's mouth or nose of mucus. To use the bulb syringe, squeeze the bulb with one hand while holding the baby's head steady with the other. Insert the bulb syringe into the sides of the mouth or nose and release pressure on the bulb syringe. The suction will remove the mucus. Repeat several times if necessary; however, overuse will result in bleeding or increased mucus production. Clean the bulb syringe with soapy water by squeezing and squirting out the water several times. Rinse with clear water and allow to dry.

Choking

Babies may occasionally choke as they are learning to coordinate sucking, swallowing, and breathing. If your baby is choking, sit him or her up and pat on the back to clear the nose, mouth, or throat. If your baby is spitting up mucus or milk, tilt the baby downward with the head positioned lower than the stomach and firmly pat his or her back. Use the bulb syringe to clear the nose and mouth.

SAFETY AND ENVIRONMENT

Relatives, visitors, and friends want to hold, feed, and play with the baby. Unfortunately, some of these people may be sick or just coming down with an illness that has not yet made them feel ill. Allow viewing of the baby from the crib, bassinet, or your arms, but do not pass the baby around for everyone to hold. Crowds are also not healthy places for babies. Protect your baby from infection by limiting exposure to crowds, sick people, or toddlers in the first month of life. Anyone who touches the baby should wash their hands first.

Car Safety

Car seats are vital to a baby's safety. All 50 U.S. states have laws requiring a child to ride in a car in a car restraint device. Babies and children who are not properly secured in a car can become "flying objects" in even minor accidents and can be seriously injured or killed by hitting windshields or dashboards or by being thrown from the car.

An infant restraint device must be used properly. It is important to read the instructions that accompany the restraint for proper use and installation in the car. It is never safe for the child to ride in the parent's arms, even if the parent is restrained by a seat belt.

Toys

Examine toys for small, loose parts on which the child may choke. Beware of older siblings' toys that may not be appropriate for a younger child. Remove toys that may cause injury from the baby's environment.

Siblings

Expect sibling rivalry. Since siblings may not understand that a baby is fragile, they may inadvertently injure or harm the baby. Do not leave the baby unattended with a sibling.

Pets

Pets may be curious or jealous of the new baby. A pet may consider the baby an intruder and harm the baby. Do not leave the baby alone with pets.

Smoking

Smoking is harmful to smokers and nonsmokers. Baby's lungs are delicate and can be irritated by second-hand smoke. Infants who are exposed to smoke are more likely to develop frequent upper respiratory infections. Do not smoke in the house, because smoke absorption by infants occurs even when smoking is done in another room of the house. Smoking should be done outside the house. Never smoke in the car when the infant is present.

Sun

Weather permitting, you make take the baby outdoors. Protect the baby from direct exposure to the sun, wind, or cold by using appropriate clothing, hats, and/or blankets. Avoid direct exposure to the sun on bare arms. Babies sunburn easily, which can be very dangerous.

Pacifier

If a pacifier is needed, purchase a commercial one-piece unit with a shield that is at least $1\frac{1}{2}$ inches in diameter. Do not put the pacifier on a string around baby's neck, because it could strangle your baby. Rinse off the pacifier after your baby finishes using it or drops to the floor.

Medications and Breast-Feeding

This appendix is intended to provide the health care professional with a quick reference list of maternal medications and breast-feeding issues. This list has been compiled from several sources (refer to reference list). The reader should refer to these and other sources if detailed information is needed.

DRUGS THAT ARE CONTRAINDICATED DURING BREAST-FEEDING
Ampethamines

Benzedrine, Dexedrine, Obetrol
Neonatal effects may include irritability, poor feeding, sleep disturbances.

Antineoplastics

No data are available for most agents, but it is likely that all are excreted into breast milk. The American Academy of Pediatrics (AAP) considers cyclophosphamide, doxorubicin, cyclosporine, and methotrexate to be contraindicated during breast-feeding because of possible immune suppression, neutropenia, carcinogenic effects, and an unknown effect on growth.

Generic Name	Trade Name
Bleomycin	Blenoxane
Busulfan	Myleran
Carboplatin	Paraplatin
Carmustine	BiCNU
Chlorambucil	Leukeran
Cisplatin	Platinol
Cyclophosphamide	Cytoxan
Cytarabine	Cytosar
Dacarbazine, dactinomycin	Cosmegen
Daunorubicin	Cerubidine
Doxorubicin	Adriamycin
Etoposide	VP-16; VePesid
Fludarabine	Fludara
Fluorouracil	5-FU
Hydroxyurea, idarubicin	Idamycin
Ifosafmide	Ifex
Lomustine	CeeNU

Mechlorethamine	Mustargen
Melphalan	Alkeran
Mercaptopurine	6-MP; Purinethol
Methotrexate, mitomycin	Mutamycin
Mitoxantrone	Novantrone
Pentostatin	Nipent
Pipobroman	Vercyte
Pilcamycin	Mithracin
Procarbazine, streptozocin	Zanosar
Teniposide	Vumon
Thioguanine, thiotepa, vinblastine	Velban
Vincristine	Oncovin

Other Drugs

- **Bromocriptine** (Parlodel): Given to suppress milk production in women who do not want to breast-feed. Breast-feeding is not possible when taking this medication.
- **Cocaine:** Cocaine intoxication, irritability, vomiting, diarrhea.
- **Cyclosporine** (Sandimmune): possible immune suppression.
- **Heroin:** Tremors, restlessness, vomiting, poor feeding, addiction.
- **Lithium:** Potential for lithium-induced toxicity.
- **Marijuana:** Long-term exposure unknown.
- **Nicotine:** Shock, vomiting, diarrhea, rapid heart rate, restlessness; decreased milk production.
- **Phencyclidine** (PCP): Potent hallucinogen.

POTENTIALLY HARMFUL MEDICATIONS FOR BREAST-FEEDING INFANTS

The safety of these drugs and the effects on the infant are unknown

Generic Name	Trade Name
Antianxiety Drugs	
Diazepam	Valium
Lorazepam	Ativan
Midazolam	Versed
Parxepam	None
Perphenazine	Trilafon
Quazepam	Dormalin
Temazepam	Restoril
Antidepressants	
Amitriptyline	Elavil, Endep
Amozapine	Asendin
Desipramine	Norpramin, Pertofrane
Doxepin	Sinequan
Fluvoxamine	Luvox
Fluxoetine	Prozac
Imipramine	Tofranil, Janimine
Sertraline	Zoloft
Trazadone	Desyrel
Antipyschotics	
Chloropromazine	Thorazine
Chloroprothixene	Taractan

Haloperidol	Haldol
Mesoridazine	Serentil
Others	
Chloramphenicol	Chloromycetin
Metoclopramide	Reglan
Metronidazole	Flagyl, Protostat
Tinidazole	Fasigyn, Simplotan

DRUGS THAT HAVE BEEN ASSOCIATED WITH SIGNIFICANT EFFECTS ON SOME BREAST-FEEDING INFANTS

These drugs should be used by nursing mothers with caution:

Generic Name	Trade Name
Acebutolol	Sectral
Aspirin (salicylates)	Many over-the-counter products
Clemastine	Tavist
Ergotamine	Bellergal-s, Cafergot, Ergomar
Phenobarbital	None
Primidone	Mysoline
Sulfasalazine, salicylazosulfapyridine	Azulfidine

MATERNAL DRUGS THAT ARE COMPATIBLE WITH BREAST-FEEDING

Generic Name	Trade Name
Alpha-Blockers, Beta-Blockers, and Other Sympatholytics	
Atenolol	Tenormin
Labetalol	Normodyne
Metoprolol	Lopressor
Propranolol	Inderal
Timolol	Blocadren, Timoptic
Anesthetics (Local)	
Lidocaine	Xylocaine
Anticoagulants	
Warfarin	Coumadin, Panwarfin
Antidepressants	
Clomipramine	None
Antigout Drugs	
Allopurinol	Lopurin, Zyloprim
Colchicne	ColBENENID
Antihistamines	
Dexbrompheniramine maleate with *d*-isoephedrine	Disophorol, Dirxoral
Triprolidine	Actifed
Anti-infectives	
Aminoglycosides	
Kanamycin	Kantrex
Streptomycin	None

Anti-infectives

Clindamycin	Cleocin
Erythromycin	E.E.S., E-Mycin, ERYC, Erythrocin
Trimethoprim	Bactrim, Septra

Antimalarials

Hydroxychloroquine	Plaquenil
Pyrimethamine	Daraprim
Quinidine	None
Quinine	Quinamm

Antituberculosis Drugs

Cycloserine	Seromycin
Ethambutol	Myambutol
Isoniazid	INH
Rifampin	Rifadin, Rimactane

Antivirals

Acyclovir	Zovirax

Penicillins

Amoxicillin	Amoxil
Ticarcillin	Timentin

Cephalosporins

Cefadroxil	Duricef
Cefazolin	Ancef, Kefzol
Cefotaxime	Calforan
Cefoxitin	None
Ceftazidime	Fortaz
Ceftriaxone	Rocephin
Moxalactam	Moxam

Tetracyclines

Tetracycline	Achromycin

Urinary Germicides

Nalidixic acid	NegGram
Nitrofurantoin	Furadantin, Macrodantin

H_2-Receptor Antagonists

Cimetidine	Tagamet

Antihypertensives

Captopril	Capoten
Enalapril	Vasotec
Hydralazine	Apresoline
Methyldopa	None
Minoxidil	Loniten, Rogaine
Oxprenolol	Trasicor

Antinausea/Anti–Motion Sickness Drugs

Scopolamine	Dallergy, Donnagel-PG, Donnatal, Ru-Tuss, Transderm Scop

Cardiac Agents

Digoxin	Lanoxin, Lanoxicaps
Diltiazem	Cardizem
Disopryamide	Norpace
Flecainide	Tambocor
Mexiletine	Mexitil

Nadolol	Corgard
Nifedipine	Procardia
Procainamide	Proestyl
Quinidine	None
Sotalol	None
Verapamil	Calan

Central Nervous System Agents

Analgesics

Acetaminophen	Tylenol, Anacin-3, Panadol, Tempra,
Phenaphens	
Propoxyphene	Darvon, Darvocet

Anticonvulsants

Carbamazepine	Tegretol
Ethosuximide	Zarontin
Magnesium sulfate	None
Phenytoin	Dilantin
Valproic acid	Depakene

Narcotic Analgesics

Butorphanol	Stadol
Codeine	None
Fentanyl	Sublimaze
Methadone	Dolophine
Morphine	None

Nonsteroidal Anti-Inflammatory Drugs

Ibuprofen	Advil, Motrin
Indomethacin	Indocin
Naproxen	Naprosyn
Phenylbutazone	Azolid, Butazolidin
Piroxicam	Feldene
Tolmetin	Tolectin

Sedatives/Hypnotics

Chloral hydrate	None
Ethanol (alcohol)	None
Secobarbital	Seconal

Stimulants

Caffeine	None

Diuretics

Acetazolamide	Diamox
Bendroflumethiazide	Naturetin
Chlorothiazide	Diuril, Chlotride
Chlorthalidone	Hygroton
Hydrochlorothiazide	HydroDIURIL
Spironolactone	Aldactone

Gastrointestinal Agents

Loperamide	Imodium
Danthron	Dorbane, Istizin
Magnesium sulfate	None
Senna	Senokot

Hormones

Contraceptive pill with estrogen/progesterone	Multiple brands

Estradiol	Delestrogen, Estrace
Levonorgestrel	Norplant
Medroxyprogesterone	Provera
Methimazole	Tapazole
Prednisone	Deltasone, Merticorten, Sterapred
Progesterone	None
Propylthiouracil	None
Tolbutamide	Orinase
Muscle Relaxants	
Atropine	None
Baclofen	Lioresal
Methocarbamol	Robaxin
Parasympatholytic	
Parasympathomimetics (Cholinergics)	
Dyphylline	Lufyllin, Dilor
Pyridostigmine	Mestinon
Spasmolytics	
Theophylline	Bronkodyl, Elixophyllin, Slo-Phyllin,
Theo-Dur	
Sympathomimetics (Adrenergics)	
Pseudoephedrine	Actifed, Afrinol, Benadryl Decongestant, Clor-Trimetron Decongestant, Comtrex, Drixoral, Novahistine DMX, PediaCare, Sinutab, Sudafed, Tylenol Cold Medication, Vicks Formula 44D Decongestant Cough Mixture, Vicks NyQuil Nighttime Cold Medicine
Terbutaline	Bricanyl, Brethine
Vitamins	
Folic acid	Fero-Folic-500, Folvite, Materna
Riboflavin (B_2)	B-C Bid, Glutofac, Mega-B, Ribo-2
Thiamine (B_1)	Belaline S
Vitamin B_{12}	Betalin 12, Cobex, Cyanoject, Cyomin
Vitamin D	Calciferol, Vitamin D capsules

REFERENCES

American Academy of Pediatrics: The transfer of drugs and other chemicals into human milk: a statement from the American Academy of Pediatrics, *Pediatrics* 108(3):776-89, 2001.

Briggs GG, Freeman RK, Yaffee SJ: *Drugs in pregnancy and lactation,* ed 6, Baltimore, MD, 2001, Williams & Wilkins.

Hale T: *Medications and mother's milk,* ed 10, Amarillo, TX, 2002, Pharmasoft Medical Publishing.

Lawrence RA, Lawrence RM: *Breastfeeding: a guide for the medical profession,* ed 5, St Louis, 1999, Mosby.

Murray SS, McKinney ES, Gorrie TM: *Foundations of maternal newborn nursing,* ed 3, Philadelphia, WB Saunders, pp 969-977.

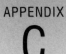

APPENDIX

C

Normal Laboratory Values and Conversion Guides

● TABLE C-1
● **Temperature—Fahrenheit (F) to Centigrade (C)***

° F	° C	° F	° C	° F	° C	° F	° C
95.0	35.0	98.0	36.7	101.0	38.3	104.0	40.0
95.2	35.1	98.2	36.8	101.2	38.4	104.2	40.1
95.4	35.2	98.4	36.9	101.4	38.6	104.4	40.2
95.6	35.3	**98.6**	**37.0**	101.6	38.7	104.6	40.3
95.8	35.4	98.8	37.1	101.8	38.8	104.8	40.4
96.0	35.6	99.0	37.2	102.0	38.9	105.0	40.6
96.2	35.7	99.2	37.3	102.2	39.0	105.2	40.7
96.4	35.8	99.4	37.4	102.4	39.1	105.4	40.8
96.6	35.9	99.6	37.6	102.6	39.2	105.6	40.9
96.8	36.0	99.8	37.7	102.8	39.3	105.8	41.0
97.0	36.1	100.0	37.8	103.0	39.4	106.0	41.1
97.2	36.2	100.2	37.9	103.2	39.6	106.2	41.2
97.4	36.3	100.4	38.0	103.4	39.7	106.4	41.3
97.6	36.4	100.6	38.1	103.6	39.8	106.6	41.4
97.8	36.6	100.8	38.2	103.8	39.9	106.8	41.6

*The metric system replaces the term *centigrade* with *Celsius* (the inventor of the scale).
Note: $° C = (° F - 32) \times 5/9$. Centigrade temperature equivalents rounded to one decimal place by adding 0.1 when second decimal place is 5 or greater.

Weight (Mass)—Pounds and Ounces to Grams

Example: To obtain grams equivalent to 6 lb 8 oz, locate "6" on top scale and "8" on side scale; then find their intersection. The equivalent is 2948 g.

	0	1	2	3	4	5	6	7	8	9	10	11	12	13	14
0	0	454	907	1361	1814	2268	2722	3175	3629	4082	4536	4990	5443	5897	6350
1	28	482	936	1389	1843	2296	2750	3203	3657	4111	4564	5018	5471	5925	6379
2	57	510	964	1417	1871	2325	2778	3232	3685	4139	4593	5046	5500	5953	6407
3	85	539	992	1446	1899	2353	2807	3260	3714	4167	4621	5075	5528	5982	6435
4	113	567	1021	1474	1928	2381	2835	3289	3742	4196	4649	5103	5557	6010	6464
5	142	595	1049	1503	1956	2410	2863	3317	3770	4224	4678	5131	5585	6038	6492
6	170	624	1077	1531	1984	2438	2892	3345	3799	4252	4706	5160	5613	6067	6520
7	198	652	1106	1559	2013	2466	2920	3374	3827	4281	4734	5188	5642	6095	6549
8	227	680	1134	1588	2041	2495	2948	3402	3856	4309	4763	5216	5670	6123	6577
9	255	709	1162	1616	2070	2523	2977	3430	3884	4337	4791	5245	5698	6152	6605
10	283	737	1191	1644	2098	2551	3005	3459	3912	4366	4819	5273	5727	6180	6634
11	312	765	1219	1673	2126	2580	3033	3487	3941	4394	4848	5301	5755	6209	6662
12	340	794	1247	1701	2155	2608	3062	3515	3969	4423	4876	5330	5783	6237	6600
13	369	822	1276	1729	2183	2637	3090	3544	3997	4451	4904	5358	5812	6265	6719
14	397	850	1304	1758	2211	2665	3118	3572	4026	4479	4933	5386	5840	6294	6747
15	425	879	1332	1786	2240	2693	3147	3600	4054	4508	4961	5415	5868	6322	6776

Note: 1 lb = 453.59237 g; 1 oz = 28.349523 g; 1000 g = 1 kg. Gram equivalents have been rounded to whole numbers by adding 1 when the first decimal place is 5 or greater.

● TABLE C-3
Length—Inches to Centimeters

1-inch increments—Example: To obtain centimeters equivalent to 22 inches, read "20" on top scale, "2" on side scale; equivalent is 55.9.

Inches	0	10	20	30	40
0	0	25.4	50.8	76.2	101.6
1	2.5	27.9	53.3	78.7	104.1
2	5.1	30.5	55.9	81.3	106.7
3	7.6	33.0	58.4	83.8	109.2
4	10.2	35.6	61.0	86.4	111.8
5	12.7	38.1	63.5	88.9	114.3
6	15.2	40.6	66.0	91.4	116.8
7	17.8	43.2	68.6	94.0	119.4
8	20.3	45.7	71.1	96.5	121.9
9	22.9	48.3	73.7	99.1	124.5

One quarter (1/4)-inch increments—Example: To obtain centimeters equivalent to 14 $\frac{3}{4}$ inches, read "14" on top scale, "3/4" on side scale; equivalent is 37.5 cm.

10–15 INCHES

0	10	11	12	13	14	15
0	25.4	27.9	30.5	33.0	35.6	38.1
$\frac{1}{4}$	26.0	28.6	31.1	33.7	36.2	38.7
$\frac{1}{2}$	26.7	29.2	31.8	34.3	36.8	39.4
$\frac{3}{4}$	27.3	29.8	32.4	34.9	37.5	40.0

16–21 INCHES

0	16	17	18	19	20	21
0	40.6	43.2	45.7	48.3	50.8	53.3
$\frac{1}{4}$	41.3	43.8	46.4	48.9	51.4	54.0
$\frac{1}{2}$	41.9	44.5	47.0	49.5	52.1	54.6
$\frac{3}{4}$	42.5	45.1	47.6	50.2	52.7	55.2

Note: 1 inch = 2.540 cm. Centimeter equivalents rounded one decimal place by adding 0.1 when second decimal place is 5 or greater; for example, 33.48 becomes 33.5.

● TABLE C-4
Chemistries in Term Infants*

Determination	Cord	1–12 hr	12–24 hr	24–48 hr	48–72 hr
Sodium, mEq/L[†]	147 (126–166)	143 (124–156)	145 (132–159)	148 (134–160)	149 (139–162)
Potassium, mEq/L	7.8 (5.6–12)	6.4 (5.3–7.3)	6.3 (5.3–8.9)	6.0 (5.2–7.3)	5.9 (5.0–7.7)
Chloride, mEq/L	103 (98–110)	100.7 (90–111)	103 (87–114)	102 (92–114)	103 (93–112)
Calcium, mg/dL	9.3 (8.2–11.1)	8.4 (7.3–9.2)	7.8 (6.9–9.4)	8.0 (6.1–9.9)	7.9 (5.9–9.7)
Phosphorus, mg/dL	5.6 (3.7–8.1)	6.1 (3.5–8.6)	5.7 (2.9–8.1)	5.9 (3.0–8.7)	5.8 (2.8–7.6)
Blood urea, mg/dL	29 (21–40)	27 (8–34)	33 (9–63)	32 (13–77)	31 (13–68)
Total protein, gm/dL	6.1 (4.8–7.3)	6.6 (5.6–8.5)	6.6 (5.8–8.2)	6.9 (5.9–8.2)	7.2 (6.0–8.5)
Blood sugar, mg/dL	73 (45–96)	63 (40–97)	63 (42–104)	56 (30–91)	59 (40–90)
Lactic acid, mg/dL	19.5 (11–30)	14.6 (11–24)	14.0 (10–23)	14.3 (9–22)	13.5 (7–21)
Lactate, mmol/L[‡]	2.0–3.0	2.0			

*From Schaffer AJ: *Diseases of the newborn*, ed 3, Philadelphia, 1971, WB Saunders.
[†]Acharya PT, Payne WW: *Arch Dis Child* 40:430, 1965.
[‡]Daniel SS, Adamsons KJ, James LS: *Pediatrics* 37:1942, 1966.

● TABLE C-5
Normal Blood Values in Premature and Term Infants

Value	Gestational Age (wk) 28	34	Full-Term Cord Blood	Day 1	Day 3	Day 7	Day 14
Hgb (g/dL)	14.5	15.0	16.8	18.4	17.8	17.0	16.8
Hematocrit (%)	45	47	53	58	55	54	52
Red cells (mm^3)	4.0	4.4	5.25	5.8	5.6	5.2	5.1
MCV (μ^3)	120	118	107	108	99	98	96
MCH (pg)	40	38	34	35	33	32.5	31.5
MCHC (%)	31	32	31.7	32.5	33	33	33
Reticulocytes (%)	5–10	3–10	3–7	3–7	1–3	0–1	0–1
Platelets (1000 s/mm^3)			290	192	213	248	252

MCV, mean corpuscular volume; *MCH*, mean corpuscular hemoglobin; *MCHC*, mean corpuscular hemoglobin concentration.
From Klaus MH, Fanaroff AA: *Care of the high risk neonate,* ed 3, Philadelphia, 1986, WB Saunders.

● TABLE C-6
Normal Leukocyte Values in Premature and Term Infants

Age (hr)	Total White Cell Count	Neutrophils	Bands/Metas	Lymphocytes	Monocytes	Eosinophils
TERM INFANTS						
0	10.0–26.0	5.0–13.0	0.4–1.8	3.5–8.5	0.7–1.5	0.2–2.0
12	13.5–31.0	9.0–18.0	0.4–2.0	3.0–7.0	1.0–2.0	0.2–2.0
72	5.0–14.5	2.0–7.0	0.2–0.4	2.0–5.0	0.5–1.0	0.2–1.0
144	6.0–14.5	2.0–6.0	0.2–0.5	3.0–6.0	0.7–1.2	0.2–0.8
PREMATURE INFANTS						
0	5.0–19.0	2.0–9.0	0.2–2.4	2.5–6.0	0.3–1.0	0.1–0.7
12	5.0–21.0	3.0–11.0	0.2–2.4	1.5–5.0	0.3–1.3	0.1–1.1
72	5.0–14.0	3.0–7.0	0.2–0.6	1.5–4.0	0.3–1.2	0.2–1.1
144	5.5–17.5	2.0–7.0	0.2–0.5	2.5–7.5	0.5–1.5	0.3–1.2

Data modified from Xanthou (1970) by Glader (1977).
From Oski FA, Naiman JL: *Hematologic problems in the newborn,* ed 3, Philadelphia, 1982, WB Saunders.

● TABLE C-7
Normal Laboratory Values (Cerebrospinal Fluid)

Cell count		
Preterm mean	9.0 (0–25.4 WBC/mm³)	57% PMNs
Term mean	8.2 (0–22.4 WBC/mm³)	61% PMNs
>1 mo	0–7 WBC/mm³	0% PMNs
Glucose		
Preterm	24–63 mg/dL	(mean 50)
Term	34–119 mg/dL	(mean 52)
Child	40–80 mg/dL	
CSF glucose/blood glucose		
Preterm	55%–105%	
Term	44%–128%	
Child	50%	
Lactic acid dehydrogenase		
Mean	20 (5–30 U/L), or about 10% of serum value	
Myelin basic protein	<4 ng/mL	
Opening pressure		
Newborn	80–110 (<110 mm H_2O)	
Infant/child	<200 mm H_2O (lateral recumbent)	
Respirations	5–10 mm H_2O	
Protein		
Preterm	Mean 115 (65–150 mg/dL)	
Term	Mean 90 (20–170 mg/dL)	
Child		
Ventricular	5–15 mg/dL	
Cisternal	5–25 mg/dL	
Lumbar	5–40 mg/dL	

From Greene MG: *The Harriet Lane handbook,* ed 12, St Louis, 1991, Mosby, p.53.

● TABLE C-8
Thyroid Function Tests: Routine Studies

Test	Age	Normal	Comments
T_4RIA (μg/dL)	Cord	7.4–13.0	Measures total T_4 by radioimmunoassay; values for
	1–3 days	11.8–22.6	premature infants below
	1–2 wk	9.8–16.6	
	2–4 wk	7.0–15.0	
T_3RU		25–35%	Measures thyroid hormone binding, not T_3
T index		1.25–4.20	T_4RIA x T_3RU
Free T_4 (ng/dL)	1–10 days	0.6–2.0	Metabolically active form
	>10 days	0.7–1.7	
T_3RIA (ng/dL)	Cord	15–75	Measures triiodothyronine by radioimmunoassay
	1–3 days	32–216	
	2–4 wk	160–240	
TSH–RIA	Cord	<17.4	Best sensitivity for primary hypothyroidism; TSH
(MIU/mL)	1–3 days	<13.3	surge peaks at 80–90 MIU/mL in term newborn by
	2–4 wk	<10.0	30 min after birth

From Greene MG: *The Harriet Lane handbook,* ed 12, St Louis, 1991, Mosby, p.104.

Standard Normal Newborn Orders

STANDARD ORDERS FOR THE NORMAL NEWBORN

1. Admit to transition care.
2. Obtain axillary temperature, heart rate, and respiratory rate at 30 minutes of age until stable and within normal limits ×2; then hourly while in transition care. Temperature, heart rate, and respiratory rate every 8 hours thereafter until discharge.
3. Weigh in grams and measure head and length in centimeters.
4. Complete gestational age assessment and plot measurements on the Colorado intrauterine growth chart.
5. Whole blood glucose screen and peripheral hematocrit per nursery protocol.
6. Vitamin K, 1 mg IM by 4 hours of age after infant bath.
7. Antibiotic ophthalmic ointment, one half-inch ribbon both eyes by 1 hour of age.
8. Hepatitis B vaccine (dose per facility policy) after infant bath and parental consent obtained. Administer by 4–12 hours of age unless vaccine is deferred by parental waiver.
9. Apply 70% alcohol to umbilical cord every 8 hours and PRN.
10. Feed every 2 to 4 hours at breast, or every 2 to 5 hours with formula using physician's or parents' choice of formula.
11. Lactation consult as needed.
12. Discharge from transition when infant is stable and a minimum of 4 hours has elapsed. Notify physician if satisfactory transition is not complete by 6 hours of age.
13. Cord blood: Clot to hold ×7 days; type and Rh if mother is type O or Rh-negative or if blood type unknown; direct Coombs test if mother is Rh-negative and infant is Rh-positive or if mother is blood type O and baby is blood type A or B.
14. Total bilirubin ×1 if jaundice is observed.
15. Newborn genetic screen at 48 hours of age or just before discharge, whichever occurs first.
16. Blood pressure prn *and* in right arm and right leg before discharge.
17. Notify physician of any deviations from normal limits.

E Parent Education and Postdischarge Care Forms

Patient Education Sheet

Follow-up appointment scheduled _____

DATE / INITIAL	TEACHING INTERVENTION	RESPONSE TO TEACHING						REINFORCEMENT			COMMENTS
	Include content taught/ handouts used	Teaching Method	States Understanding	Can Return Demonstrate	Routinely Performs	No Evidence of Learning	Other	Reinforce Content	Routinely Performs		
	Temperature Taking										
	Diapering										
	Holding/Handling										
	Feeding: Breast, Formula										
	Bathing										
	Skin Care										
	Cord Care										
	Dressing										
	Fingernail Trimming										
	Bulb Suctioning										
	Safety										
	Car Seat										
	Development										
	Immunizations										
	Fever										
	Vomiting										
	Diarrhea										
	Color Changes										
	Respiratory Changes										
	Temperament Changes										
	Rashes										
	General Illness										

(Rows Fever through General Illness grouped under "Signs and Symptoms of Illness")

Parent/Guardian _____
(Signature)

From University Hospital, Denver, Colorado, with permission.

*Teaching method code   A = audiovisual   D = demonstration
N/A = Not Applicable   R = role play   H = handout
E = explanation   G = group class

NEWBORN FOLLOWUP VISIT

Date:_____Time:_____
Baby's name:_____
Birthdate:_____
Birthplace:_____
Primary Care Provider:_____
Medical Record #:_____

HISTORY

Mother's Name:_____ Age:_____
Mother's Blood Type:_____
Baby Blood Type:_____ Coombs:_____
Delivery: Vaginal _____ C/S _____
Prenatal Labs: Hep B _____ VDRL _____ Rubella ___
Apgars:_____ 1 min._____ 5 min.
Significant PG/L&D problems:_____
_____
_____
Transition complications:_____
_____
_____
Other complications:_____
_____
_____
Labs:_____
Hep B Vac:_____ Hearing: Pass ☐   Fail ☐
Newborn Genetic Screen: #1 ☐   #2 ☐

FEEDINGS

Breast:_____ Formula:_____
Breastfeeding
    Frequency:_____
    Time at Breast:_____
    Milk in:_____
Problems:_____
_____
_____
Recommendations:_____
_____
_____

Formula Feeding
    Type of formula:_____
    Volume per feed:_____
    Frequency:_____
Problems:_____
Recommendations:_____
_____

ELIMINATION

Voids past 24 hrs:_____
Stools past 24 hrs:_____
Color & consistency of stools:_____
_____

PHYSICAL EXAMINATION

Birth WT._____Current WT._____
% Change from birthweight: ↑_____ ↓_____
TPR ____/_____/_____ BP _____
General Appearance:_____
_____
Skin:_____
HEENT:_____
_____
Cardiovascular/Pulses:_____
_____
Respiratory:_____
_____
Abdomen/Cord:_____
_____
GU:_____
Circ. Site:_____
Neuro:_____
_____
Other:_____
_____
Labs:_____
_____
Parent Concerns:_____
_____
Teaching Needs:_____
_____

ASSESSMENT/PLAN:_____
_____
_____

FOLLOWUP RECOMMENDATIONS:
_____
_____
Primary Care Provider Notified: ☐ Fax ☐ Mail ☐ Call

SIGNATURE:_____

From University Hospital, Denver, Colorado, with permission.

HEALTH MAINTENANCE VISIT
2 WEEKS — 2 MONTHS

Date: _____ Time: _____

Mother's Name: _____

Infant's Name: _____

Past Medical History: _____
_____
_____

Parental Concerns/Interim Problems: _____
_____

RECENT ILLNESSES _____
_____

CURRENT STATUS

Diet/Feeding: _____
_____
_____

Elimination: _____
_____
_____

Sleep Patterns: _____
_____

Allergies: _____

Medications: _____

DEVELOPMENT

Smiles: _____ Coos: _____

Head Control: _____

Vision/Tracking: _____

Hearing: _____

Crying: _____

General Activity: _____

SOCIAL

Family Structure: _____
_____

Family Stress: _____
_____

Support Systems: _____
_____

Integration of child into family: _____
_____

Sibling Rivalry: _____
_____

TPR ____ /____/_____ BP _____

Birthweight: _____ gms. _____ %

Current Wt: _____ gms. _____ %

Height: _____ cm _____ %

OFC: _____ cm _____ %

PHYSICAL EXAM	NL	ABNL	COMMENTS
Gen Appearance			
Skin			
Head/Fontanel			
Eyes/RR			
Ears/Nose/Mouth			
Neck			
Chest/Lungs			
Cardiovascular/Pulses			
Abdomen			
Genitalia			
Musculoskeletal/Hips			
Neuro/Reflexes			

Additional PE comments: _____
_____

TEACHING CHECKLIST

Nutrition
- ☐ Feeding technique
- ☐ No solids
- ☐ Vit/Fe supplements
- ☐ Bottle propping
- ☐ Burping

Family
- ☐ Sibilings
- ☐ Working mother
- ☐ Father's role
- ☐ Babysitter/daycare
- ☐ Discipline

Safety
- ☐ Car seat
- ☐ Crib
- ☐ 1st aid/911
- ☐ Falling
- ☐ Pets
- ☐ Bathing
- ☐ Sleeping position
- ☐ Pacifiers

Development
- ☐ Stimulation
- ☐ Sleeping at night

Health Promotions
- ☐ Immunizations
- ☐ Bulb syringe
- ☐ Stooling pattern
- ☐ Diaper rash
- ☐ Cradle cap
- ☐ Heat rash
- ☐ Temp taking
- ☐ Smoking side effects
- ☐ Sunscreen
- ☐ Resp season

IMMUNIZATIONS NEEDED:

Hep B_____ IPV_____ DTP_____ Hib _____

NEWBORN GENETIC SCREEN

#1 ☐ NI ☐ Abnl #2 ☐ Not needed ☐ Pending ☐ Needs

ASSESSMENT: _____
_____

PLAN: _____
_____
_____

NEXT FU APPOINTMENT: _____

SIGNATURE: _____

From University Hospital, Denver, Colorado, with permission.

Index

Note: Page numbers followed by b indicate boxes; f, figures; t, tables.